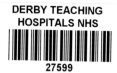

TRANSITIONS
IN NURSING
PREPARING FOR PROFESSIONAL PRACTICE

Fourth Edition

CONTENTS

PREFACE

Welcome to the fourth edition of *Transitions in Nursing: Preparing for Professional Practice*. As with the first, second and third editions, this book has been developed to assist undergraduate students, new registered nurses and other professionals interested in issues and challenges associated with the transition from higher education to practice. For the majority of new graduates this rite of passage is associated with a degree of stress, strain and culture shock. These are issues that have existed in nursing, internationally, for decades. The literature shows that this transition is a multidimensional and complex process. Intensive socialisation brings to the surface many challenges and opportunities for new registered nurses as they assimilate into their professional work roles. Research has shed much light on the issues associated with transition and has uncovered knowledge, including strategies that can be useful in negotiating the process.

The book has been designed to provide comprehensive information on key issues associated with transition. Readers will find viewpoints that are challenging and sometimes disconcerting, but at the same time motivating and thought-provoking. The fourth edition is divided into three sections. Section 1 examines issues from student to graduate nurse. Section 2 looks at skills for dealing with the world of work. Section 3 discusses the organisational environments. This edition also includes three new chapters in the area of evidence-based practice/knowledge translation: a practical guide; establishing and maintaining a professional identity: portfolios and career progression; and transition into practice: the regulatory framework for nursing. Understanding the context in which we work is crucial to effective functioning in the workplace. Knowing how to provide care for patients and their families in the health system is not sufficient: we need to learn how to care for ourselves in order to care for our patients effectively. The exercises and learning activities that appear throughout the book offer readers a range of helpful suggestions in understanding the nursing context, managing stress and caring for themselves. In addition, each chapter includes recommended readings, case studies and reflective questions for further exploration.

Our intention was to involve clinicians and academics in producing a resource that is scholarly, accessible, reality-based and practical. More importantly, it is a resource for every student, practising nurse, educator and administrator in understanding the issues of transition for new registered nurses. By reading the book, reflecting on the issues and posing possible answers, readers should be able to gain a comprehensive view of the issues, challenges and opportunities that lie ahead of them. The journey during this period can be rewarding, with implications for a long-term career for new nurses, particularly when educators, administrators and clinicians collaboratively anticipate and manage the socialisation process.

We extend our sincere appreciation to the contributors to the book for their shared interest in and concern for the issues and challenges of transitioning from student to registered nurse. This book would not be possible without them. We would like to extend our special appreciation to Natalie Hamad, Libby Houston, Karthikeyan Murthy, Robyn Flemming and the rest of the team at Elsevier for their encouragement and support. Elsevier Australia joins us in thanking the reviewers for their feedback on the manuscript. We would also like to thank our partners and families for their support. Finally, we wish to dedicate this text to our past, present and future students.

Esther Chang and John Daly

CONTRIBUTORS

Amanda Adrian RN, LLB, BA, FACN
Principal, Amanda Adrian and Associates
NSW, Australia

Susan Alexander RN, PhD, BN (Hons), GCTE, GDCounsel, MACN
Lecturer, School of Nursing and Midwifery
University of Western Sydney, NSW, Australia

Christine Ashley FACN, MACMHN, RN, RM, GC Ethics & Legal Studies, BHlthSc, MN
Director, Christine Ashley Consulting
Canberra, ACT, Australia

Alan Barnard RN, BA, MA, PhD
Senior Lecturer, School of Nursing
Queensland University of Technology, Qld, Australia

Professor Esther Chang RN, CM, DNE, BAppSc(AdvNur), MEdAdmin, PhD, FACN
Professor of Nursing, School of Nursing and Midwifery
University of Western Sydney, NSW, Australia

Professor Mary Chiarella RN, RM, LLB (Hons), PhD (UNSW), FACN
Professor of Nursing, Sydney Nursing School
The University of Sydney, NSW, Australia

Tiffany Conroy RN, BN, MNSc, DipBusFLM, FACN
Program Coordinator, School of Nursing
University of Adelaide, SA, Australia

Professor Jane Conway RN, BHSc, BNurs (Hons1), Grad Cert HRM, Grad Dip FET, DEd
Professor Teaching, Learning and Scholarship, School of Health
University of New England, NSW, Australia

Elizabeth Crock PhD, MPH, BSc, Grad Dip Ed, RN, ACRN
Clinical Nurse Consultant – HIV
Royal District Nursing Service, Vic, Australia

Professor Patrick Crookes PhD, BSc (Nursing), Cert Ed, RN, RNT, MCNA
Director, Wollongong Academy for Tertiary Teaching and Learning Excellence (WATTLE)
Professor, School of Nursing, University of Wollongong, Australia
Visiting Professor, University of Huddersfield (UK) and University of Stavanger (Norway)

Professor John Daly PhD, RN, FACN, FAAN
Dean, Faculty of Health
Head, World Health Organization Collaborating Centre for Nursing, Midwifery and Health Development
University of Technology, Sydney, NSW, Australia

Professor Patricia M Davidson RN, PhD, FACN, FAAN
Dean and Professor, School of Nursing
Johns Hopkins University, Baltimore, United States
and University of Technology, Sydney, NSW, Australia

Professor Gary E Day DHSM, MHM, BNurs, DipAppSc (Nursing Mgt), RN, EM, FCHSM, FGLF
Professor of Health Services Management and Director of the Centre for Health Innovation
School of Medicine, Griffith University, Gold Coast, Qld, Australia

Kathleen Dixon PhD, MHA, BA, CFH (cert), RN
Senior Lecturer, School of Nursing and Midwifery
University of Western Sydney, NSW, Australia

Professor Christine Duffield RN, PhD, FACN, FAAN
Director, Centre for Health Services Management (UTS) and
Professor of Nursing & Health Services Management UTS and Edith Cowan University
University of Technology, Sydney, NSW, Australia

Associate Professor Bronwyn Everett RN, PhD
Associate Professor, School of Nursing and Midwifery
University of Western Sydney, NSW, Australia

Professor Mary FitzGerald RN, MN, Cert Ed(FE), PhD
Professor of Nursing, School of Nursing, Midwifery and Indigenous Health
Charles Sturt University, Wagga Wagga, NSW, Australia

Professor Kim Foster RN, DipAppSc, BN, MA, PhD, MACN, FACMHN
Professor and Head, Disciplines of Nursing and Midwifery, Faculty of Health
University of Canberra, ACT, Australia

Deborah Hatcher PhD, MHPEd, BHlthSc(N), DipTeach(PhysEd), RN
Senior Lecturer, School of Nursing and Midwifery
University of Western Sydney, NSW, Australia

Professor Megan-Jane Johnstone PhD, BA, RN, FACN
Professor of Nursing, School of Nursing and Midwifery, Faculty of Health
Deakin University, Burwood, Melbourne, Vic, Australia

Cathy Jones BAppSci (SpPath) (Hons), MBA
National Manager Quality & Compliance, Healthscope, Vic, Australia

Professor Judy Lumby AM, FCN, DipNed, BA, MHPEd, PhD
Emeritus Professor, University of Technology, Sydney, NSW, Australia
Honorary Professor, The University of Sydney
Honorary Professor, University of Adelaide

Paul McLiesh RN, BN, GDip Orth, MNSc
Lecturer, School of Nursing
University of Adelaide, SA, Australia

Professor Margaret McMillan RN, PhD, M Curr St (Hons), BA, DNE, Grad Cert Management
Emeritus Professor, School of Nursing and Midwifery
University of Newcastle, NSW, Australia

Annette Moore RN, BN, Graduate Diploma in Nursing
Clinical Nurse Educator – Transition to Practice
Centre for Education & Research; Nursing & Midwifery
Royal Hobart Hospital, Tas, Australia

Professor Paul Morrison RMN, RN, BA (Hons), PhD, PGCE, GradDip Counselling, AFBPsS, CPsychol, MAPS
Dean, School of Health Professions
Murdoch University, Perth, WA, Australia

Alison Natera RN, BN, Grad Cert Critical Care, Graduate Diploma in Nursing
Clinical Nurse Educator – Transition to Practice
Centre for Education & Research; Nursing & Midwifery
Royal Hobart Hospital, Tas, Australia

Associate Professor Stephen Neville RN, PhD, FCNA (NZ)
Associate Professor of Nursing and Head of Department, Department of Nursing
Auckland University of Technology, Auckland, New Zealand

Steve Outram BA (Hons) Sociology, MA Deviancy and Social Policy, PGCE
Visiting Fellow, University of Liverpool
Consultant in Academic Practice
UK Higher Education Academy, York, United Kingdom

Jan Sayers PhD, MA (Educational Administration), Grad Dip Adult Ed, RN
Lecturer and Deputy Director Research, School of Nursing and Midwifery
University of Western Sydney, NSW, Australia

Professor Jane Stein-Parbury RN, BSN, MEd, PhD, FCNA
Professor of Mental Health Nursing, Faculty of Health
University of Technology, Sydney, NSW, Australia

Lyn Stewart RN, RM, BHScN, MEd(Adult Ed), Cert1V (Teaching Conversational English), FACN
Lecturer, School of Nursing and Midwifery
University of Western Sydney, NSW, Australia

Professor Debra Thoms RN, RM, BA, MNA, Grad Cert Bioethics, Adv Dip Arts, FACN(DLF), FACHSE (Hons)
Chief Executive Officer, Australian College of Nursing
Adjunct Professor, University of Technology, Sydney, NSW, Australia

Professor Kim Usher RN, RPN, A/DipNEd, BA, DipAppSc (Nsg), MNSt, PhD, FACN, FACMHN
Dean and Head of School
School of Health, University of New England, Armidale, NSW, Australia

Professor Kenneth Walsh RPN, RGN, BNurs, PhD
Fellow of the Joanna Briggs Institute
Professor of Translational Research in Nursing and Midwifery
School of Health Sciences, Faculty of Health
University of Tasmania, and The Tasmanian Health Organisation South
Hobart, Tas, Australia

Professor Jill White AM, RN, RM, BEd, MEd, PhD, FACN
Professor of Nursing and Midwifery
Faculty of Nursing and Midwifery
The University of Sydney, NSW, Australia

Rick Wiechula RN, BA, OrthoCert, BN, MNSc, DNurs
Senior Lecturer
Post Graduate Coordinator,
School of Nursing, University of Adelaide, SA, Australia

Professor Denise Wilson RN, PhD, FCNA(NZ)
Professor Māori Health; Director Taupua Waiora Centre of Māori Health Research
School of Public Health & Psychosocial Studies
Auckland University of Technology, Auckland, New Zealand

REVIEWERS

Jessica Biles RN, Masters of Health Sciences Education, PhD Candidate
Lecturer, School of Nursing, Midwifery and Indigenous Health
Charles Sturt University, Albury, NSW, Australia

Sue Floyd RN, BM, MN, MCNA (NZ)
Nursing Practicum Manager, School of Nursing
Eastern Institute of Technology, Napier, New Zealand

Eleanor Horton RN, Ad Dip (Nsg), B Hlth Sc (NSg), M Hlth Sc (Nsg), PhD
Senior Lecturer, School of Nursing and Midwifery
University of the Sunshine Coast, Maroochydore, QLD, Australia

Helen Kelly BN (Hons), Grad Cert Cardiac Nursing, Grad Cert University Teaching
Lecturer, School of Nursing
University of Notre Dame, Sydney, NSW, Australia

Rebekkah Middleton RN, BN, MN (Res), Grad Cert Emergency Nursing, Grad Cert Clinical Management, PhD candidate
Lecturer, School of Nursing
University of Wollongong, NSW, Australia

Gloria Thompson RN, BHealth, MNLead, GCAP, MACN, MGKIHS, MIIWI
Lecturer, School of Nursing
Queensland University of Technology, Caboolture, Qld, Australia

SECTION 1
FROM STUDENT TO GRADUATE

CHAPTER 1

Managing the transition from student to graduate nurse

Esther Chang and John Daly

LEARNING OBJECTIVES

When you have completed this chapter you will be able to:

- describe the process of transition from student to graduate nurse
- appreciate a range of factors and issues that influence the transition from student to graduate nurse
- consider strategies to ease the tension associated with adjustment to the realities of nursing practice for new registered nurses
- recognise the importance of a positive, proactive approach to managing transition on an individual level
- identify and access resources which have been shown to facilitate adjustment to nursing practice for new registered nurses.

KEYWORDS: transition, role stress, strategies, students, new graduate nurse

INTRODUCTION

Nursing attracts people from many walks of life, motivated largely by a concern and a desire to understand and help people who are confronted by a range of actual or potential health problems and challenges. Many of these experiences cause major disruption in people's lives – for example, illness, suffering, loss, grief and trauma. According to Englert,[1] 'such experiences are both the privilege and burden of nurses and of others who share the drama, the humour and the tragedy of other people's lives' (p 1). Englert, a leader in administration of nursing services, encouraged members of the nursing profession to 'reflect for a moment ... to recall some of those high and low points of the beginning years as a registered nurse' (p 1). She went on:

> I believe that the situation of our nursing students and new graduates today is not so very
> different. Their motivations in entering nursing are much the same as were ours. They too

share an idealism based on the desire to help their fellow human beings, an apprehension that they will be found wanting when the crisis occurs, a certain awkwardness in accepting advice, however kindly given, and an admiration for those whom they see as epitomising the best of nursing.[1]

The nursing profession in Australia and elsewhere continues to be concerned with the process of transition for graduates of undergraduate nursing courses on entry to the world of clinical practice.[2-9] This concern exists for several reasons: (1) it has remained an issue of concern in nurse education in Australia because of ongoing changes in the clinical practice environment; (2) research data continue to show that this period of transition can be stressful;[5] (3) professional, service and economic issues can impact recruitment and retention; and (4) there are related questions about adequate preparation of new graduate nurses.

One key issue here is the relevance and quality of clinical education in undergraduate courses. Indeed, in recent times, access to an adequate number of quality clinical placements has become a serious challenge to educators in nursing, medicine and allied health. This has fostered a number of innovations, including the development of more sophisticated clinical simulation teaching and learning environments.[10] The impact of such innovations on clinical competence of graduates in the health professions will require ongoing research and evaluation.

These challenges are international, particularly in developed countries that are struggling with health sector reforms, cost containment challenges, the growing burden of chronic disease, ageing populations and human resources for health issues. In the United States, a provocative and scholarly report for the Carnegie Foundation for the Advancement of Teaching called recently for a reinvention of preregistration nursing education.[11] The authors' argument is based on a number of factors, one dimension being the relevance of current models of undergraduate nursing education in the present-day context of health system re-engineering. The Council of Australian Governments established Health Workforce Australia (HWA) in 2010, which had a role to play in creating solutions to clinical education challenges (www.hwa.gov.au). HWA had a concern with 'improving and expanding access to quality clinical training for health professionals in training across the public and private and non-government sectors. This will be achieved through funding programs which expand capacity, improve quality, reform delivery systems and offer diversity in learning opportunities' (p 2).[12]

However, the Australian federal government closed HWA in 2014 and transferred its role and functions to the Commonwealth Department of Health. Undoubtedly, challenges will persist with supply of and access to quality clinical placements across health professional education, including undergraduate nursing.

In addition, recruitment and retention of new graduates are issues from time to time, both nationally and internationally. Demand for, and supply of, registered nurses is cyclical, and occasionally healthcare systems are confronted by a shortage of nurses. Such shortages can reach crisis proportions, a phenomenon that is seen in Australia and overseas from time to time as a result of an ageing workforce and the undersupply of graduates in many areas.[13] Recent HWA predictions pointed to a likely workforce shortage of 109,225 registered nurses by 2025 due to demographic changes in society and the profession of nursing.[14]

Other reasons for this concern with the experience of transition include changing attitudes in society towards nursing as a career, a decline in the number of people choosing to enter undergraduate nursing courses, and the need to create sustainable nursing. It also appears that healthcare system reform has created an environment that has a negative impact on the quality of worklife for nurses and other health professionals, and on the quality of patient care. Nursing leaders are currently investigating these issues and searching for strategies to enhance the quality of undergraduate clinical education, the image of nursing as a career, transition for new graduates, quality of worklife, and the recruitment and retention of qualified staff in the nursing workforce.

There is a large amount of literature on the process of transition from senior student to graduate nurse. It is clear from this literature that transition is multifaceted and complex, and that problems often described and discussed in relation to the process are not new.[7,15,16] In Australia, nursing education has undergone rapid transformation since the late 1980s. The system of basic nurse education (BNE) is now university-based with 3-year degree programs leading to eligibility to register as a nurse. In addition, the national healthcare system has undergone radical change in the last decade in particular. Much of this system change has been driven by the shift to an economic model for designing and managing health services. This has led to changes in the nursing practice environment that have implications for new graduates entering employment.

To date, the Australian government has commissioned two national reviews[2,17] of undergraduate nurse education since the national shift of BNE from hospital schools of nursing to the higher-education sector. The second review (the Heath report) was published in 2002.[2] Two major matters of concern uncovered by the first national review committee were 'the adequacy of clinical education provided during pre-registration nursing courses and the best means of facilitating the transition from higher education to work' (p 4).[17] The first national review of BNE made a number of recommendations designed to enhance the quality of educational endeavours in both these areas and outcomes for course graduates and nursing services providers. These concerns remain and were also considered by the second national review[2] and the Australian Senate inquiry into nursing.[3] The National Nursing and Nursing Education Taskforce, which was established to implement the recommendations of the Heath report[2] and which concluded its work in 2006, also considered the issue of transition.[4] In the Heath report,[2] transition was addressed through recommendation 14, standards for transition programs. It was recommended that:

> to ensure consistency and quality in the development and delivery of transition programs a national framework be developed for transition to provide guidelines and standards for institutions. State and territory nursing registration boards should accredit transition programs; employing institutions should be responsible for meeting the standards (p 22).[2]

Preregistration nursing courses today need to prepare graduates for a work environment that has undergone enormous change in the last decade. The practice environment is constantly changing, and this has implications for the type of knowledge and skills that new graduates will require. University schools of nursing are constantly challenged to ensure that their courses are designed to give graduates the best possible preparation for entry to nursing practice as new registered nurses, and to optimise their ability to move through the transition process confidently and successfully. Experience has shown that this is best done in cooperation with nursing service leaders and providers. Preparation of new graduates in nursing is best viewed as a shared responsibility between the universities and nursing service sectors.[18]

University schools of nursing aim to prepare flexible, critical thinkers for the practice of professional nursing. They emphasise individual client- or patient-centred holistic care and lifelong learning as key values. All preregistration nursing courses are required to provide a clinical education component to ensure that course graduates meet the clinical competency expectations of beginning registered nurses. In many surveys, however, new graduates report that the clinical practice and clinical education components of their undergraduate course were too short and that the course was too theoretical.[16] Other research work has found that, on entry to the workforce, graduates perceive that employers do not understand what they actually know and are capable of doing.[19]

Nursing service providers often report that new graduates 'are inadequately prepared for clinical practice in that they are deficient in certain skills' (p 17).[18] This reflects a clear mismatch in expectations of new graduate nurses between the education and service sectors.

Preregistration nursing courses do not aim to produce expert practitioners on graduation. Research has demonstrated that development of clinical expertise requires some years of constant immersion in clinical experience following entry to nursing practice as a registered nurse.[20] It would be ideal if newly registered nurses could meet all expectations required by the healthcare settings immediately following entry to the workforce. Experience has shown that few individuals are able to perform at this level, and for the majority of new graduates this is an unrealistic and difficult expectation.

Nursing has a long history of anti-intellectualism,[21] and at one time it was believed that nurses who are too academic tend to be hamstrung when it comes to clinical practice. Paradoxically, many authorities argue that contemporary nursing requires intelligent, flexible, critical thinkers and problem solvers who are able to demonstrate the ability to deliver safe, competent care in a range of environments. Many of the environments in which nurses work are highly complex and demand higher-order cognitive skills. The ability to 'do' is prized in clinical nursing – this is understandable to a large degree, but there has to be acceptance of some middle ground in debates about these issues. Nursing requires adequate theoretical preparation and competence in clinical practice. Conway and McMillan[22] argue that the transition from student to graduate and practitioner requires the development of the ability to examine critically our own and others' practice and be accountable for our own actions. These abilities are often linked to the idea of being a lifelong learner and are seen as increasingly important to professional nursing practice in the 21st century.

It is important, therefore, that new graduates are provided with support, tolerance, patience and encouragement as they learn to assimilate values, beliefs and practices acquired in their undergraduate education with the practice values and beliefs that are dominant in the clinical work world. It is no surprise that in this context the transition process presents many challenges and potential rewards for the new graduate in nursing. The first 3–6 months as a new registered nurse have been identified as potentially the most challenging and stressful period in professional adjustment.[5,15,18,23–26] This period is 'crucial in determining new graduates' commitment to nursing as well as their acquisition of technical, clinical and patient management skills' (p 20).[18] Perhaps the key to successful negotiation of this phase is anticipation and psychological preparation. This requires you to be adequately informed of what is known about the process and what you can do to ease your transition into practice as a new registered nurse. In addition, nurses in service need to place greater emphasis on the clinical area as a place where learning is ongoing[27] and a lifelong process.

A survey of the table of contents in this book will show that component chapters are concerned with preparation for entry into the nursing workforce and the development of a successful, sustainable and rewarding career in nursing. Chapter topics can be classified according to a number of themes: managing self in clinical practice; caring for self; understanding the forces that shape the practice environment; learning to manage different approaches to nursing care delivery; collaborating and working with colleagues and patients/clients; and professional development strategies.

TRANSITION: A PROCESS

The transition from student to graduate nurse is characterised by a period of intense socialisation into the culture of the clinical work world. Socialisation, in this context, may be defined as 'a reciprocal process by which the neophyte nurses learn what others will demand of them in a specific role and, in turn, learn to exert control over their new environments' (p 1).[28] Myers and Arbor describe this process as one of 'give and take', a process through which new registered nurses 'learn to behave as nurses in the hospital setting'. It is through this process that the new nurse learns to behave 'according to the culturally prescribed rules and standards' of the clinical work world (pp 120–1).[28] Corwin[29] believes there is a 'turning point' between graduating from a nursing school and induction into employment for students. This turning point in a career produces role conflict between professional (idealised) role conceptions and bureaucratic (actualised) role conceptions in the working environment. Consequently, a sense of conflicting loyalties towards bureaucratic and professional systems of work organisation emerges.

The gap between what students are taught to expect and what is actually experienced in the early stages of work has been termed 'reality shock'.[30] Marlene Kramer, a nurse researcher, first recognised the problem in 1966. The difference between professional and bureaucratic role conceptions is a source of conflict for the nurse.[26,30,31] The strong dissimilarity in the expectations of these two systems often gives rise to nursing role conflicts.

Most studies of transition for new registered nurses have shown that there are challenges and difficulties associated with the process.[15,16,18,28,29,31,32–40] Common reactions to initial employment as a registered nurse include:

> physical and emotional exhaustion; a sense of inadequacy; frustration; loss of ideals and, at the extreme, the abandonment of nursing as a career. In other cases, where they [new graduates] have received support and encouragement and advice from more experienced nurses and from their own peers and families, initiation into the world of nursing is reported to be less stressful (p 3).[16]

Common problems that surface during transition include the theory–practice gap[41] (where theory learnt in the classroom does not match the theory said to be required in clinical practice),[16] limited proficiency in managing and executing technical procedures, time management, drug administration, patient assessment and report-writing skills.[1] Other issues include:

- managing nursing care responsibilities for a number of patients simultaneously
- working in teams
- coping with a beginning level of skill as a new registered nurse relative to job demands and workload
- the acceptance of accountability
- independently taking action and making decisions
- coping with unexpected events
- supervising other nurses
- shift work
- learning how to collaborate with other nurses and health professionals, including liaison and discussion about the total care of patients
- developing competence in planning and organising.[15,32,36,42–47]

In some research studies, heavy patient loads were found to create excessive tiredness in many new graduate nurses because they were often allocated high-dependency patient loads. This was further affected by low staffing ratios, which resulted in additional stress for the graduates as they attempted to adjust to their new culture (p 56).[35] A common issue for new graduates in many studies was having inadequate staff and time to complete all client care.[15,36,42,43] Many new registered nurses were also having to adjust not only to their own role, but also to the health service organisation. Because of the pressures in hospitals, many new nurses felt they lacked a receptive climate in which to enact many of the aspects of what they perceived should comprise a professional nurse's role, such as having autonomy and more responsibility to assess and plan care. This need to care for others well has been found to be related to personal satisfaction, as has appreciation for one's efforts.[48]

Role Ambiguity and Role Overload

Role ambiguity and role overload have also been identified as sources of stress during role transition and have been linked to organisational dynamics and subsequent job dissatisfaction and turnover. Many research studies, as far back as the 1970s, show a relationship between role ambiguity and voluntary turnover.[49–51] According to some authors, role ambiguity was more influential than role conflict in an individual leaving the organisation. In general, role ambiguity is defined as the lack of clear, consistent information about the behaviour expected in a role (p 23).[52]

There are two types of role ambiguity in relation to the uncertainty felt by the individual: (1) objective ambiguity, which arises from lack of the information needed for role definition and role performance; and (2) subjective ambiguity, which is related to the social–psychological aspects of role performance. This occurs where individuals are concerned about how others perceive them in relation to attainment of their personal goals.[52] Studies with registered nurses have shown, in all relationships, that role conflict or role ambiguity was a basis of negative influence, causing decreased job satisfaction.[15,48,53,54]

Role ambiguity is often increased by the fact that each ward is a specialty unit in an organisation, and has different personnel and unique patient management. New graduates not only have to adjust to the nursing role, but also adapt to the transition within complicated social networks. Role ambiguity can be further compounded by role overload, when graduates lack skills in handling role demands, establishing priorities and allocating their time wisely.[15,55,56]

Chang[15] conducted two longitudinal surveys on role stress. The first survey showed that role overload and ambiguity were negatively related to job satisfaction in the first few months of employment. However, in the second survey role overload was not significantly related to job satisfaction. In spite of the overload prevalent in the role of registered nurses, many of the graduates did not relate this to job satisfaction after 11–12 months of employment. It appears to be easier for graduates to deal with role overload after 1 year of employment. This may be a reflection of the graduates' coping abilities and experience gained in their role, which can ultimately make a difference in dealing with problems in the work environment (p 140).[57]

Factors Affecting Role Transition

According to a major Australian study undertaken by Madjar and colleagues in 1997:

> how well and how quickly newly graduated nurses are able to demonstrate mastery of their new role, acting in a safe, competent, sensitive, and confident manner, depends on a range of factors. In broad terms these may include:
> - personal qualities of each beginning registered nurse, including age, maturity, previous work experiences, motivation, aspirations, and availability of personal supports;
> - the quality and extent of the educational preparation, including the nature and duration of structured clinical experiences during the pre-registration course, and the quality and rigour of formative and summative assessments within the course;
> - the quality and duration of orientation/transition programs for new graduates provided by employing institutions;
> - the expectations, attitudes, reactions, and behaviour of more experienced clinical nurses, nurse managers and other staff toward new graduates, the role modelling of expected behaviour by more senior nurses, and the prevailing ethos of the institution;
> - the exigencies of clinical situations, staffing levels, and other demands placed on the registered nurse (p 3).[16]

The complexity of the process of transition is illustrated by the many factors that can influence individual experience. For most new graduates this is a time of stress and strain, learning and assimilation. It is also a time of upheaval and adjustment affecting all aspects of life (p 79).[16] During this time decisions are made about a long-term commitment to nursing. It is reassuring to note, however, that the majority of participants in the study reported that the transition process was worthwhile and culminated in 'a sense of satisfaction and personal achievement' (p 79).[16]

NEW GRADUATES: SKILLS AND STRENGTHS

Against this background of challenges and difficulties it is important to acknowledge the skills and strengths that new graduates have on entry to the workforce.[15,58] In a major longitudinal study of new graduates by Chang[15] conducted in New South Wales, Australia, both nursing unit managers and graduates believed that the graduates were well prepared in three main areas: (1) communication skills with patients; (2) psychosocial assessment skills; and (3) accountability for their actions.

These areas of strength were consistent with the findings of several other researchers who found that graduates excelled in identifying patients' psychological needs and in communicating with them. Even though more was thought to be needed in the development of technical and clinical skills, both graduates and their managers considered the overall performance to be adequate and felt that their education had been quite sufficient in preparing them for the job. Over time, graduates felt more confident and demonstrated significant improvement in performance. This may well have been expected, but strong significant improvement was observed across all areas of their role. In addition, nursing unit managers rated the overall performance of the graduates more positively compared with hospital-trained nurses. The graduates had mostly positive feelings about their tertiary program, and perceived that it had provided them with a theoretical background to care for the multidimensional needs of their patients – not only physical needs, but economic, spiritual and psychosocial needs as well.[15,35,58,59]

Other research studies[36,43] show that, over a period of time, graduates were working more autonomously, establishing relationships with their clients and coping with their new role. They saw the importance of their professional role, including being a health teacher, a provider of care, a communicator, an advocate, a coordinator of care, a decision maker and making suggestions for change in practice. These values are consistent with findings from studies in Australia and overseas which have examined the professional or value systems of graduates.[15,35,60,61] There is also evidence of greater skill acquisition in relation to assessing clients more quickly and in giving advice to other staff (p 41).[36] Skill acquisition was an important issue for many graduates as they progressed from novice to advanced beginner.[20]

STRATEGIES TO FACILITATE TRANSITION

Several strategies have been shown to be of use in easing the transition from student to new registered nurse. Cooperation between service and education plays a key role in the success or otherwise of many of these strategies. Many experts in nursing believe that:

> the key to bringing respective expectations [i.e. those of providers of BNE and clinical nursing services] into line with each other ... [is] the establishment of a more cooperative framework in which higher education and health agencies both contribute to improvements in clinical practice and in the graduate's transition to work (p 5).[17]

In relation to specific strategies, a positive preceptor relationship, adequate support systems and assignment congruence have been shown to have positive outcomes in the first 6 months of employment as a new registered nurse.[62] Preceptorship programs are one practical strategy offered to reduce culture shock and to assist new registered nurses in the integration of theory and practice. There is extensive literature on preceptorship programs.[34,63–67] One version of this strategy is called the professional nurturance preceptorship program, which can be jointly sponsored by healthcare and tertiary institutions. Reports of graduate nurse preceptorship programs have demonstrated that these programs are an effective means of facilitating the transition process for new graduates, including clinical learning. Such programs could also be incorporated as a subject in the final year of undergraduate nursing courses. During the preceptorship experience, the student is guided by the registered nurse preceptor in caring for appropriate patients. Initially, preceptor and student work closely together; as students develop greater confidence and competence, they are given more autonomy in patient care. A similar approach can be used with the experienced nurse preceptor and the new registered nurse.

Many important variables make the work environment either positive or negative for graduates. The key factors that appear to facilitate successful transition include a supportive environment that accommodates incremental development in clinical skill acquisition and patient management skills.[7,18] A graduate nurse who is assigned too many patients within a short timeframe may not be proficient enough to provide for patients' physical and psychosocial care. It is crucial that the workload is structured to provide opportunities for newly registered nurses to see the effective outcomes of their work.

In the practice environments that accept new graduates in nursing there needs to be ready recognition of, and support for, the fact that learning, especially clinical learning, is a lifelong process. Another positive influence on transition is preparedness and commitment by experienced registered nurses to value and nurture new registered nurses as they move through the transition process. The first national review of nurse education carried out in Australia (in 1994) made specific recommendations about transition support for beginning graduates of nursing. Relevant recommendations include that:

> graduates be provided with employer-funded assistance for transition to employment, including appropriate induction and orientation activities, peer support and mentoring as appropriate, and introduction to specific clinical requirements ... [and] ... where relevant infrastructure is not available (for example in rural and remote areas), funds be made available to provide appropriate levels of support (p 21).[17]

Some employers appear to be high performers in the way they manage new graduates entering employment. Consequently, a number of hospitals and community settings appear to function as 'magnets' for new registered nurses on the basis of the reputation they have built up for supporting and developing new graduate nurses. Other research has found that the attitudes of staff and a welcoming and positive environment also encourage graduates to adjust to the workplace.[68,69]

Knowing how to provide patient care is not enough for new graduates, although this, in itself, is a complex process requiring appropriate exposure and clinical learning. It is important that nurses are able to manage job stressors successfully. Health professionals, including nurses, need to learn how to care for themselves in order to care effectively for their patients. This requires a balanced approach to all facets of life and stress management skills.[2]

It is important to raise issues of concern during transition with appropriate colleagues and support systems. Discussion of these issues will lead to the identification of appropriate ways of managing problems early. This approach can be invaluable in reducing anxiety and stress, and facilitating successful adjustment to nursing practice.

Quality of worklife is a concept that is gaining currency, and health service providers need to address it to ensure adequate recruitment and retention of nursing staff. Sources of dissatisfaction in clinical nursing have been found to include inadequate staffing patterns, conflict with other healthcare providers, lack of support in dealing with death and dying, unresponsiveness in leadership, poor communication among staff and poor administration.[70,71] There is a clear need for leaders in nursing education to work with leaders in nursing service to develop short- and long-term strategies to promote and ensure sustainable nursing. This will require attention to a number of factors and processes that influence commitment to nursing; for example, socialisation programs affect the general satisfaction of staff and their feelings of autonomy and personal influence.

Other factors known to facilitate transition include:

- formal unit orientation programs that incorporate realistic goals[17,69]
- a unit climate of open communication and timely provision of constructive feedback on performance[69,72,73]
- assignment congruence – that is, not being given tasks beyond the new graduate's sphere of competence[65]
- participative, democratic governance[74,75]
- appropriate guidance from senior staff[76,77]
- continuing staff development opportunities[78]
- the provision of support and counselling for new employees[73]
- using personal strategies such as exercise or recreational activity to reduce stress levels.[57]

It is important that senior students in undergraduate nursing courses and new registered nurses anticipate the issues and challenges associated with transition. By building knowledge and understanding of these phenomena it is possible to plan to manage the transition period.[16] Managing involves the selection of a range of strategies designed to facilitate positive adjustment to the professional registered nurse role.

CONCLUSION

All graduates of nursing courses will experience a degree of culture shock on entry to the world of clinical practice. This experience is complex and multidimensional. Research has uncovered a number of issues and challenges that confront new graduates on entry to the workforce as registered nurses. In addition, a number of strategies have been found to be useful in easing the stress and strain associated with transition. Careful planning and use of resources in the practice environment can also facilitate positive adjustment to employment as a registered nurse. Nursing education and nursing service need to monitor the transition process continually to optimise the number of new registered nurses who manage this phenomenon successfully and go on to enjoy fulfilling, rewarding careers in their chosen profession.

CASE STUDY 1.1

Jane, a final-semester third-year student in a Bachelor of Nursing program, is preparing a plan to assist her in moving into a registered nurse role. She is apprehensive and anxious to excel in her new role. She knows that she can prepare for transition by drawing on the literature and other resources available to her. In this situation, Jane considers the following questions in preparing to develop her transition plan.

REFLECTIVE QUESTIONS

1. What do we know and understand from the literature about factors influencing transition?
2. What strategies have been found to be successful in enhancing transition to practice?
3. What types of resources can be accessed to facilitate individual transition?

CASE STUDY 1.2

Geoff, a nursing unit manager in a cardiac step-down unit, has a number of new graduate registered nurses starting work in his clinical area. He needs to develop an orientation program that will assist them in adjusting to their new roles and responsibilities. What advice could you give him regarding the needs of the new graduates?

REFLECTIVE QUESTIONS

1. What specific topics could be covered in the program, and why?
2. How could Geoff prepare his senior registered nurse colleagues to meet the support needs of the new graduates?

CASE STUDY 1.3

Mary Anne is a new graduate registered nurse who has worked in an aged care unit for 6 months. She is keen to enhance and extend her level of competence in the area of dementia care.

REFLECTIVE QUESTIONS

1. What professional competency frameworks can Mary Anne access to meet her needs?
2. How can she document and validate her learning needs and develop competence for this area of practice?

RECOMMENDED READING

Chang E, Hancock K. Role stress and role ambiguity in new nursing graduates in Australia. *Nursing and Health Sciences* 2003;**5**:155–63.

Ebert L, Hoffman K, Levett-Jones T, Connor G. 'They have no idea of what we do or what we know': Australian graduate's perceptions of working in a health care team. *Nurse Education in Practice* 2014. Online. Available: <http://dx.doi.org/10.101016/j.nep.2014.06.005/>.

Hinton A, Chirgwin S. Nursing education: reducing reality shock for graduate Indigenous nurses – it's all about time. *Australian Journal of Advanced Nursing* 2010;**28**:60–6.

Laschinger HK, Grau AL. The influence of personal dispositional factors and organizational resources on workplace violence, burnout and health outcomes in new graduate nurses: a cross sectional study. *International Journal of Nursing Studies* 2012;**49**:282–91.

Missen K, McKenna L, Beauchamp A. Satisfaction of newly graduated nurses enrolled in transition-to-practice programs in their first year of employment: a systematic review. *Journal of Advanced Nursing* 2014;2419–33.

REFERENCES

1. Englert J. *From the president. NRB Board Works: Newsletter of the Nurses Registration Board of New South Wales. November 2000.* Sydney: Nurses Registration Board of New South Wales; 2000.

2. Heath P. *National review of nursing education 2002: our duty of care.* Canberra: Commonwealth of Australia; 2002.

3. Department of Education, Science and Training. *The patient profession: a time for action. Senate Inquiry Report.* Canberra: Department of Education, Science and Training; 2002.

4. Australian Health Minister's Advisory Council. National Nursing and Nursing Education Taskforce. Online. Available: <www.nnnet.gov.au/> [2 April 2007].

5. Clare J, White J, Edwards H, et al. *Curriculum, clinical education, recruitment, transition and retention in nursing. Final Report for the Australian Universities Teaching Committee (AUTC).* Adelaide: Flinders University; 2002.

6. Theobald K, Mitchell M. Mentoring: improving transition to practice. *Australian Journal of Advanced Nursing* 2002;**20**:27–33.

7. Missen K, McKenna L, Beauchamp A. Satisfaction of newly graduated nurses enrolled in transition-to-practice programs in their first year of employment: a systematic review. *Journal of Advanced Nursing* 2014;2419–33.

8. Weng RH, Huang CY, Tsai WC, Chang LY, Lin SE, Lee MY. Exploring the impact of mentoring functions on job satisfaction and organizational commitment of new staff nurses. *BMC Health Services Research* 2010;**10**(240):1–9.

9. Hinton A, Chirgwin S. Nursing education: reducing reality shock for graduate Indigenous nurses – it's all about time. *Australian Journal of Advanced Nursing* 2010;**28**:60–6.

10. Kelly M, Flanagan B. Trends and developments in the use of health care simulation. *Collegian (Royal College of Nursing, Australia)* 2010;**17**:101–2.

11. Benner P, Sutphen M, Leonard V, et al. *Educating nurses: a call for radical transformation.* San Francisco: Jossey Bass; 2010.

12. Health Workforce Australia Workplan December 2010. Online. Available: <www.hwa.gov.au/>.

13. Preston B. Nurse workforce futures [electronic resource]: development and application of a model of demand for and supply of graduates of Australian and New Zealand pre-registration nurses and midwifery courses to 2010. Burwood, Victoria: 2007 Online. Available: <http://nla.gov.au/anbd.bib-an000041213952/> [2 April 2007].

14. Health Workforce Australia. *Health Workforce 2025 – Doctors, nurses and midwives*, vol. 2. Adelaide: Health Workforce Australia.

15. Chang EML. The socialisation of tertiary graduates into the workforce. PhD dissertation. School of Education Administration, University of New South Wales, Sydney; 1993.

16. Madjar I, McMillan M, Sharke R, et al. *Report of the project to review and examine expectations of beginning registered nurses in the workforce.* Sydney: Nurses Registration Board of New South Wales; 1997.

17. Reid J. *Nursing education in Australian universities: report of the national review of nurse education in the higher education sector 1994 and beyond.* Canberra: Australian Government Publishing Service; 1994.

18. Greenwood J. Critique of the graduate nurse: an international perspective. *Nurse Education Today* 2000;**20**:17–23.

19. Ebert L, Hoffman K, Levett-Jones T, Connor G. 'They have no idea of what we do or what we know': Australian graduate's perceptions of working in a health care team. *Nurse Education in Practice* 2014. Online. Available: <http://dx.doi.org/10.101016/j.nep.2014.06.005/>.

20. Benner P. *From novice to expert: excellence and power in clinical nursing practice.* Menlo Park, CA: Addison-Wesley; 1984.

21. Walker K. On philosophy: nursing and the politics of truth. In: Daly J, Speedy S, Jackson D, editors. *Contexts of nursing: an introduction.* Sydney: Elsevier; 2006. pp 60–72.

22. Conway J, McMillan M. Connecting clinical and theoretical knowledge for practice. In: Daly J, Speedy S, Jackson D, editors. *Contexts of nursing: an introduction.* Sydney: Elsevier; 2006. pp 317–31.

23. Godinez G, Schweiger J, Gruver J, et al. Role transition from graduate to staff nurse: a qualitative analysis. *Journal for Nurses in Staff Development* 1999;**13**:97–110.

24. Dobbs KK. The senior preceptorship as a method for anticipatory socialisation of baccalaureate nursing students. *Journal of Nursing Education* 1988;**2**:67–71.

25. Fisher JA, Connelly CD. Retaining graduate nurses: a staff development challenge. *Journal of Nursing Staff Development* 1989;**5**:6–10.

26. Kramer M. Role conceptions of baccalaureate nurses and success in hospital nursing. *Journal of Nursing Research* 1970;**19**:428–39.

27. Jarvis P. The practitioner-researcher in nursing. *Nurse Education Today* 2000;**20**:30–5.

28. Myers LC. *The socialization of neophyte nurses.* Ann Arbor, MI: UMI Research Press; 1979.

29. Corwin R. Role conception and mobility aspirations: a study in the formation and transformation of nursing identities. PhD dissertation. Sociology Department, University of Minnesota, Minneapolis; 1960.

30. Kramer M. *Reality shock.* St Louis, MO: Mosby; 1974.

31. Kramer M. *Some effects of exposure to employing bureaucracies on the role conceptions and role deprivation of neophyte collegiate nurses. PhD dissertation.* School of Education, Stanford University, Stanford, CA; 1966.

32. Horsburgh M. Graduate nurses' adjustment to initial employment: natural fieldwork. *Journal of Advanced Nursing* 1989;**14**:610–17.

33. Perry J. Theory and practice in the induction of five graduate nurses: a reflexive critique. Masters thesis. Massey University, Palmerston North, New Zealand; 1985.

34. Prebble K, McDonald B. Adaptation to the mental health setting: the lived experience of comprehensive graduates. *Australian and New Zealand Journal of Mental Health Nursing* 1987;**6**:30–6.

35. Kilstoff K. Evaluation of the process of transition from college student to beginning nurse practitioner. Masters dissertation. School of Education, Macquarie University, Sydney; 1993.

36. Walker W. The transition to registered nurse: the experience of a group of New Zealand graduates. *Nursing Praxis in New Zealand* 1998;**13**:36–43.

37. Troskie R. Critical evaluation of the newly qualified nurse's competency to practise: part 2. *Curationis: South African Journal of Nursing* 1993;**16**:56–61.

38. Dufault M. Personal and work milieu resources as variables associated with role mastery in the novice nurse. *Journal of Continuing Education in Nursing* 1990;**21**:73–8.

39. Kapborg ID, Fischbein S. Nurse education and professional work: transition problems? *Nurse Education Today* 1998;**18**:165–71.

40. van Vorst S. New graduate nurses' perceptions of their experience in mental health nursing. Masters dissertation. Faculty of Nursing, Midwifery & Health, Sydney University of Technology, Sydney; 1999.

41. Speedy S. Theory–practice debate: setting the scene. *Australian Journal of Advanced Nursing* 1998;**6**:12–19.

42. Jasper M. The first year as a staff nurse: the experience of a first cohort of project 2000 nurses in a demonstration district. *Journal of Advanced Nursing* 1996;**24**:779–80.

43. Kelly B. Hospital nursing: it's battle! A follow-up study of English graduate nurses. *Journal of Advanced Nursing* 1996;**24**:1063–9.

44. Mackay L, Brooke A, Bruni N. *The first working year in nursing: an evaluation of a group of college students.* Canberra: Commonwealth Tertiary Education Commissioner; 1981.

45. McArthur J, Brooke A, Bruni N. *Further comparative evaluation of students and graduates.* Canberra: Commonwealth Tertiary Education Commissioner; 1983.

46. Nichols G. Important satisfying and dissatisfying aspects of nurses' jobs. *Supervisor Nurse* 1974;**5**:10–15.

47. Rotkovich R. Fifty golden years of education and service: a marriage of convenience or necessity? *Journal of Nursing Administration* 1973;**Sep/Oct**:10–12.

48. Crout T, Crout J. Care plan for retaining the new nurse. *Nursing Management* 1984;**15**:30–3.

49. Johnson T, Graen G. Organisation assimilation and role rejection. *Organisational Behaviour and Human Performance* 1973;**10**:72–87.

50. Lyons F. Role clarity, need for clarity, satisfaction, tension and withdrawer. *Organisational Behaviour and Human Performance* 1971;**6**:99–110.

51. Rizzo JR, House RJ, Lirtzman SI. Role conflict and ambiguity in complex organisations. *Administrative Science Quarterly* 1970;**15**:1150–69.

52. Kahn R, Wolfe D, Quinn R, et al. *Organizational stress: studies in role conflict and ambiguity.* New York: Wiley; 1964.

53. Rogers DL, Molnar DL. Organisational antecedents of role conflict and ambiguity in top level administrators. *Administrative Quarterly* 1976;**21**:598–610.

54. Szilagyi A. An empirical test of causal inference between role conceptions, satisfaction with work, performance and organisational level. *Personnel Psychology* 1977;**30**:43–71.

55. Hardy M. Role stress and role strain. In: Hardy ME, Conway ME, editors. *Role theory: perspectives for health professionals.* New York: Appleton-Century-Crofts; 1978.

56. McCloskey JC, McCain BE. Satisfaction, commitment, and professionalism of newly employed nurses. *Image: Journal of Nursing Scholarship* 1987;**19**:20–4.

57. Chang E, Hancock K. Role stress and role ambiguity in new nursing graduates in Australia. *Nursing and Health Sciences* 2003;**5**:155–63.

58. Chang E, Kilstoff K. Implications for professional practice: reflections of issues that impact on nursing education. Paper presented at 6th National Nursing Education Conference, Canberra; 1994.

59. Chang EML. Surveying the professional socialisation of tertiary graduates into the workforce. In: Macpherson RJL, Weeks J, editors. *Pathways to knowledge in educational administration.* Armidale, NSW: Australian Council for Educational Administration; 1990.

60. Carroll E, Dwyer L. *What kind of crisis? The nursing shortage in NSW.* Canberra: Australian Public Policy Case Library; 1988.

61. Goldsworthy A, Pickhaver A, Young W. *They seem different.* Adelaide: Sturt College of Advanced Education; 1984.

62. Seed A. Crossing the boundaries – experiences of neophyte nurses. *Journal of Advanced Nursing* 1995;**21**:1136–43.

63. Allanach BC, Jennings BM. Evaluating the effects of a nurse preceptorship programme. *Journal of Advanced Nursing* 1990;**15**:22–8.

64. Brasler ME. Predictors of clinical performance of new graduate nurses participating in preceptor orientation programmes. *Journal of Continuing Education in Nursing* 1993;**24**:158–65.
65. Boyle DK, Popkess-Vawter S, Taunton RL. Socialisation of new graduate nurses in critical care. *Heart and Lung: Journal of Acute and Critical Care* 1996;**25**:141–54.
66. Santucci J. Facilitating the transition into nursing practice: concepts and strategies for mentoring new graduates. *Journal for Nurses in Staff Development* 2004;**20**:274–84.
67. Pickens JM, Fargostein B. Preceptorship: a shared journey between practice and education. *Journal of Psychosocial Nursing* 2006;**44**:1–5.
68. Butts BJ, Witmer DM. New graduates: what does my manager expect? *Nursing Management* 1992;**23**:46–8.
69. Wootton RM. *Orientation of newly registered comprehensive nurses for work in the health care service*. Christchurch: Christchurch Polytechnic, Department of Nursing Studies; 1987.
70. Smyth E. *Surviving nursing*. Menlo Park, CA: Addison-Wesley; 1984.
71. Bailey JT. Job stress and other stress-related problems. In: Claus KE, Bailey JT, editors. *Living with stress and promoting well-being*. St Louis, MO: Mosby; 1980.
72. Hart G, Rotem A. The best and the worst students' experiences of clinical education. *Australian Journal of Advanced Nursing* 1994;**11**:26–33.
73. Feldman DC. A practical program for employee socialisation. *Organisational Dynamics* 1976;**5**:64–80.
74. Ellis BH. Nurses' communicative relationships and the prediction of organizational commitment, burnout, and retention in acute care settings. PhD dissertation. Michigan State University, East Lansing, MI; 1991.
75. Leveck ML, Jones CB. The nursing practice environment, staff retention and quality of care. *Research in Nursing and Health* 1996;**19**:331–43.
76. Vance C. Managing the politics of the workplace. *Imprint* 1992;**39**:16–19.
77. Coeling HV. Commentary on supportive communication among nurses – effects on commitment, burnout, and retention. *AONE's Leadership Perspectives* 1995;**3**:13.
78. Kiat KT. NYP nursing graduates in the first year. *Professional Nurse (Singapore)* 1996;**23**:22–3.

CHAPTER 2

Becoming a competent, confident, professional registered nurse

Jill White

LEARNING OBJECTIVES

When you have completed this chapter you will be able to:

- ▲ develop an understanding of the complexity of the development of practice knowledge
- ▲ appreciate the deeply contextual nature of professional practice knowledge
- ▲ understand the transformation in skill acquisition from novice to expert
- ▲ construct a personal plan for reflective practice
- ▲ develop a positive perception of yourself as being on a career-long journey of refining understandings of nursing practice.

KEYWORDS: competent, competencies, confidence, reflection, professional development

INTRODUCTION

On graduation one of the hardest things to come to terms with is the apparent discrepancy between the way you, as a new graduate, see a clinical situation and the way an expert nurse might see it. At university the focus seemed to be on understanding the signs, symptoms and diagnoses, and making decisions through the exercise of 'clinical judgment'. This usually involves breaking the situation down into understandable, 'bite-sized' pieces and then reintegrating them. Experienced nurses rarely seem to do this in their practice. *How do I get from where I am now to that sort of confidence and competence?* is a question that, as a new graduate, you may sometimes find yourself asking. *Why didn't my university studies prepare me properly for the real world? And what is this competent/competence/competency anyway?*

COMPETENCE IN NURSING PRACTICE

At university, nursing programs focus on the development of competence as meaning the 'skills, knowledge, attitudes, values and abilities that underpin effective ...

performance in a profession/occupational area' as defined in the Nursing and Midwifery Board of Australia competencies document, *National Competency Standards for the Registered Nurse*, commonly referred to as the Australian Nursing and Midwifery Council competencies.[1] These are a set of minimum competencies accepted by the national registration authority in Australia as core standards for registration. They are a means by which expectations of standards of nursing practice can be communicated within the profession, across health professions and to consumers.

There are currently ten competency standards involving responsibilities related to four domains. These domains are: (1) professional practice (including practising ethically and within the law); (2) critical thinking and analysis (including professional development, and valuing and using evidence and research); (3) provision and coordination of care (including coordination, organisation, comprehensive assessment, and the provision and evaluation of care); and (4) collaborative and therapeutic practice (including professional relationships with individuals and groups, and communication and collaboration within interdisciplinary healthcare teams). By now you will be familiar with these as they will have been the benchmarks against which you will be, or will have been, assessed in the clinical environment to be competent prior to graduation.

University, however, can only do part of the job of preparing a confident, competent professional nurse. It is in the nature of the acquisition of practice understanding that it takes layer upon layer of personal clinical experiences to move towards competence in the practice reality of nursing, as opposed to assessment of 'competence' following graduation from university and the beginning of practice as a registered nurse.

SKILL ACQUISITION

The cardinal work of Patricia Benner[2] provides us with a useful map for understanding the notion of skill acquisition within practice. Benner's work was a refinement and application of the work on skill development by Dreyfus and Dreyfus,[3] who developed this schema by studying airline pilots and chess players. From this study, Dreyfus and Dreyfus came up with five levels of skill acquisition: (1) novice; (2) advanced beginner; (3) competent; (4) proficient; and (5) expert. (Yes, there is that word again. It's very confusing when the word 'competent' is used by so many to mean so many different things.)

The novice in Benner's work has no experience of a situation and requires context-free rules to be available in order to make sense of what would otherwise be an impenetrably messy, undifferentiated situation. Remember what it felt like when you approached your first few clinical practice experiences?

The advanced beginner has coped with sufficient clinical situations to have grasped what to do in a global sense and can demonstrate what Benner[2] describes as 'marginally acceptable performance'. It is still difficult for advanced beginners to be really sure of what is important in a situation, and rapidly changing situations or subtle changes often elude them. This time the question is not 'Do you remember this?', but 'Do you recognise this?'. Benner suggests that new graduates are advanced beginners and that they remain so until they have spent upwards of a year-and-a-half in one type of clinical setting, at which time they reach Benner's level of skill acquisition of 'competent'.[4] She further states that transferring to a very different clinical environment brings the nurse quickly back to advanced beginner status, despite expertise in another field of nursing.

The biggest jump in practice skill development occurs between the competent nurse and the proficient one, as this represents a move in cognitive grasp from perceiving aspects of a situation to perceiving the situation as a whole. It is at this stage that it becomes easier to tell whether a patient is moving along an expected path, or is moving subtly into difficulties.

The movement through the levels of skill acquisition is characterised by:

> ... a movement from reliance on abstract principles to the use of past
> concrete experiences; a change in the learner's perception of the demand of
> the situation, in which the situation is seen as less and less a compilation
> of equally relevant bits, and more and more as a complete whole in which
> certain parts are more relevant; and a passage from detached observer to
> involved performer.[2]

The expert involved performer is defined by Benner[2] as one who:

> ... no longer relies on an analytic principle to connect her or his
> understanding of the situation to an appropriate action. The expert – with
> an enormous background of experience – now has an intuitive grasp of
> each situation.

But hang on, isn't intuition the thing that we have without formal education – the 'just knowing' that is demonstrated so well by adolescents?

INTUITION

Two of the most confusing words that are constants of the new environment of work are 'competence' and 'intuition', and trying to gain a sense of shared understanding about them seems difficult.

'Intuition' is an often used, frequently misunderstood word – we use it colloquially to mean 'undifferentiated gut feeling' and at other times very specifically to mean 'expert clinical judgment'. One of the main confusions in looking at this concept is that we do not often stop to explore and ensure that our use of the word is received with shared meaning.

In a systematic review of the literature on intuition within the discipline of nursing from 1981 to 2006, Rew and Barrow[5] devised the following definition from the literature:

> A way of knowing something immediately as a whole that improves with
> experience, informs their judgements and decisions, and leads them to take
> action within the caring relationship.

We have all heard people say they 'just knew' something, that they had a 'gut feeling', but what is it that distinguishes the type of intuition ascribed to the expert practitioner and that 'knowing' that we refer to as naive, mystical thinking or simple prejudice? Intuition is not something commonly regarded as descriptive of expert behaviour, and yet in the clinical literature it is often seen as the hallmark of expert practice. Perhaps if we look at the practice-focused literature on intuition we may find a clue.

The term 'intuition' appears to have entered the clinical literature in the 1980s with the work on skill development in practice by Dreyfus and Dreyfus[3] and Schon,[6] and within nursing by Benner and others.[2,4]

The key aspects that Dreyfus and Dreyfus[3] saw as representing this intuitive judgment were:

- pattern recognition – similarities and links with previous experiences
- similarity recognition – 'fuzzy' resemblances, similarities despite differences
- common-sense understanding – knowing the practice setting and its patterns
- skilled know-how – mastery of the job
- sense of salience – recognition of some events as more important than others
- deliberative rationality – exploring what might stand out as significant if one's perspective were changed.

It is obvious when we look at these aspects of intuitive judgment that they are predicated on deep contextual knowing of a practice situation. So, it is time to be kind to yourself, and to think of this as an opportunity to look at how you can take best advantage of your new clinical access to begin to gather and mentally file your repertoire of pictures of clinical situations, rather than being harsh with yourself about what you do not know.

If we accept that there is an important component of expert practice that has, for good or ill, been called intuition, we return to the question of how we differentiate this from the more colloquial use of the term. The work of Belenky and colleagues, in *Women's Ways of Knowing*,[7] may be helpful here. This research was influenced by the work of Kohlberg[8] and Perry,[9] two key figures in our understanding of psychological development, and by Gilligan's[10] critique of these works as gender-distorted, as they were developed studying only men.

As a result of their extensive research with women, Belenky and colleagues[7] found that the women's positions were better represented as five – rather than Perry's four – ways of knowing, and that women have a position previous to Perry's first level. The researchers called this level 'silence', where women perceive themselves as having no voice at all. The five ways of knowing are:

1. Silence: nothing worth saying.
2. Received knowledge: listening to the voices of others and holding them as 'true' – 'black-and-white' thinking.
3. Subjective knowledge: the inner voice – personal opinion.
4. Procedural knowledge: the voice of reason, of what is known.
5. Constructed knowledge: integrating the voices. Here it is possible to hold a personal opinion, having considered the available literature and being aware of the multiple other positions that might be held on the subject.

The reason for introducing this work here is that it provides us with a strong point of differentiation between the various ways in which the word 'intuition' is used. The chapter in *Women's Ways of Knowing* on subjective knowledge begins with the words of a young mother, Inez:

> There's a part of me that I didn't know I had until recently – instinct, intuition, whatever. It helps me and protects me. It's perceptive and astute. I just listen to the inside of me and I know what to do.[7]

In this stage of subjective knowledge things cease to be clear-cut, and personal freedom and personal opinions are asserted. Inez continues:

> I can only know with my gut. I've got it tuned to a point where I think and feel at the same time and I know what is right. My gut is my best friend – the one thing in the world that won't let me down or lie to me or back away from me.[7]

We do not wish to denigrate this powerful personal knowing. It is a deep point of inner strength on a journey of knowing, but it is a private knowing and, as such, has the limitations of 'small sample size and limited generalisability'; it also suffers the inevitable influences of potency of an experience and recency of experience. First-hand experience and the intergenerational stories of those in close private spaces are critical to the development of this knowing. It is the 'feel-right' component of knowing, for example, one's children. It seems not dissimilar to the knowing described by Tanner and colleagues[11] in their early work on 'knowing the patient', with its in-depth knowledge of the patterns of responses and the knowing of the patient as a person. (We return to knowing the patient later.)

Such personal knowing is the agency of maternal authority and is therefore not to be ignored. It is the unwise nurse or doctor who does not listen to the mother's report on her child's condition and, particularly, on subtle changes in condition. The mother knows her own child, but would not be in a position to make a judgment on the child of another mother. The knowing needs to be understood and responded to as highly contextually confined.

As an aside, an interesting difference in the wording of subjective knowledge and Perry's second level – called 'multiplicity' – is the masculine assertion, 'I have a right to my opinion', contrasted with the less confrontational position, 'It's just my opinion.' The qualification 'just' characterises women's description of their intuitions, as does the description of the 'feeling' component.

In moving to procedural knowledge there is a profound shift – a shift to appreciating the fallibility of gut feelings and of the importance of shared knowledge and understanding which can be gained without direct experience of an event. Seeing outside our own frame of reference characterises this stage – setting personal experience within the context of extant knowledge of an informed community.

How, then, do we gain access to understanding something that we have not or could not experience directly? This is the research and theory base of the procedural knowledge of Belenky and colleagues[7] and represents the theoretical and research base provided by formal education. It includes work such as the meta-analyses being undertaken by groups like the Cochrane Collaboration with their user-friendly outcome summaries, detailing those practices that reduce negative outcomes, those that appear promising, those that have unknown effects and, most importantly, those that should be abandoned.

The issue for practice and practitioners here is not necessarily the lack of research and theory but the issue of having practitioners incorporate the research findings into practice, particularly those identified as 'should be abandoned'. Procedural knowledge gives the novice-to-competent nurse a basis for determining: What can be wrong? What can go wrong? What can be done? This then allows the nurse to enter the clinical field with a framework of generalised knowledge from which to personalise and contextualise for a specific patient: What should be done for this person, at this time, in this circumstance? Inherent in this is an element that we might call 'knowing the patient'. This, importantly, is where you find yourself now.

KNOWING THE PATIENT

In later refinements of the concept of expert practice, Tanner and colleagues[11] took Benner's notion of 'involved performer' and explored it further through what they called 'knowing the patient'. They saw this as a precursor to the exercise of intuitive judgments and therefore to moving from the stage of competent to that of proficient or expert nurse. Two specific elements to 'knowing the patient' were found: 'in-depth knowledge of the patient's responses' and 'knowing the patient as a person'. In-depth knowledge of the patient's patterns of responses included responses to therapeutic measures, routines and habits, coping resources, physical capacities and endurance, and body typology and characteristics.

This was illustrated by the following clinical exemplar:

> ... you look at this kid, because you know this kid and you know what he looked like two hours ago. It's a dramatic difference to you but [it] is hard to describe that to someone in words.[11]

Knowing the patient as a person, on the other hand, was seen as the need to be able to know the person outside his or her present situation, particularly where the patient was a baby or an unconscious adult.

> I had never ever spoken to this man, but I grew to know him because of the family, because I became real close to his wife and son and knew what he was like before.[11]

An extension of this work by Liaschenko and Fisher[12] gave even greater clarity to this notion. They suggest there are three types of knowledge, which they call 'case', 'patient' and 'person' knowledge. *Case knowledge* is that generalised knowledge which we were just discussing. The two types of particular interest here are patient and person knowledge. These are differentiated as follows.

Patient knowledge includes knowledge of how the individual is identified as a patient, the individual's responses to therapeutics, how to get things done for the person within and between institutions, and a knowledge of other providers involved in the care of the person. This places the person in the context of healthcare and treatment as an individual.

Person knowledge is knowledge of personal biography. Person knowledge is a potent reminder that the life lived is the life of the recipient of care. Nurses use their person knowledge to defend their arguments for an alternative management of disease trajectories and to justify their actions when those actions support an individual's agency, even though this can conflict with established biomedical or institutional courses of action.

Stein-Parbury and Liaschenko[13] took this concept further when exploring the collaborative work of nurses and doctors in the intensive care context. They used the classifications of case, patient and person knowledge to analyse situations in which interprofessional collaboration broke down. They found that 'collaboration broke down when doctors dismissed nurses' concerns because they did not fit into a schema of case knowledge'. Managing the confused patient was seen as a problem to be solved by nurses, as it requires 'knowing the patient' in order to be able to respond to the person's particular behaviour, and 'making sense' of behaviour is made possible when one could put it in the context of the specific person – that is through having patient knowledge.

Liaschenko and Fisher[12] elaborated on the importance of social knowledge that links patient knowledge to person knowledge. They stressed the importance of understanding illness trajectories that go beyond the health system and into the world of the person who is the patient. This includes knowledge of:

- the social conditions in which the recipient lives
- the impact of the particular disease on the individual's ability to function and manage his or her disease in a variety of contexts
- the stigma attached to a given disease
- the degree to which the individual takes up the dominant cultural discourse about his or her particular disease.

This type of knowing is helped by providing opportunities to walk in the shoes of the other, and can be accessed through storytelling, by novels or books of accounts of illness experience, through poetry and in movies. These sources provide us with profound glimpses into the experiences of others, and increase our personal repertoire of knowing and therefore our readiness to interact appropriately with others. This knowing can be elaborated by narrative analysis, and by research using a variety of interpretive methodologies.

Understanding culture and its relationship to power, politics, language, identity, family and land connection is an essential part of knowing the person. It includes exploration of whose voices are privileged and whose voices are silenced. It seeks to expose and explore alternative conceptions of reality. Ramsden's[14] ground-breaking work on cultural safety developed in New Zealand (*kawa whakaruruhau*) offers nursing the opportunity to explore its practice in relation to cultural recognition, respect and nurture. This dimension of our nursing knowledge is now being developed in Australia and presents much in the way of a challenge.[15,16] This challenge is posed to all nurses by the Council for Aboriginal and Torres Strait Islander Nurses and Midwives (CATSNaM). We can enhance our cultural/political understandings through research grounded in critical theory such as action research, by critical ethnography, by feminist studies or by discourse analyses, but the fundamental element of cultural understanding is knowing oneself and challenging 'taken-for-granteds'. Brookfield,[17] although writing over two decades ago now, makes the point in a way we have not seen bettered when he states: 'coming to realise that every belief we hold, every behaviour we cherish as normal, every social or economic arrangement we perceive as fixed and unalterable can be and is regarded by others as bizarre, inexplicable, and wholly irrational.'

Knowing the patient at all three levels of case, patient and person allows the nurse to accrue layer upon layer of clinical pictures and patient responses which, on reflection, enable the nurse to have a body of experience on which to draw 'intuitively' when faced with any of Dreyfus and Dreyfus's aspects of intuition – that is, pattern recognition; similarity recognition; common-sense understanding; skilled know-how; sense of salience; and deliberative rationality.

This is the experience described by Benner[2] and Schon.[6] It is experience that incorporates reflective practice. They both speak of experience as not simply being time spent in a situation, but rather as new understandings that come with a disturbing of the taken-for-granted and expected happenings through reflection in action or reflection on action. In Benner's[2] words, experience results when 'preconceived notions and expectations are challenged, refined, or disconfirmed in the actual situation'[2] or, as she and her colleagues elaborate in a later text:

> Experience, as defined here, is not the mere passage of time but rather is an active transformation and refinement of expectations and perceptions in evolving situations. The nurse shifts from exclusive use of objective characteristics and quantitative measures as guides to understanding and action with particular patients. Clinical reasoning is based on understanding patient changes through time – that is reasoning through transitions.[4]

This work has clear implications for organisational work practices of relevance to new graduates, particularly in terms of consistency of work environment and stable ward staffing to facilitate the development of collegial trust and the authority that comes with trust. It holds implications, too, for the introduction of models of care delivery that enhance opportunities for continuity of care and carer, a continuity that enables very thorough 'knowing [of] the person'.

McCormack and McCance[18] have developed a theoretical framework for person-centred nursing which is predicated on the work of Benner, Tanner and colleagues, Liaschenko and others, and captures these organisational and staffing issues as well as those of nursing skill acquisition. The framework has four central constructs:

- prerequisites, which focus on what they call the 'attributes' of the nurse
- the care environment, which focuses on the care context
- person-centred processes, which focus on the activities through which care is delivered
- expected outcomes, which come from effective person-centred nursing.

The attributes of the nurse which form McCormack and McCance's[18] prerequisites include 'being professionally competent; having developed interpersonal skills; being committed to the job; being able to demonstrate clarity of beliefs and values; and knowing self'.

The care environment elements that affect person-centred nursing include 'appropriate skill mix; systems that facilitate shared decision-making; the sharing of power; effective staff relationships; organisational systems that are supportive; the potential for innovation and risk-taking; and the physical environment'. These elements are heavily dependent on skilled nursing leadership and an open and inquiring organisational culture. They influence the nurse's ability to know the patient and to observe and gain feedback from skilled colleagues.

Person-centred processes require working with the person's beliefs and values, sharing decision making and the provision of holistic care. With the above in place the outcomes should be manifest by the creation of a therapeutic environment within which the patient and family are satisfied with their care.

It is clear, then, that if the goal of nursing is the creation of a therapeutic environment in which patients receive safe, appropriate and quality care with which they are satisfied, developing the attributes described above is an essential step – that is, becoming a competent, confident, professional registered nurse.

REFLECTIVE PRACTICE

This brings us to perhaps the most potent of all aspects of your continued learning – reflective practice, the key to learning from experience. Much has been written about the importance of reflection to the developing practitioner, most notably by Schon,[6] but it has been elaborated on within nursing by many. Reflective practice is the subject of a chapter of its own (Chapter 18) but is referred to briefly here as it is critical to practise skill acquisition and movement towards expert practice. Johns[19] provides an excellent example of the transformation of novice to expert learning from practice through reflection by using Belenky and colleagues' ways of knowing, as described earlier. This will give you a clear exemplar of this movement in thinking to the constructed voice or, as Johns calls it, 'whole brain stuff using both hemispheres to marry logic, reason [and] analysis with creativity, curiosity and perception'. Rolfe[20] is also helpful here, as he provides a framework for different levels of sophistication of reflective thinking. These he calls 'descriptive', 'theory–knowledge building' and 'action-oriented' reflection. *Descriptive reflection* asks: What? What happened? What was my role? What was the response? *Theory–knowledge building reflection* asks: So what? What does this teach me? What was I thinking? What could or should I have done better? *Action-oriented reflection* asks: Now what? What do I need to do to improve care?

There are many texts that will assist you in gaining reflective practice skills. Two of the most accessible 'how to' books are Bev Taylor's[21] *Reflective Practice for Health Professionals* and Lioba Howatson-Jones's *Reflective Practice in Nursing,*[22] where the skill development options are extensively laid out. Both books assist you to write, draw, meditate, use a diary – to do whatever will help you look back critically on what you did and how you did it, on how it may have affected people and on what else could have been done, on what you would do differently next time and what you have learnt from the experience.

Deep engagement in clinical practice, deep connection with patients in their circumstances and deep reflection on the process are the essential ingredients of what Belenky and colleagues[7] call 'constructed knowledge'. *Constructed knowledge* is the integration of the voices, obliterating the spaces between private and public knowing: 'weaving together the strands of rational and emotive thought and of integrating objective and subjective knowing'. The real learning of artful practice is through the intelligent watching of the practice of ourselves and others and reflecting in and on that practice. This highest level of knowing, necessary for the development of expert practice, allows the very difficult work of the experienced, expert nurse who is often called upon to make judgments with imperfect and often contradictory information and to do so in a time-bound manner.

CONCLUSION

Bringing together intuition from our private life experiences (subjective knowing) and theoretical understanding through research undertaken in the public domain (procedural knowing) in their fullness through practice-based experience gains the other type of intuition (expert clinical practice). But let us call it what it is, the best of constructed knowledge in action – practice wisdom.

Bring forward the best of your theoretical learning as it has been modified and tested through your clinical experiences to date. Bring them together with the layer upon layer of clinical pictures you are beginning to collect and collate, enrich these through reflection on what you have learnt and are learning, deeply engage with your patients and colleagues, and be open to changing your current understandings of the meaning of illness, pain and suffering. You are ready. You are at the beginning of the rest of your journey towards being a competent, confident, professional registered nurse. Here is the best bit. The journey can last for as long as you choose to practise. The gaining of wisdom is a never-ending journey. Go well.

CASE STUDY 2.1

Sally is the senior nurse on the general medical surgical ward to which Jane has been allocated for her second new graduate rotation. After dinner one evening, Mr Falter in bed 1 appears unwell and is complaining of epigastric pain but says it is just his heartburn playing up again. Jane reports this to Sally, who moves quickly into assessment action and appears to be taking the situation very seriously. And indeed, within a matter of minutes Mr Falter has suffered a heart attack. When Jane and Sally have time to debrief later during the shift, they discuss the differences in what they saw, what it may have signalled and what action they would have planned.

REFLECTIVE QUESTIONS

1. Take a few minutes at the end of a shift to write a brief account of a critical incident in which you were involved that day, one in which an experienced nurse also took part.
2. When you have finished your account, ask the experienced registered nurse to recount his or her recollection of the event and what he or she saw as the most significant aspects. How did your accounts differ? Why might this be so?

CASE STUDY 2.2

Harriet Preacher is a 35-year-old woman from Roseville in Sydney. She was admitted to your hospital last night and is currently in the intensive care unit. She was admitted via ambulance after an episode of lack of consciousness, followed on arousal by complaints of severe neck and head pain. On scan she was diagnosed as having had a small bleed from an aneurysm, which was clipped in theatre prior to admission to the ward. Mrs Preacher has a picture of two children beside her bed and they appear to be a boy and girl in their early teens. She is currently being visited by her husband Sean, who tells you that she is very upset at missing the children's school drama production this evening and that she has asked Sean to bring her in some food to replace the hospital food, which she says is flavourless.

REFLECTIVE QUESTIONS

1. Which pieces of the above information are examples of 'knowing the patient' using Liaschenko and Fisher's topology: case knowledge, patient knowledge and person knowledge?
2. Explore your clinical work on your next shift and note examples of case knowledge, patient knowledge and person knowledge.
3. In what ways do these different ways of 'knowing the patient' help you to determine the basis for your care?

CASE STUDY 2.3

Asham has been a registered nurse for 4 years and loves his job. He consistently volunteers to help mentor new graduates and staff who are new to the area. Patients really respond well to him, and the feedback the nursing unit manager receives is always that Asham is a nice person and an excellent communicator. He leads the 'essentials of care' team in the values clarification exercises, having already completed the facilitator's course, of which introspection and personal values clarification are inherent parts.

REFLECTIVE QUESTIONS

1. Assess Asham in terms of his attributes for engaging in person-centred nursing. What other information would you want to know before completing this assessment?
2. In McCormack and McCance's[17] patient-centred nursing framework, give yourself a score out of five for the 'prerequisites' or 'attributes' of the nurse:
   - professional competence
   - interpersonal skills
   - commitment to the job
   - clarity of beliefs and values
   - self-knowledge.
3. Studying these results, what actions might you take to increase your score so that it is closer to 5 out of 5?

RECOMMENDED READING

Benner P. *From novice to expert: excellence and power in clinical nursing practice.* Menlo Park, CA: Addison-Wesley; 1984.

Benner P, Tanner C, Chesla C. *Expertise in nursing practice.* 2nd ed. New York: Springer; 2009.

Howatson-Jones L. *Reflective practice in nursing.* 2nd ed. Thousand Oaks, CA: Sage Publications; 2013. (E-book)

McCormack B, McCance T. *Person-centred nursing: theory and practice.* Oxford, UK: Wiley Blackwell; 2010.

Taylor B. *Reflective practice for health professionals.* 3rd ed. McGraw-Hill International (UK) Ltd; 2010. (E-book)

REFERENCES

1. Australian Nursing and Midwifery Council. *National competency standards for the registered nurse.* 4th ed. Canberra: Australian Nursing and Midwifery Council; 2006. Available: <www.nursingmidwiferyboard.gov.au/Codes-Guidelines-Statements/Codes-Guidelines.aspx#practiceguide>.

2. Benner P. *From novice to expert: excellence and power in clinical nursing practice.* Menlo Park, CA: Addison-Wesley; 1984.

3. Dreyfus H, Dreyfus S. *Mind over machine: the power of human intuition and expertise in the era of the computer.* New York: Free Press; 1986.

4. Benner P, Tanner C, Chesla C. *Expertise in nursing practice.* 2nd ed. New York: Springer; 2009.

5. Rew L, Barrow E. State of the science: intuition in nursing, a generation studying the phenomenon. *ANS. Advances in Nursing Science* 2007;**30**:E15–25.

6. Schon D. *The reflective practitioner.* New York: Basic Books; 1983.

7. Belenky M, Clinchy B, Goldberger N. *Women's ways of knowing.* New York: Basic Books; 1986.

8. Kohlberg L. *The philosophy of moral development.* New York: Harper & Row; 1981.

9. Perry W. *Forms of intellectual and ethical development in the college years.* New York: Holt, Rinehart & Winston; 1970.

10. Gilligan C. *In a different voice: psychological theory and women's development.* Cambridge, MA: Harvard University Press; 1982.

11. Tanner C, Benner P, Chesla C. The phenomenology of knowing the patient. *Image* 1993;**25**:273–80.

12. Liaschenko J, Fisher A. Theorizing the knowledge that nurses use in the conduct of their work. *Scholar Inquiry Nurse Pract* 1999;**13**(1):29–41.

13. Stein-Parbury J, Liaschenko J. Understanding collaboration between nurses and physicians as knowledge at work. *American Journal of Critical Care* 2007;**16**:470–7.

14. Ramsden I. *Kawa whakaruruhau: cultural safety in nursing education in Aotearoa.* Wellington: Ministry of Education; 1990.

15. Adams K. Indigenous cultural competence in nursing and midwifery practice. *Australian Nursing Journal* 2010;**17**:35–8.

16. Van der Berg R. Cultural safety in health for Aboriginal people: will at work in Australia. *The Medical Journal of Australia* 2010;**193**:136–7.

17. Brookfield S. *Developing critical thinkers.* Milton Keynes, UK: Open University Press; 1987.

18. McCormack B, McCance T. *Person-centred nursing: theory and practice.* Oxford, UK: Wiley Blackwell; 2010.

19. Johns C. *Becoming a reflective practitioner.* 4th ed. Wiley-Blackwell; 2013. (E-book)

20. Rolfe G. Models and frameworks for critical reflection. In: Rolfe G, Jasper L, Freshwater D, editors. *Critical reflection in practice.* 2nd ed. Basingstoke, UK: Palgrave Macmillan; 2010. pp 31–51.

21. Taylor B. *Reflective practice for health professionals.* 3rd ed. McGraw-Hill International (UK) Ltd; 2010. (E-book)

22. Howatson-Jones L. *Reflective practice in nursing.* 2nd ed. Thousand Oaks, CA: Sage Publications; 2013. (E-book)

CHAPTER 3

Becoming part of a team

Mary FitzGerald, Annette Moore and Alison Natera

LEARNING OBJECTIVES

When you have completed this chapter you will be able to:

- ▲ identify realistically the challenges facing new graduates of nursing
- ▲ identify the significant characteristics of a nursing team and match them to personal and professional values and career aspirations
- ▲ recognise the importance of clarifying responsibility, accountability and authority within role boundaries
- ▲ understand the importance of self-awareness in order to assess reliably one's contribution to the team
- ▲ know the appropriate sources of critical feedback on performance.

KEYWORDS: teamwork, team profile, reflective practice, performance management, mentorship

INTRODUCTION

Introducing the concept of 'becoming part of a team' is hard without resort to platitudes, rhetoric and, frankly, more of the same old stuff. Ideals and theories surrounding teamwork abound; they sound moral (create and maintain mutual respect), sensible (choose the team carefully) and supportive (have a preceptor) – yet the reality is not so clear for many who join a team for the first time as registered nurses. Graduate nurse transition programs (GNTPs) of one type or another are the norm in Australia. The landscape of graduate nurse placement has changed significantly in recent years, due to an increased number of nursing graduates across the country that has occurred in line with workforce planning. This has resulted in non-traditional graduate nurse placements; for example, graduate nurses are now placed in acute specialty areas, primary healthcare, mental health and rural/remote settings.

While the GNTP nurse may be assigned a mentor or preceptor, there is no guarantee of how often they will work together; and, in order to gain a range of experience, new graduates may be allocated to teams as temporary members, rendering the notion of 'choosing your team' obsolete.

This chapter is written for both the GNTP and the first-year post-GNTP nurse. Following the program, with experience and more confidence, registered nurses are in a good position to find a team to suit their career aspirations and settle down to nurse successfully.

We write here about some of the 'old stuff', but hopefully it is with a measure of common sense born of experience in the health system. There is plenty of evidence (both anecdotal and research-based) that the first year can be both 'tough' and 'tremendous'.[1-9] We hope to write in a way that prepares the reader to dodge or ride the tough, and appreciate and capitalise on the tremendous. This involves:

■ considering the make-up of any team, beginning with overt and covert values held by the team
■ defining the new role, responsibilities and accountability mechanisms
■ learning to assess as accurately as possible one's contribution to the team
■ planning and organising in order to maximise chances of success in the new team.

In short, the process of transition from nursing student to registered nurse is one of socialisation.[10] The new member of the team learns the knowledge, skills and behaviours of the group in order to become part of the team.[7] The process is not automatic, and wise graduates will approach the transition with healthy amounts of common sense complemented by an ability to draw on prior learning, question the status quo and assess their place within the team.

CAREER OR JOB ASPIRATIONS

During the years of undergraduate study the goal is crystal clear – to register as a nurse and graduate from university. Longer-term plans may seem unreal, but it is expedient to spend some time questioning and clarifying career aspirations. If nurses have social priorities, they may ultimately choose an area that offers regular hours or one that is conveniently situated for travelling to work. Some nurses may have plans to travel. For these nurses, experience in areas that would make them a valuable casual employee overseas is the right choice. A few may want to become academics in the future and begin this course by enrolling in a GNTP that offers an Honours degree and later work in areas where they have a clinical research interest.[11] Many will know of an area of specialisation that they would like to work in and should seek advice on the best experience that will make them attractive employees in that specialist area. For example, theatres may prefer new team members to have had experience in a surgical ward; a nursing home may prefer staff to have worked in a general medical ward. Some nurses may want to be leaders in nursing and choose areas where there is the likelihood of early promotion.

Although not specifically relating to teams, Glover and colleagues,[12] in a survey of newly registered nurses, found that the reasons for choosing hospitals related to the following: the hospital's reputation, the location of the hospital, the conditions of employment, personal preferences and familiarity. Since that survey was conducted there has been a change in nurse labour force numbers and opportunities for newly registered nurses to capitalise on projected nursing shortages do exist, particularly in rural, mental health and elderly care.[13] Be aware that there are very different versions of GNTPs across the country.[14]

Clear aspirations may help nurses to make convincing applications for a particular type of experience, even where managers allocate places. Acknowledgment of such aspirations may also help nurses to locate their own frustration in a particular, and possibly unwanted, allocation and to accept that the fault does not lie with the new team. Nurses who find themselves in an area that does not suit their plans are well advised to recognise that there is a range of generic nursing technologies that need to be practised and there is always something to be gained during an allocation. Any post-registration experience is considered valuable, and reports that nurses collect describing their ability to adapt and work well within a team are likely to impress future selection committees.

THE TEAM PROFILE

Some teams have readily available information that describes the area, the service, the people (clients and multidisciplinary team), work systems, evaluation techniques, goals, values and beliefs about nursing. The information may be found in printed mission/ philosophy statements and locally prepared documents and protocols.[15] It is possible for new nurses to judge from these documents the degree to which the team matches their own ideas and ideals of how nursing should be and the degree to which they might 'fit in'.

Surveys of new nursing graduates have shown that they tend towards having strong professional ideals[5,16] which may or may not wane as they become socialised. These ideals also appear high in more experienced staff when they are asked about nursing as it should be.[16,17] However, it may be difficult for both new and experienced nurses to translate ideals into practice in contemporary health service organisations. This particular point is shown in a study by Pearson and colleagues[17,18] of patterns of nursing care in a fairly typical large Australian hospital. Comparisons were made between:
- stated philosophies
- verbal accounts of beliefs, values and work practices
- actual practice.

In theory the teams espoused current nursing ideology such as care of the individual, holistic nursing, preserving human dignity, advocacy and health promotion. The nurses' practice was observed using a work-sampling technique that showed that ideals, in terms of time allocated to various aspects of nursing work, were not on the whole translated into practice. Proportionally, little time was spent in health promotion or social care of patients, and continuity of care was provided through reporting mechanisms rather than allocation of nurses to the same patients each day. Direct patient care time was spent predominantly in physical care of patients, rather than attending to social or psychological problems with either the patients or their families. When challenged, the nurses, quite reasonably, argued that with increasing acuity and shorter stays in hospital physical care is a priority for both nurses and patients.

From the taste of practice that most newly qualified nurses have had during undergraduate clinical placements they realise that it is not always possible to achieve idealistic standards of nursing. Philosophies and mission statements are indicators that allow new members to know how the team would like practice to be and the way towards improvement through change. New team members will not be popular if they are openly critical of custom and practice, especially before they have some experience of working in an area. They do, however, bring a fresh view to the area and their impressions may remind the team of their stated values and purposes. It is possible to adopt small changes, in line with the stated philosophy, to make improvements – for example, asking to look after the same group of patients, getting to know their families and improving discharge planning. Once individual nurses are established as permanent, trusted and respected members of the team it is more likely that they will be able to influence substantial change.

Nursing is hierarchical and it is worth working out who the different members of the team are and how much experience they have, so that it is known which staff member can help in specific circumstances and to whom the new team member should account. One GNTP nurse from the intensive care unit said:

> ... but the thing I found good in the first few weeks was the support from senior staff. I felt comfortable really from day one, in knowing, that if I was in trouble, I could just sing out, and there would be someone. And I asked a lot of questions.[3]

In the early days some kind of preceptorship or mentorship is essential. While traditional methods of one-to-one preceptorship continue, new models of preceptorship are emerging as clinical areas are faced with periods of instability. Workplace staff shortages, differing skill levels and increased patient acuity all have an impact on the success of individual preceptorship.[19] The lack of structure and continuity between a preceptor/allocated nurse and novice/graduate nurse can have a negative impact upon the novice nurse's experience of the environment and can affect patient–nurse rapport, critical care skill development, clinical competence and confidence.[20,21] Effective preceptorship models must be implemented to ensure nurses in transition to practice remain appropriately supported.[22] Clinical areas may adopt the use of a team preceptorship model to support nurses new to clinical practice. Nurses in transition to practice can benefit from the support of expert nurses as well as less experienced preceptors who are often able to demonstrate support and empathy for the new nurse due to their own recent postgraduate experience.[23] Newly registered nurses gain exposure to a broader and more diverse range of resources by the approach of different nurses within the team to preceptorship.[23] In turn the novice nurse new to preceptorship can learn from experienced practitioners as they work in a collaborative relationship.[23] Team preceptorship can facilitate effective socialisation of new nurses as it engenders a more supportive environment.[23]

Some areas – and some preceptors – are a lot better than others at providing this type of support. Determine what you want of the preceptor, make sure to capitalise on the shifts worked together, and determine how to get essential support if your preceptor is not on every shift that you work. It is worth remembering that a great deal is learnt when working alone. This forces the practitioner to work things out for himself or herself and to watch carefully to see the results of any decisions taken. Reid,[24] drawing on the work of Daloz,[25] contends that too much support can impede progress while a few challenges can promote progress.

In any organisation where there are obvious power differentials between staff there is the possibility that the more powerful will make the less powerful feel uncomfortable. The behaviour of some team members may intimidate new staff members and this will adversely affect their experience in the team. Much seemingly unreasonable behaviour is more understandable if there is a fair attempt to see the incident from the other person's perspective. Remember that the pace of work in some areas of nursing, coupled with the acuity of the patients and the added responsibility that comes with seniority, makes nursing stressful for more experienced nurses too. In these situations, think through the incident carefully and try not to take it personally – unless, that is, it was meant personally!

Madeline demonstrates how she settled down after she found confidence:

> I found the first two or three months really, really stressful. Um, I found staff – half the staff, to be really supportive, and the other half of the staff didn't want to have a bar to do with you. So I found that really upsetting and what not. Umm ... but the last three months, when everything started to fall into place, I really enjoyed myself.[3]

More than 10 years later new graduates are saying similar things.[7] However, when people are encountered who abuse their power, a practical response is to find a neutral person who will talk through the situation with either party or both parties. There is evidence that bullying is rife in the nursing profession, and most worrying is that one's response is to become acculturated and in time mimic the bullying behaviour oneself.[26,27] Griffin[28] has studied bullying in nursing and offers practical advice to nurses about what constitutes bullying behaviour and how to respond assertively. Formal complaint processes are cumbersome, have serious repercussions and can be extremely stressful for the complainant. Nevertheless, if the behaviour amounts to bullying, a formal process should be pursued. The longer it takes for corrective measures to be taken, the worse the behaviour is likely to become. Bullies typically pick on people in the organisation who are perceived to have no power, and this makes the new nurse particularly vulnerable.

KNOWLEDGE FOR PRACTICE

Deborah Mitchell wrote about her first placement after graduating that 'the learning curve went straight up!'.[2] Predominantly, learning will be from experience. The opportunity to rehearse new skills until they become almost like second nature is extremely rewarding. The techniques of critical reflection on practice, learnt in most undergraduate schools of nursing and detailed in Chapter 18, should help the new graduate to make sense of what is going on and to gain confidence.

Routines and procedures in any area of nursing are essential early learning because supervision is required until they are mastered. Although it sounds obvious, until new nurses know where stocks are kept they will have to interrupt other people's work to be shown, or waste time looking for themselves. Most nurses are busy and it will be appreciated if the new nurse is considerate and tries to save others time, but this has to be balanced against the risk of being perceived as slow and/or inefficient if you do not ask – it is a fine balancing act!

Watson[29] describes the core and trim of nursing. Core nursing comprises those elements relevant to nursing, irrespective of specialty, and is organised by Watson into 12 carative factors. These elements of nursing will be familiar to new graduates, for they are the very substance of most nursing curricula. Trim, on the other hand, 'refers to the practice setting, the procedures, the specialised clinical focus, and the techniques and specific terminology surrounding the diverse orientations and preoccupations of nursing'. New members of any team need to concentrate on trim skills and knowledge for, once they have mastered the specialist knowledge, they will be more confident about refining and extending their expertise in core skills such as nursing assessment, establishing and maintaining therapeutic relationships, health promotion and communication.[30] All of the latter are covered in the undergraduate curriculum and therefore all new graduates are expected to be reasonably competent.

Nursing is becoming so specialised these days that there are bound to be equipment or procedures in each new area that the nurse has not encountered before. Mitchell[2] said of her early experiences:

> I had never encountered central lines and many of the oncology drugs and procedures mentioned in that first ward report. During the next few weeks I experienced stress as high as any I'd known ... I am relieved to report that by week seven and eight, I was no longer overwhelmed. I knew enough to be reasonably confident, cheerful and more relaxed.

In our experience of undertaking 'Fears, Hopes and Expectation' exercises with graduate nurses on commencement of their first year, they most commonly cite medication management as being stressful and concerning; this is regardless of how educationally prepared they may feel. The successful socialisation to a team can have a direct impact on the graduate nurse's ability to manage patient medication safely, with feelings of isolation, and not wanting to bother busy colleagues and/or to question the decisions of senior nurses, all contributing to potential medication errors. However, safety cannot be compromised and therefore medication management should not deviate from the rules. This may mean that the new nurse needs to be assertive.[9]

It will be time to reopen the books and read about physiology and pathophysiology, medical treatments, pharmacology and best practice in the form of systematic reviews of available research and summary sheets available on the evidence-based practice sites listed. Watch the experienced clinicians as they perform procedures, ask questions, and relate their practice to theory in order to understand the processes. The following extract is from a GNTP nurse in the intensive care unit talking about her early experiences:

> ... you follow other nurses around, watch what they do, get their habits, and do the same thing ... how someone might do this, or do a turn, or how someone might do suction, and how someone might check the ventilators ... any little procedure, CVC [central venous catheter] lines, using the pumps.[3]

The multidisciplinary team members are also valuable sources of knowledge and expertise. Mitchell[2] advises other nurses on graduate nurse programs to ask questions and to make frequent notes in a journal.

RESPONSIBILITY AND ROLES

Although hierarchies are thought by some to obstruct the autonomy required for professional practice, in the early days of practice it is probably an advantage to be part of an organisation with predetermined spheres of work and authority.[31] Newly registered nurses may retain a degree of control by determining their specific role in the team and thereby confidently deciding what they should be doing and what there is to be learnt. There are formal and informal clues to the precise nature of the role. Informally, nurses who are new team members but with slightly more experience can be valuable in terms of sharing experiences and giving advice about team membership and cooperative working. The ward clerk or administrative assistant in any unit can be a mine of information, as can some of the longer-term patients who will 'look out for' the new nurse.

Formally, the senior nurse in any team should agree with new team members what their job involves and how they fit into the routine. By delegating these duties the senior nurse is offering certain responsibilities to the new nurse. The senior nurse is accountable for this decision. In turn the new nurse makes a decision to accept the responsibility and is then accountable for actions and decisions that he or she makes in the specified area of practice. The important factor is that both decisions (the delegator's and delegatee's) are reasonable in light of each individual delegatee's experience and knowledge to date. The Australian Nursing and Midwifery Council's decision-making framework[32] is an invaluable resource regarding scope of practice for all clinicians.

Two hypothetical situations may demonstrate this: a new graduate is asked to receive a patient back to the ward following cardiothoracic surgery; the patient arrests while the monitors are being set up and recognition of ventricular fibrillation and consequent defibrillation is delayed. It is not reasonable for the new nurse to be delegated this responsibility and the senior nurse will be held accountable for the decision. There is an onus on all nurses to refuse a responsibility for which they are not qualified. On the other hand, if a new nurse who was asked to take and record the observations of a patient with congestive heart failure failed to report that the patient's blood pressure had dropped from 120/80 to 85/40 mmHg, this nurse would be accountable for the error. The person who gave the nurse the responsibility should not have a problem convincing people that, in light of the nurse's education and training to date, it was reasonable to ask the new nurse to undertake this task and to expect her to report a significant change.

There is a degree of autonomy in the role of the new nurse as long as the freedom is exercised within the boundaries of the role. The definition of autonomy is: 'freedom to make discretionary and binding decisions consistent within [sic] one's scope of practice and freedom to act on these decisions'.[33] 'Discretionary' refers to decisions made based on wisdom, 'binding' refers to accountability, and 'scope of practice' refers to the role within specific boundaries. It is not necessary for newly registered nurses to defer to seniors on every matter. There are areas of practice where they have been assessed and deemed competent. As new nurses gain experience and confidence, autonomous decision making within their role will become both challenging and very rewarding. It will increase independence and thereby the contributions made by the nurse to the team's work.

The job description is the document that is used to define roles, responsibilities and boundaries. Some of these documents are precise and extremely helpful, while others are frankly obtuse. Irrespective of the standard of the documentation, it is important to talk with someone senior about the job and what is expected from the new team member. New nurses who demonstrate an appreciation of their role and work well within its boundaries may quickly gain the trust and respect of the rest of the team.

ASSESSING PROGRESS

> I was looking after this dialysis, while this guy was out at lunch. And, he had, sort of, explained it all to me, umm … beforehand. Which way the fluid was going, which way that fluid was going. And, umm … I seemed to be doing really well. As long as it didn't really beep, I was fine. [smiles] He thought I did really well.[3]

It is not difficult to pick up from others whether you are 'doing OK' or not, and this is an important daily marker for the new nurse. However, as can be seen from the quotation above, this kind of feedback is not particularly reliable and depends, to some extent, on the personalities involved and the way the day is going generally. New nurses need constructive critique of their work and progress in order to know how they are doing, what next to learn and what new responsibilities they may reasonably be able to accept. Van Hooft and colleagues[34] remind readers that critique is not criticism; rather, it is a rational examination of, in this case, the new nurse's work and may or may not produce praise. Critique, because it is a rational process, provides reasons for judgments and this lends authority to appraisals. Remember that it is as informative and helpful to receive negative feedback on performance as it is to receive positive information. The new nurse can encourage others to provide constructive feedback by receiving it in a professional manner. Floods of tears or loud remonstrations, either face to face or behind a person's back, are difficult to handle and some people will avoid the future possibility of such episodes by saying nothing when improvement is needed. Johns[35] writes of the myth of the 'harmonious team' in which problems are never approached for the sake of keeping the peace. He recommends that professionals learn to give and receive rational feedback in order to maintain high standards of nursing work in any nursing team.

The obvious person to provide new nurses with constructive feedback is the preceptor. Both parties may find it tempting, if things feel as if they are going 'well enough', not to bother. At the end of a shift all people want to do is go home. One nurse who experienced this laissez-faire attitude said:

> I think feedback should be a regular thing … I didn't know what stage I was at. I thought I was progressing. The other[s] [graduate nurses] that I talked to felt the same way as I did. They were having trouble, struggling, things like that … once I started applying myself, I ended up really loving it

there. I didn't want to leave. My attitude towards the nurses changed and I was much happier within myself.[3]

Times for detailed feedback and planning do need to be arranged with transition nurses, clinical nurse educators or the nursing unit manager so that this important process is not ad hoc or hurried. Some type of framework helps. The performance appraisal processes used by health services differ; however, we would recommend that regular formal written feedback and plans for professional development are recorded. Using the appraisal system means that it may be more likely that nurses, once they have completed a transition program, will continue to ask for a performance agreement each year. Whatever the framework, both parties need to know about it beforehand. At the end of the session the main points should be summarised and agreement on these reached. Together, decide what the targets are for the next period of practice and how these might be achieved. The experience and the study required to meet the targets should also be discussed and planned.

Patients are a source of feedback. It is not always spoken, but observant nurses watch carefully to gauge the impact their nursing has had. The man who sleeps because he has been positioned comfortably after the administration of pain relief, the discharge that has gone smoothly because it was planned well, and the elderly woman who is dry because she was walked to the toilet on time are all indicators of good nursing.

Colleagues who work alongside the new nurse on a shift, or take over their patients on the next one, are seldom used to providing critique and yet they are in an excellent position to judge the work of all members of the team. In particular, they can tell how the nurse is blending into the team. Peer review is a well-known but little-used form of performance appraisal in Australia.[36] Of course, this appraisal or critique is not exclusively one-way. The new nurse will be capable of judging the behaviour of team members, particularly in terms of their ability to help new graduate nurses settle into the team. It is probably wise, however, to wait until constructive feedback is solicited before giving it. When members of the team have been helpful it is appropriate to give them positive feedback on their behaviour and to acknowledge their help to the rest of the team.

An ability to make a sound estimate of one's own strengths and weaknesses is something everyone should consciously work towards. Pearson and colleagues[37] were told by a range of nurses in their study, intended to identify indicators of continuing competence, that nurses with performance problems commonly have a problem with insight. They simply cannot see where their work is substandard. The reverse is probably true of nurses who lack insight into their strengths, as they are likely to be less confident than they might be and probably slower to reach their full potential.

Maintaining a journal is one way to practise critical reflection and to learn from experience. If this is too laborious, then some time after a shift should be taken for critical thinking about the decisions and actions that have occurred at work and the contribution the individual is making to the work of the team.

PLANNING AND MANAGEMENT

To keep control of progress and to optimise opportunities, systematic planning is essential. With the help of the preceptor, or a number of the more experienced nurses in the team, it is quite possible to plan specific learning opportunities to help new nurses gain the experience they require to become confident level-one nurses. There are several methods that can be used to help with this planning process. A written plan will enable nurses to pace their learning and experience, and ensure that these are comprehensive. This type of learning is proactive, but of course a great deal of learning from experience is reactive in so far as it is opportunistic. That is, opportunities arise without warning and the astute nurse will make the most of them. For example, a patient who has been cared for over several shifts by a new nurse dies when she is on duty. It may be quite appropriate that, with the right support from a senior nurse, this nurse breaks the bad news to the family. The preceptor and the new nurse may not have planned for this experience but at the time it seems to be appropriate for both the nurse and the family. Remember that these opportunities are as valuable in terms of learning as those that are planned.

Time management is another skill that, once acquired, will make the new nurse feel a part of the team. Almost by definition nurses are busy and a feeling of constant pressure to get through tasks is extremely stressful.[38] An analysis of the routine tasks undertaken each day and some estimation of the time required to do them will allow nurses to calculate how much time there is to deal with unforeseen tasks and emergencies. An ability to prioritise demands on time and to ask for help when it is all getting too much is worth acquiring. The difficulty is that the day the new nurse is busy is likely to be the day when the whole team is just as stretched.

Good time management practice is as valuable as it is difficult to develop. Worse still, it is difficult to apply consistently to nursing work because so much of what occurs during the day is not predictable. However, it is possible to reduce work by being organised. Truthful nurses will admit that when they spend their day just responding to the next request a great deal of work fails to get done. Even though routines and rituals are lampooned by some, in terms of managing busy nursing schedules they have some merit.[39] Once routine physical care is given, the nurse can be assured that all the patients are safe and comfortable. There is then time for some of the work that can be neglected, such as psychological support, health promotion and discharge planning.

CONCLUSION

At the beginning of the chapter we referred to long-term plans and careers in nursing. However, most of the learning in the first year is necessarily focused on the job and the acquisition of specialist knowledge, language and skills. To become accepted as part of the team, new nurses are usually required to demonstrate to members of the team that they can do the job or, in other words, be useful and take a share of the workload. Mastering a set of skills for which the employer remunerates the new nurse is a requirement of employment. Experiences in the first year are likely to elicit a mixture of emotions – stress, distress, frustration, pride and satisfaction. The more positive emotions tend to dominate as confidence and a feeling of belonging to the team develop.

Our advice is similar to Mitchell's:[2]

- Be honest: admit your mistakes.
- Ask questions: no question is a stupid question – it is better to ask beforehand than to blunder in, then try to fix up a mess afterwards.

- Make frequent notes in a journal to improve your problem-solving skills.
- Spend a few minutes of quality time with your patients at the beginning of the shift – this can make them your allies and not your opponents.
- Practise friendly assertiveness.
- Try hard not to make enemies.

Beyond Mitchell's good advice, we reiterate that it is possible to control the situation from a position of limited power by good planning and by getting agreement from team members to the plan. This is a time to appreciate knowledge and to become aware of the synergy there is between the intellectual training you received at university and the problem-solving skills required in practice; the evidence generated from research and applied in practice; and the theories that explain and make sense of nursing.

CASE STUDY 3.1

Tina had been on her new ward for around 3–4 weeks when information started to filter through the nursing team to the transition office that she was not 'coping' or at the 'expected level' in her clinical practice that the team thought she should be. A performance management plan was set in place between Tina, her preceptor and the certified nurse educator from the transition office to facilitate Tina's learning needs and to provide her with extra clinical support.

REFLECTIVE QUESTION

How would you assist Tina with her performance management plan?

CASE STUDY 3.2

Despite the performance plan, Tina's development progressed very slowly and at times it seemed that, as hard as she tried, she could not do a thing right. Although Tina did have some areas of clinical practice that required improvement, it became evident that her cultural background was a factor interfering with two-way communication and acceptance into the ward culture. A way forward was chosen to ensure that Tina was culturally safe and to help her to learn more about different ways of working and communicating. She attended cultural diversity workshops and was moved to another clinical area. Workshops were set up and were well attended by staff from the wards and nurse educators. There were no preconceived ideas about Tina when she moved to her new ward; she assimilated into the team very quickly and as her confidence grew, so did her standards of practice. Tina is now a valued and respected team member of her ward and has secured employment to remain there beyond her graduate placement.

REFLECTIVE QUESTIONS

1. How would the areas of clinical practice that required improvement be communicated effectively to Tina, taking into account her cultural background and the ward culture?
2. How would Tina have benefited from attending these cultural diversity workshops, and what would she be able to take back to the workplace?

CASE STUDY 3.3

Jenny burst into tears during the first week of orientation. She was very disappointed about her placement in the aged-care assessment wards. She wanted to learn to nurse in the acute hospital and to become a confident practitioner. She was surrounded by friends who had places in intensive care, emergency and cancer services, and she felt she was being left behind.

After some sound advice from the transition office staff and her family, Jenny started work on the ward. She put on a brave face and was pleasantly surprised at the welcome she received from both patients and the ward staff. She very quickly began to appreciate how the different skill mix on the elderly care ward meant that she was challenged to take a leadership role much earlier than were some of her friends. The work that she was asked to do related well to the preparation she had had at university and every day she felt as if she had really stretched herself. Soon she found herself offering advice to enrolled nurses and enjoyed taking responsibility for a team of nurses. The patients' needs were very complex and she learnt a great deal about discharge planning and the realities of social and physical support for people with continuing care needs in the community. When, after 6 months, she began work on a general medical ward, she found she was more confident than her peers at leading a team, supervising the practice of enrolled nurses and providing holistic care to patients with complex needs. She would advise any new nurse to start work on the elderly care assessment unit.

REFLECTIVE QUESTIONS

1. How could Jenny have overcome her initial disappointment with regard to her placement?
2. What processes could Jenny put into place once she was capable of leading a team of her peers in this area to assist future staff who are experiencing these difficulties?

EXERCISE 3.1

1. Write a career plan for the next 10 years. Start with the general objective and then plot the steps you will need to take to get there. In particular, make a note of the opportunities you require in the first year of practice to set you on track. Remember that when you go for interviews it is always impressive if you can refer to things that you have achieved.
2. Take a trip to the library in the institution in which you work. Locate and browse through the specialist journals relating to the types of patients you are nursing. Ask the librarian for help if you are unfamiliar with the library.
3. At the end of each shift make some time to reflect and note down at least five things that you have learnt during the day.

RECOMMENDED READING

FitzGerald M. Meeting the needs of individuals. In: Daly J, Speedy S, Jackson D, editors. *Contexts of nursing: an introduction.* 2nd ed. Sydney: MacLennan & Petty; 2006. pp 240–51.

Joanna Briggs Institute for Evidence Based Practice. Best Practice Information Sheets. Online. Available: <www.joannabriggs.edu.au>.

Levett-Jones T, Bourgeois S. *The clinical placement: an essential guide for nursing students.* Sydney: Elsevier; 2007.

Malouf N, West S. Fitting in: a pervasive new graduate nurse need. *Nurse Education Today* 2011;**31**:488–93.

Pearson H. Transition from nursing student to staff nurse: a personal reflection. *Paediatric Nursing* 2009;**21**:30–2.

REFERENCES

1. Maben J, Macleod J. Project 2000 diplomates' perceptions of their experiences of transition from student to staff nurse. *Journal of Clinical Nursing* 1998;**7**:145–53.
2. Mitchell D. Riding the learning curve roller-coaster. *Nursing Review* 2000;**June**:44.
3. Amadio J. *The experience of being a new graduate nurse in intensive care [MNSc].* Adelaide: Adelaide University; 1997. p 92.
4. Kelly B. Hospital nursing: it's a battle! A follow-up study of English graduate nurses. *Journal of Advanced Nursing* 1996;**24**:1063–9.
5. Boyle D, Popkess Vawter S, Taunton R. Socialization of new graduate nurses in critical care. *Heart & Lung: The Journal of Critical Care* 1996;**25**:141–54.
6. Cubit K, Ryan B. Tailoring a graduate nurse program to meet the needs of our next generation of nurses. *Nurse Education Today* 2010;**31**:65–71.
7. Malouf N, West S. Fitting in: a pervasive new graduate nurse need. *Nurse Education Today* 2011;**31**:488–93.
8. Kelly J, Ahern K. Preparing nurse for practice: a phenomenological study of the new graduate in Australia. *Journal of Clinical Nursing* 2009;**18**(6):910–18.
9. Ostini F, Bonner A. Australian new graduate experiences during their transition program in a rural/regional acute care setting. *Contemporary Nurse* 2012;**41**(2):242–52.
10. Goslin D. *Handbook of socialization theory and research.* Chicago: Rand McNally; 1969.
11. Hawes C, Schmitz K. A model for the future. Integration of the bachelor of nursing honours degree with the graduate nurse program. *Collegian: Journal of the Royal College of Nursing Australia* 2000;**7**:10–13.
12. Glover P, Clare J, Longson D, et al. Should I take my first offer? A graduate nurse survey. *Australian Journal of Advanced Nursing* 1998;**15**:17–25.
13. Australian Institute of Health and Welfare, 2006. *Nursing Labour Force 2004.* Canberra: AIHW (National Health Labour Force Series); 1999.
14. Levett-Jones T, FitzGerald M. A review of graduate nurse transition programs in Australia. *Australian Journal of Advanced Nursing* 2005;**23**:40–5.
15. FitzGerald M. A unit profile. In: Vaughan B, Pillmoor M, editors. *Managing nursing work.* London: Scutari Press; 1989. pp 81–95.
16. McCloskey J, McCain B. Variables related to nurse performance. *Image: Journal of Nursing Scholarship* 1988;**20**:203–7.
17. Pearson A, FitzGerald M, Walsh K, et al. *Patterns of nursing care*, vol. 5. Adelaide: Department of Clinical Nursing, Adelaide University; 1999.

18. FitzGerald M, Pearson A, Walsh K, et al. Patterns of nursing: a review of nursing in a large metropolitan hospital. *Journal of Clinical Nursing* 2003;**12**:326–33.
19. DeWolfe J, Laschinger S, Perkin C. Preceptors' perspectives on recruitment, support, and retention of preceptors. *Journal of Nursing Education* 2010;**49**:198–206.
20. Proulx DM, Bourcier BJ. Graduate nurses in the intensive care unit: an orientation model. *Critical Care Nurse* 2008;**28**:44–52.
21. Myer E, Lees A, Humphris D, et al. Opportunities and barriers to successful learning transfer: impact of critical care skills training. *Journal of Advanced Nursing* 2007;**60**:308–16.
22. Scott E, Smith S. Group mentoring: a transition-to-work strategy. *Journal for Nurses in Staff Development* 2008;**24**:232–8.
23. Beecroft P, Hernandez A, Reid D. Team preceptorship: a new approach for precepting new nurses. *Journal for Nurses in Staff Development* 2008;**24**:143–8.
24. Reid B. The role of the mentor to aid reflective practice. In: Burns S, Bulman C, editors. *Reflective practice in nursing: the growth of the professional practitioner.* 2nd ed. Oxford, UK: Blackwell Science; 2000. pp 79–102.
25. Daloz L. *Effective teaching and mentoring.* London: Jossey-Bass; 1986.
26. Randle J. Bullying in the nursing profession. *Journal of Advanced Nursing* 2003;**43**:395–401.
27. Hutchinson M, Vickers M, Jackson D, et al. Workplace bullying in nursing: towards a more critical organizational perspective. *Nursing Inquiry* 2006;**13**:118–26.
28. Griffin M. Teaching cognitive rehearsal as a shield for lateral violence: an intervention for newly licensed nurses. *Journal of Continuing Education in Nursing* 2004;**35**:257–64.
29. Watson J. *Nursing – the philosophy and science of caring.* Boulder, CO: Colorado Associated University Press; 1985.
30. FitzGerald M. Educational preparation for primary nursing. In: Ersser S, Tutton E, editors. *Primary nursing in perspective.* London: Scutari; 1991. pp 49–61.
31. Singleton E, Nail F. Role clarification: a prerequisite to autonomy. *Journal of Nursing Administration* 1984;17–22.
32. Australian Nursing and Midwifery Council. *National framework for the development of decision-making tools for nursing and midwifery practice.* Canberra: Australian Nursing and Midwifery Council; 2007.
33. Batey M, Lewis F. Clarifying autonomy and accountability in nursing service: part I. *Journal of Nursing Administration* 1982;13–17.
34. van Hooft S, Gillam L, Byrnes M. *Facts and values: an introduction to critical thinking for nurses.* Sydney: MacLennan & Petty; 1995.
35. Johns C. Ownership and the harmonious team: barriers to developing the therapeutic nursing team in primary nursing. *Journal of Clinical Nursing* 1992;**1**:89–94.
36. Wainwright P. Peer review. In: Pearson A, editor. *Nursing quality measurement: quality assurance methods for peer review.* Chichester, UK: John Wiley; 1987. pp 15–25.
37. Pearson A, FitzGerald M, Borbasi S, et al. *Study to identify the indicators of continuing competence in nursing, final report.* Adelaide: Australian Nursing Council; 1999. p 139.
38. Huber D. *Leadership and nursing care management.* Philadelphia: WB Saunders; 1996.
39. Ford P, Walsh M. *New rituals for old.* Oxford, UK: Butterworth Heinemann; 1994.

CHAPTER 4

Understanding organisational culture in the community health setting

Deborah Hatcher and Kathleen Dixon

LEARNING OBJECTIVES

When you have completed this chapter you will be able to:

- describe the features of organisational culture
- define the general structure and role of community health services in Australia and New Zealand
- discuss the importance of primary healthcare to the organisational culture of community health services
- describe the role of health promotion in community nursing practice
- discuss how the functions of organisational culture serve community health services.

KEYWORDS: culture, organisational culture, community nursing, community health, primary healthcare, health promotion

INTRODUCTION

Nurses work across a variety of settings, including the community. With an increasing ageing population, the associated growth in chronic health conditions and the current focus of government health policies targeting primary healthcare, nurses will be at the forefront of providing support and care to a growing number of clients in the community. The organisational culture of community health settings is ever changing in response to the health needs of people in the community. Nurses require an understanding of ways in which the provision of community health services (CHS) are structured in order to practise effectively and in collaboration with other health professionals and service providers. It is from this understanding that the healthcare needs of people in the community can most effectively be assessed, planned for and responded to by community health nurses.

The organisational structure of CHS in Australia and New Zealand is complex. With this in mind, the intent of this chapter is to provide an overview of organisational culture and to explore the organisational culture of community nursing, its history, governance and funding. Within this chapter, particular emphasis is placed on exploring the role of primary healthcare and health promotion and their importance to the culture and organisation of community health nursing. The chapter concludes with a discussion of the roles of community health nurses.

ORGANISATIONAL CULTURE

Organisational culture can be described as the shared values, norms, understandings and beliefs of people belonging to an organisation or group.[1] Historically, research and writing on culture arose from the fields of anthropology and social sciences; more recently, leaders in management and organisations have examined culture from an organisational perspective.[2] This trend is also reflected in healthcare, with increasing interest and focus on the organisational culture of health services. Recognition of the importance of organisational culture to client quality and safety in healthcare has been highlighted recently through public inquiries such as the Special Commission of Inquiry into Acute Care Services in NSW Public Hospitals[3] and in the United Kingdom with the Francis Report.[4]

For organisations, culture represents a set of shared values and customs that can be seen as a unifying factor for a group of people who have a common language and belief system. Organisational culture has two important functions: (1) to provide a means for members of the group to integrate in order to function cohesively; and (2) to ensure that organisations are responsive to the external environment.[1]

COMMUNITY NURSING AND ORGANISATIONAL CULTURE

Community nurses work in organisations in the community that have their own sets of values and beliefs. Within the community, development of a community culture happens gradually over time.[5] However, culture is also dynamic and may change in response to external influences or events. In order to understand the organisational culture of CHS and community nursing practice, it is necessary to have an understanding of global and national influences. Australia and New Zealand do not create healthcare policy in a vacuum. Both countries seek direction from organisations that provide international expertise and leadership, including the World Health Organization (WHO), the United Nations (UN) and the World Bank. At a national, state and territory level, professional organisations providing policy advice include, among others, the Public Health Association Australia and the Australian College of Nursing; and in New Zealand, the College of Nurses Aotearoa New Zealand. In addition, there have been a number of reports that have had a significant influence on community health nursing policy and practice. They include:

- 1974 WHO Technical Report on Community Health Nursing[6]
- 1978 WHO Declaration of Alma-Ata[7]
- 1986 WHO Ottawa Charter for Health Promotion[8]
- 1998 WHO Report on Primary Health Care in the 21st Century[9]
- 2000 UN Millennium Declaration from which arise the Millennium Development Goals[10]
- 2008 WHO World Health Report, *Primary Health Care, Now More Than Ever.*[11]

The Australian government through the Department of Health and Ageing, and the New Zealand government through the Ministry of Health, formulate policies in relation to community health. These policies are supported through federal, state, territory and local governments in Australia and regional areas in New Zealand, and are then implemented throughout Australia and New Zealand in a variety of practice settings. Community health nurses play a key role in the implementation of community health policies.

Of particular importance to understanding the culture of community nursing are two reports: (1) the Alma-Ata declaration for its focus on primary healthcare as an approach to the provision of healthcare; and (2) the Ottawa Charter for its focus on health promotion. These two reports have had a major impact on shaping the provision of health services by community nurses, with nurses providing health services such as education and community-based clinical care specifically targeted at individuals, localised groups or whole communities[12] using both primary healthcare and health promotion approaches. Health promotion is discussed in more detail later in the chapter.

EXERCISE 4.1

Take some time to review the two reports, the Declaration of Alma-Ata and the Ottawa Charter for Health Promotion.

Primary Healthcare

Organisational culture and governance of CHS vary and are broadly influenced by a range of social, cultural and political factors such as history, geographical location, the cultural milieu of the local community, the availability of general health services and government policy. Despite the range of influences on CHS, the principles of primary healthcare are a common factor underpinning all health planning and service provision in the community.[12]

EXERCISE 4.2

Review the 2008 WHO World Health Report, *Primary Health Care, Now More Than Ever.* Think about how primary healthcare is relevant to community health.

Primary healthcare is a social model of health providing an integrated approach to health service delivery through a multidisciplinary environment. The principles of primary healthcare (Box 4.1) originally described in the Declaration of Alma-Ata resulted in a shift of focus from acute healthcare settings to community-based settings, because it was widely recognised that health and wellbeing are dependent upon the social, environmental and economic determinants of health.[13] This understanding of the

BOX 4.1 The principles of primary healthcare[14]

Accessible healthcare
Community participation
Intersectoral collaboration
Health promotion
Appropriate technology
Cultural sensitivity

BOX 4.2 The social determinants of health[15]

Social gradient
Stress
Early life
Social exclusion
Work
Unemployment
Social support
Addiction
Food
Transport

importance of primary healthcare resulted in a new direction in the health policies of Australia and New Zealand. This was marked in Australia in 2010 with the release of Australia's First National Primary Health Care Strategy[16] and in New Zealand in 2009 with the strategy known as 'Better, Sooner, More Convenient Health Care in the Community'.[17]

Primary healthcare is both a philosophy and a social model of health that underpins the practice of nurses in the community health setting. The primary healthcare model was endorsed by the WHO in 1978, the aim of which was to achieve equity across healthcare systems globally by providing health for all in a cost-effective and efficient way. Both Australia and New Zealand have adopted primary healthcare as the means to achieve health and wellbeing in the community.

In a community health setting, these principles can be represented as:

- a shift of health resources from acute care to the community, including relocating healthcare professionals to work with clients and communities in the community health sector
- creating healthy environments through addressing the social and environmental conditions affecting health and wellbeing.

It is recognised under the primary healthcare model that health and wellbeing are influenced by the social determinants of health (Box 4.2). The focus of health service provision is therefore directed towards political, economic, social and environmental factors. People marginalised by, for example, poverty, unemployment, addiction, culture, chronic illness or disability are those least likely to participate in their own health decisions and to have access to the care and services they need.[18] Therefore, it is important to target the social determinants of health in order to address social inequity, facilitate access to healthcare, and empower individuals and communities.[13]

EXERCISE 4.3

Review the WHO's *Solid Facts* report on the social determinants of health.[15] Think about how and why you would collect information on these determinants to guide your practice.

GOVERNANCE AND FUNDING OF COMMUNITY HEALTH SERVICES

CHS are intended to promote access for all individuals and families.[19] These services are provided by government, non-government and private not-for-profit organisations and are usually publicly funded at little to no cost to the client. A strong focus of CHS is the ongoing support for universal or population-based services such as maternal and child health, and school health services, as well as targeted services designed to meet the needs of vulnerable families with young children or older people living alone. More recently, services have been expanded to include chronic disease programs focused on early intervention, education and support for self-management.

Many of these CHS also respond to their respective government's health priorities and targets. There are currently nine National Health Priority Areas chosen by Australian governments because of their contribution to illness and injury. These are: cancer control, cardiovascular health, injury prevention and control, mental health, diabetes mellitus, asthma, arthritis and musculoskeletal conditions, obesity and dementia. In New Zealand the government has set six health targets, three of which are focused on improving consumer access to health services and three on prevention. The targets are: shorter stays in emergency departments, improved access to elective surgery, shorter waits for cancer treatment, increased immunisation, better help for smokers to quit, and more health and diabetes checks.[20]

The Australian government does not provide dedicated funds for CHS; rather, funding is a shared responsibility between federal, state and local jurisdictions.[13] An analysis of health expenditure in Australia for 2011–12 demonstrated that 38.2% ($50.6 billion) of recurrent health expenditure was spent on primary healthcare.[21] In New Zealand, District Health Boards (DHB) are the local health organisations responsible for funding and planning services in their districts; they include 20 DHB providing regional public health services delivered by regional Public Health Units and Primary Health Oganisations.[22] In New Zealand, spending on prevention and public health services for the period 2009–10 was approximately $1.39 billion; and for the period 2005–10 spending on prevention and public health services experienced an annual growth rate of 9.9%.[23]

CHS may receive funding from a range of sources to support a variety of services. For example, the general running of the CHS may be funded by the government in each state, but the podiatry or occupational therapy component of the service may be funded by the Australian government if referred by a general practitioner (GP). The CHS is accountable to each body that provides funding. The complexity of funding and governance can be illustrated by the Home and Community Care Program (HACC). In Australia, this program is an Australian government initiative designed to provide support and care for older people to enable them to continue to live in their own home. There are numerous services provided under this program, including nursing care, personal care, transport, assistance with domestic household duties, home modification and home maintenance, delivery of meals, centre-based day care, allied health services and respite care. The Australian government assumes full funding, policy and operational responsibility for services provided by HACC except in Victoria and Western Australia, which are jointly funded by the Australian government and the state. However, for people under the age of 65, or under age 50 for Aboriginal and Torres Strait Islander peoples, the state and territory governments are responsible for funding and administration of services.[24]

In New Zealand the funding of home healthcare is determined on the basis of individual need. People referred for home healthcare and support may be eligible for one of the following:

- aged care services managed and funded by the DHB on behalf of the Ministry of Health
- Disability Support Services as part of the Ministry of Health's responsibility for planning and funding disability services
- community nursing services administered by DHB and the Accident Compensation Corporation (ACC)
- support for people to return to work following an injury provided by the ACC.[25]

HISTORY OF COMMUNITY HEALTH NURSING

Prior to the early 1970s, community-based nurses in Australia were known by a range of titles, including public health nurse, school health nurse, and maternal and child health nurse. The WHO's 1974 technical report on community health nursing and the introduction of community health centres and services by the Whitlam government in the early 1970s greatly influenced state and territory health departments across Australia. It was at this time that the title 'public health nurse' was changed to 'community health nurse'. The terms 'community health' and 'community health centre' gradually became the norm across the country.

There is a long tradition in New Zealand of community nursing practice and outreach. Historically, primary healthcare services have been provided by nurses in schools, workplaces, homes and clinics. Prior to 1980 these nurses were known as 'nurses working in the community'. In New Zealand the Primary Health Care Strategy, introduced by the Ministry of Health in 2001, identified primary healthcare nurses as crucial to the implementation of the strategy. The Expert Advisory Group on Primary Health Care Nursing (2003:9) defined primary healthcare nurses as:

> ... registered nurses with knowledge and expertise in primary health care practice. Primary health care nurses work autonomously and collaboratively to promote, improve, maintain and restore health. Primary health care nursing encompasses population health, health promotion, disease prevention, wellness care, first-point-of-contact care and disease management across the lifespan. The setting and the ethnic and cultural group of the people determine models of practice. Partnership with people – individuals, whānau, communities and people – to achieve the shared goal of health for all, is central to primary health care nursing.[26]

CURRENT CONTEXT OF COMMUNITY HEALTH NURSING

Community health nursing today has a strong professional and organisational culture that is influenced by professional continuing education, regulatory and professional bodies, and special interest groups. Community nursing is characterised by a health promotion approach that engenders partnerships, collaboration and multidisciplinary team work. The focus of community nursing, however, is changing as a result of spiralling hospital costs, an ageing population and a greater prevalence of people living with chronic illness. This changing focus has also meant that the role and scope of the community nurse's practice are being transformed. However, it is the philosophy of primary healthcare that continues to have an enduring impact on the culture of community health nursing.

Community Nursing and Health Promotion

Community nurses have been involved in health promotion programs for many decades. Health promotion involves actions that foster improvement and maintenance of health in individuals and communities. The success of health promotion programs depends upon addressing the social determinants of health. The original principles of health promotion outlined in the report *Health Promotion: Concepts and Principles. Report of a Working Group* were prepared by the WHO in 1984. Together with the strategies of the Ottawa Charter for Health Promotion developed by the WHO in 1986, these frameworks for action have underpinned the policy and practice culture of community health and community nurses worldwide.

The following encapsulates the original principles of health promotion from the 1984 WHO working group:

- Health promotion involves the population as a whole in the context of their everyday life, rather than focusing on people at risk for specific diseases. It enables people to take control over, and responsibility for, their health as an important component of everyday life. This requires full and continuing access to information about health.
- Health promotion is directed towards action on the determinants of health. Health promotion, therefore, requires a close cooperation of sectors beyond health services, reflecting the diversity of factors that influence health. Government, at both local

and national levels, has a responsibility to ensure that the environment is conducive to health.

- Health promotion approaches include communication, education, legislation, fiscal measures, organisational change, community development, and response at a local level to emerging health issues.
- Health promotion aims to enhance public participation in decision making about health through the development of skills in individuals and in communities.
- Health professionals when working in health promotion utilise skills in education and health advocacy.[27]

Following this, in 1986 the Ottawa Charter was developed to address inequities in health on a global level through strategies for health promotion. Five major strategies influence the community nursing culture:

1. Build healthy public policy.
2. Create supportive environments.
3. Strengthen community action.
4. Develop personal skills.
5. Reorient health services.

Community Participation, Partnership and Collaboration

The idea of community participation and partnership in health and health promotion is not new and has been advocated since the 1980s.[28] Central to the philosophy of community health are client-centred services that not only reflect the needs of the community but are also responsive to community needs as they arise. For successful community participation, client-centred services must be provided where the recipients of care are actively engaged in the partnership and decisions about care become joint decisions. The care providers are accountable to the community for the type and range of care models delivered, and this may be achieved through community forums, community-based committees of management and regular community needs assessments. The CHS must also work within the parameters set down by local communities, including other local agencies. Examples include local government, schools and community groups (e.g. church and social welfare groups).[12] These partnerships all operate from within state, federal and international policy guidelines. Importantly, there is a need for community health nurses to create a supportive and empowering environment so that individuals and groups have the knowledge and skills to participate.

Community Nursing and the Multidisciplinary Team

Providing nursing care in the community is usually referred to as either working *in* the community or working *with* the community. Working *in* the community is community-based nursing that involves the nurse providing clinical care in the community either as a practice nurse based in a GP private practice or as a community nurse through a community health centre. The scope of practice for community nurses includes preventive healthcare, health education and health maintenance. The nursing roles include: practice nursing; district nursing; hospital in the home; chronic illness management such as cardiac, respiratory or diabetes; and community mental health nursing. In New Zealand, practice nurses conduct nurse-led clinics to support the health needs of those in the community with chronic health problems. Community-based nurses working in the community coordinate and plan care, provide case management, and promote client self-management.

Working *with* the community is community health nursing that involves the community health nurse working with high-risk populations or communities to promote health, community development and engagement.[28] The nurse's role includes primary, secondary and tertiary prevention activities such as screening, surveillance, education and rehabilitation. Nurses practise with the community to provide school health, workplace health, mental health, justice health, immunisation clinics, sexual health, and drug and alcohol services.

Traditionally, these CHS have been delivered by multidisciplinary teams, of which community nurses are an important component. Today there remains a strong focus on working in multidisciplinary teams and developing partnerships within CHS to address social inequity. Multidisciplinary teams may be comprised of a broad range of health professionals such as nurses, doctors, social workers, physiotherapists and counsellors, who work in partnership with organisations and groups such as migrant services, schools, adolescent mental health services, and drug and alcohol services. Such teams work collaboratively to provide health services required by both individuals and communities in remote, rural, regional or urban areas of Australia and New Zealand. Integrated teams are required in each of these geographical contexts to ensure that services are equitably provided to all community members. Many CHS have ongoing programs, including drug and alcohol, mental health, adolescent support groups, family planning and early childhood health services. Additionally, in response to health issues that may arise unexpectedly in communities such as outbreaks of hepatitis A or influenza, mass vaccination clinics are provided by CHS in partnership with Public Health.

From the above discussion it can be seen that in Australia and New Zealand community nurses' practice is shaped by the location, demographics and needs of their community, and that they work collaboratively with other health professionals to build the capacity and empowerment of communities and individuals.

CONCLUSION

This chapter provides you with an overview of the diversity and complexity of organisational culture in the community health setting. We introduced you to the role of the community health nurse, as well as to the underlying philosophy and policies that guide community nursing practice. We have explained the importance of the links between healthcare and the community, and why it is so important to embrace the concepts of community participation and partnerships.

CASE STUDY 4.1

You are employed as a community nurse working in a chronic and complex care team. You are assigned a new client, Dan, who is an 80-year-old Australian man with chronic respiratory disease and heart failure. He has a 40-year history of smoking and has been losing weight for the past 6 months. Dan lives at home with his wife, who has early onset dementia. He has two daughters who are married and live an hour away by car. Dan is finding it increasingly difficult to do his gardening and to move around the house.

REFLECTIVE QUESTIONS

1. Consider the social determinants of health. Identify which of these currently impact on Dan's quality of life, and describe how they are likely to impact on his future health and wellbeing.
2. Having assessed Dan's situation, what health promotion approaches would you utilise for the planning and provision of his care?

CASE STUDY 4.2

A community prevention program for rheumatic fever in children in New Zealand was developed when a GP and practice nurse identified a high number of children with sore throats. Under this program, registered nurses and GPs work in partnership with the community to provide training for people with no health qualifications. Once trained, these people visit schools and take throat swabs of children who have sore throats.

For more information, refer to the New Zealand Ministry of Health's document, *Better, Sooner, More Convenient Health Care in the Community.*

REFLECTIVE QUESTIONS

1. Identify the elements of community participation, partnership and collaboration in this program.
2. Briefly describe how this model of care fits within a health promotion framework.

CASE STUDY 4.3

You are a practice nurse working in a small general practice within a large Indigenous community. There is a high level of diabetes and, in collaboration with the GP, you plan to provide diabetes education. You contact Diabetes NSW and set up a program to provide education and support. The GP identifies patients and provides the facility for education, while your role is to conduct education sessions and monitor self-management.

REFLECTIVE QUESTIONS

1. Identify how this model of practice fits with the nurse's scope of practice.
2. Discuss the importance of the multidisciplinary team and how it fits within a primary healthcare model.

RECOMMENDED READING

Department of Health. Commonwealth (HACC) Program. Online. Available: <www.health.gov .au/hacc> [Viewed 16 September 2014].

Department of Health and Ageing. *Building a 21st century primary health care system: Australia's first national primary health care strategy. Publication no. 6594.* Canberra: Commonwealth of Australia; 2010.

Kralik D, van Loon A. *Community nursing in Australia.* 2nd ed. Brisbane: John Wiley; 2011.

McMurray A, Clendon J. *Community health and wellness: primary health in practice.* 4th ed. Sydney: Elsevier Churchill Livingstone; 2011.

Ministry of Health. *Better, sooner, more convenient health care in the community.* Wellington: Ministry of Health; 2011 Online. Available: <www.health.govt.nz/publication/better-sooner-more-convenient-health-care-community> [Viewed 16 September 2014].

REFERENCES

1. Ozanne E, Rose D. *The organisational context of human service practice.* Melbourne: Palgrave Macmillan; 2013.
2. Finkelman A. *Leadership and management for nurses: core competencies for quality care.* 2nd ed. Upper Saddle River, NJ: Pearson; 2012.
3. Garling P. *Final report of the special commission of inquiry. Acute care services in NSW public hospitals.* Sydney: NSW Department of Health; 2008.
4. Report of the Mid Staffordshire NHS Foundation Trust Public Inquiry. 2013 Online. Available: <www.midstaffspublicinquiry.com/report> [Viewed 16 September 2014].
5. Talbot L, Verrinder G. *Promoting health: the primary health care approach.* 3rd ed. Sydney: Elsevier Churchill Livingstone; 2009.
6. World Health Organization. *Community health nursing. Report of an expert committee. Technical Report Series, No. 558.* Geneva: WHO; 1974 Online. Available: <http://whqlibdoc.who.int/trs/WHO_TRS_558.pdf> [Viewed 9 March 2011].
7. World Health Organization. *Declaration of Alma Ata.* Geneva: WHO; 1978 Online. Available: <www.who.int/publications/almaata_declaration_en.pdf> [Viewed 9 March 2011].
8. World Health Organization. *Ottawa Charter.* Geneva: WHO; 1986 Online. Available: <www.who.int/hpr/NPH/docs/ottawa_charter_hp.pdf> [Viewed 9 March 2011].
9. World Health Organization. *Primary health care in the 21st century is everybody's business.* Press release WHO/89; 27 November 1998. Online. Available: <www.who.int/inf-pr-1998/en/pr98-89.html> [Viewed 9 March 2011].
10. United Nations. *United Nations millennium development goals and beyond.* 2015 Online. Available: <www.un.org/millenniumgoals/> [Viewed 16 September 2014].
11. World Health Organization. *World health report 2008: Primary health care, now more than ever.* Online. Available: <www.who.int/whr/2008/whr08_en.pdf> [Viewed 9 March 2011].
12. Kralik D, van Loon A. *Community nursing in Australia.* 2nd ed. Brisbane: John Wiley; 2011.
13. Keleher H. Primary health care. In: Willis E, Reynolds L, Keleher H, editors. *Understanding the Australian health care system.* 2nd ed. Sydney: Elsevier Churchill Livingstone; 2012. pp 55–66.
14. McMurray A, Clendon J. *Community health and wellness: primary health in practice.* 4th ed. Sydney: Elsevier Churchill Livingstone; 2011.
15. World Health Organization. *Social determinants of health. The solid facts.* 2nd ed. 2003 Online. Available: <www.euro.who.int/_data/assets/pdf_file/0005/98438/e81384.pdf?ua=1> [Viewed 16 September 2014].
16. Department of Health and Ageing. *Building a 21st century primary health care system: Australia's first National Primary Health Care Strategy. Publication no. 6594.* Canberra: Commonwealth of Australia; 2010.
17. Ministry of Health. *Better, sooner, more convenient health care in the community.* Wellington: Ministry of Health; 2011 Online. Available: <www.health.govt.nz/publication/better-sooner-more-convenient-health-care-community> [Viewed 16 September 2014].

18. Guzys D, Arnott N. The social model of health. In: Guzys D, Petrie E, editors. *An introduction to community and primary health care*. Melbourne: Cambridge University Press; 2014. p 5.

19. Edgecombe G, Stephens R. Healthy communities: the evolving roles of nursing. In: Daly J, Speedy S, Jackson D, editors. *Contexts of nursing*. 3rd ed. Sydney: Elsevier Churchill Livingstone; 2010. pp 274–86.

20. Ministry of Health New Zealand. 2014 Online. Available: <www.health.govt.nz/new-zealand-health-system/healthtargets?mega=NZ%20health%20system&title =Health%20targets> [Viewed 16 September 2014].

21. Australian Institute of Health and Welfare. Health expenditure Australia 2011–12: analysis by sector.

22. Ministry of Health New Zealand. 2014 Online. Available: <www.health.govt.nz/new-zealand-health-system/key-health-sector-organisations-and-people/district-health-boards> [Viewed 16 September 2014].

23. Ministry of Health. *Health expenditure trends in New Zealand 2000–2010*. Wellington: Ministry of Health; 2012 Online. Available: <www.health.govt.nz/publication/health-expenditure-trends-new-zealand-2000-2010> [Viewed 16 September 2014].

24. The Department of Health. *Commonwealth (HACC) Program*. Online. Available: <www.health.gov.au/hacc> [Viewed 16 September 2014].

25. Access. *Care and support for independent living*. Online. Available: <www.access.org.nz/get-started/funding-options> [Viewed 16 September 2014].

26. Cited in Primary Health Care Nurse Innovation Evaluation Team. *The evaluation of the eleven primary health care nursing innovation projects: a report to the Ministry of Health by the primary health care nurse innovation evaluation team*. Wellington: Ministry of Health; September 2007.

27. World Health Organization. *Health promotion: concepts and principles. Report of a Working Group*. Copenhagen: WHO Regional Office for Europe; 9–13 July 1984 Online. Available: <http://whqlibdoc.who.int/euro/-1993/ICP_HSR_602__m01.pdf> [Viewed 9 March 2011].

28. Guzys D. Working with or in the community. In: Guzys D, Petrie E, editors. *An introduction to community and primary health care*. Melbourne: Cambridge University Press; 2014.

CHAPTER 5

Understanding organisational culture in the hospital setting

Gary E Day

LEARNING OBJECTIVES

When you have completed this chapter you will be able to:

- ▲ describe what organisational culture is and what its impact can be on the organisation
- ▲ explain the organisational factors that can impact on the culture in the hospital setting
- ▲ understand the internal complexity of the social/task relationships in and between organisational subsystems
- ▲ understand the influences on nursing practice within healthcare organisations
- ▲ discuss the structure of authority in nursing services and its influence on the culture and areas of potential conflict within a health service.

KEYWORDS: organisational culture, organisational structures, functional design, bureaucracy, learning culture

INTRODUCTION

This chapter outlines what organisational culture is and what impact a culture can have on an organisation. Furthermore, the chapter will highlight internal organisational factors that impact upon an organisation's culture. The chapter gives an overview of the traditional bureaucratic organisational structure and examines the development of the professional bureaucratic organisational structures found in health services. Finally, the chapter discusses the structure of authority in nursing services and its subsequent influence on the organisational culture of a health service, as well as a range of issues that impact on culture, including conflict management strategies.

ORGANISATIONAL CULTURE OF A HEALTH SERVICE

The culture of an organisation can be simply described in a number of ways:

■ the unique ways we do things around here

■ our corporate or organisational 'DNA'

■ what separates us from our competitors.

Organisational culture can best be described as enduring attributes such as values, assumptions and beliefs that are unique to each organisation. Formally, Kaufman and McCaughan (p 52) articulate culture as 'a complex mixture of different elements that influence the way things are done, as well as the way things are understood, judged and valued'.[1] Scott-Findlay and Estabrook[2] suggest that organisational culture gives 'a sense of what is valued and how things should be done in an organisation'. Marquis and Huston[3] define it as the total of an organisation's values, language, history, formal and informal communication networks, rituals and 'sacred cows'. Additionally, Hemmelgarn and colleagues[4] argue that these beliefs and expectations are the basis for socialising co-workers in how to behave within an organisation, and create a social climate that shapes the tone, content and objectives of work accomplished within the organisation. In addition to the way things are done and specifically understood, the organisation's unique 'feel' is supported by particular symbols, rituals and language.[1] Simply put, new members to the organisation are taught through observation, modelling and personal experiences the 'way things are done around the organisation', as well as the rewards, punishments and expected outcomes that follow from one's work behaviour (p 77).[4] Strong cultures can take a long time to develop and an equally long time to change. Culture can affect how care is given, as well as how staff interact with each other. At their best, strong, positive workplace cultures can:

■ increase patient safety[1]

■ improve mental and physical wellbeing of healthcare staff [5,6]

■ lower patient mortality[6]

■ increase the intention of staff to stay in their jobs[6]

■ improve organisational performance.[7]

Equally, the literature demonstrates that at their weakest, poor or negative workplace cultures can:

■ lead to an increase in workplace bullying[8,9]

■ promote unethical behaviour.[10]

Given the research on the organisational outcomes of positive and negative cultures, it is evident that developing strategies to maintain a positive workplace culture has significant personal, professional and organisational benefits.

Factors Contributing to Positive Workplace Cultures

All staff, from the novice nurse to senior hospital executives, play an important role in the maintenance and improvement of an organisation's culture. While the senior executives in the hospital have a primary and pivotal role in setting the 'mood' of the organisation, all staff contribute to the overall culture. The literature outlines a number of factors that contribute to positive organisational cultures.

One factor that is highlighted in the literature is teamwork.[1,11,12] Developing strong, trusting, cooperative teams reinforces positive work practices and cultures. Second, effective and consistent leadership[1,7] drives positive workplace cultures over a period of time. Other factors identified as contributing to positive workplace cultures include:

- staff- or person-centred focus[11,12]
- open communication[12]
- positive attitudes to change[12]
- involvement, participation and collaboration[12]
- building of emotional resilience[5]
- workplace empowerment.[6]

Strategies to Deal with Counter-culture Norms

In this chapter so far, the content has covered aspects of what workplace culture is and what factors contribute to positive workplace culture. It is important to note that, in large, multidepartment organisations (such as major tertiary teaching hospitals), each department will have a slightly different but aligned subculture that makes up the overall culture of the hospital. This is quite normal, and can also be seen in other industries and organisations such as large multinational corporations and the armed forces. However, an organisation does not want to develop or support counter-cultures. A counter-culture is a subculture that directly challenges the prevailing or dominant culture of the organisation.[13] These subcultures work against the best interests of the organisation as a whole. In time, these counter-cultures can negatively impact or destroy the progress and purpose of the organisation.

Strategies used to to deal with counter-cultures include those listed earlier that help to build positive workplace cultures, namely: encouraging open communication and being staff-centred. Additionally, approaches that help to overcome these negative subcultures include:

- hospital management providing a clear outline of acceptable behaviour, standards, activities and policies
- having strong, positive leadership that promotes performance monitoring and is committed to organisational change[14]
- if the counter-culture continues, disbanding the team in question and moving the team members to other areas.

Types of Organisational Culture

Culture can be categorised or described in a number of ways. Cameron and Quinn[15] argue that any organisation's culture is based on competing values, and that the 'tension' between an organisation's (or department's) flexibility over control and internal focus over external focus creates certain cultural characteristics.

Cameron and Quinn categorised culture as being one of four types:

- clan culture
- adhocracy culture
- hierarchy culture
- market culture.

Gifford and colleagues[16] discuss these four cultural groupings in terms more helpful to healthcare. The authors account for clan culture as group culture; adhocracy culture as developmental culture; and market culture as rational culture. Hierarchy culture remains unchanged.

Group (or clan) culture can best be described as an organisation (or department) that values cohesion and high morale, with an emphasis on the training and development of its staff. This culture may be described as a human relations model.

Developmental (or adhocracy) culture is best described as an organisation that values growth, resource acquisition and external support. This type of culture is highly adaptable and ready for change. The culture can be described as an open systems model.

Rational (or market) culture describes an organisation that values productivity and efficiency. The key attribute of this type of culture is a focus on planning and goal setting. This type of culture can be categorised as a rational goal model.

Hierarchical culture describes an organisation that values stability and control. Organisations with this type of culture are driven by information management and communication processes. This type of culture can be categorised as an internal process model.

How is an Organisational Culture Spread?

There are several views about how organisational culture is spread, reproduced or changed within an organisation. The most favoured view is that there exists within an organisation a single culture that is developed or imported by its organisational members. Similar values, beliefs and perceptions are said to be shared by the members of the organisation.

Sovie[17] believes that a positive and constructive hospital culture is essential to achieve organisational goals, and thus is too important to be left simply to chance. To move to a constructive culture, the leader of the organisation must take an active role in building the type of organisational culture that will bring success to the organisation.

How organisations are internally managed and constituted has an impact on workplace culture. To better understand the development of organisations, it is important to review their history and evolution.

THE EVOLUTION OF THE BUREAUCRATIC ORGANISATION

Generally acclaimed to be the father of organisational theory, Max Weber, a German social scientist, developed in the 1920s a comprehensive formulation of the characteristics of a bureaucracy. The bureaucracy was an ideal weapon to routinise the energy of production during the Industrial Revolution. However, Weber's work did not consider the complexities of managing a dynamic organisation in the 21st century. He wrote during a time when the motivation of workers was taken for granted, and his simplification of manager and employee roles did not examine the complexities of the bilateral relationships found between employee and manager in the majority of organisations today.[3]

In his ideal bureaucracy, Weber[3] describes five main characteristics of the bureaucratic type of organisation:

1. They have a high degree of specialisation.
2. They have a hierarchical authority structure with limited areas of command and responsibility.

3. There is impersonality of relationships between organisational members.
4. The recruitment of officials is based on ability and technical knowledge.
5. There is differentiation of private and official income and fortune.

We find that modern managers have learnt about human behaviour, and now design and redesign their organisational structure in an effort to reduce rigidity and increase flexibility for their individual workers.

The other theorist who had a major impact on the early structure of organisations was Frederick Taylor. Taylor supported the system of bureaucracy but, in contrast to Weber, he was interested not so much in the organisational problems of society's power structures (general administrative management), but in the practical problem of efficiency (scientific management). His main unit of analysis was not society as a whole, but the individual workplace and the organisational productivity related to this workshop level. Taylor[18] (p 23) states: 'The principal object of management should be to secure maximum prosperity for the employer, coupled with maximum prosperity for the employee.' Taylor believed that, for every process, every task in industry, there is one best way of performing it. To discover this unique way, one has to examine the parts of the organisation in a scientific way. When they are known, they can be applied in the working situation to regulate the various activities and other factors of production in such a way that maximum productivity is achieved. Thus, scientific knowledge replaces intuition and the rule-of-thumb method in organisational behaviour.

Traditional Bureaucratic Organisations

The traditional bureaucratic organisation is found to have a hierarchy of authority and a dependence on rules and regulations. Rules govern most official business, leaving little opportunity for creativity or discretion in decision making. The repetitive and highly predictable nature of the work means it can be easily monitored. The organisation functions through coordination of work and tasks and, as the organisation grows and becomes more complex, the administration also grows to support and maintain the organisation's systems. A middle-management layer is necessary to oversee and monitor the specialised work of the core business.

In healthcare organisations there are many organisational objectives; however, the major objective is patient care. A number of professional participant groups contribute to patient care. These groups include medical, nursing, administrative, allied health and other staff. Each group has its own body of professional knowledge, and they all interpret organisational objectives according to their own value systems. Such issues can be problematic in terms of the coordination and integration of work when competing and different groups exercise legitimate authority in the same organisation with no line of authority between them. A complex organisation such as a healthcare facility requires coordination through standardisation of the skills of its employees. Such a configuration is known as a professional bureaucracy.[19]

Professional Bureaucratic Organisations

Professional bureaucratic organisations can lead to conflict. In the Australian health industry, conflict has been evident between the medical and other health professions, and hospital managers. Professionals have extensive training, which is designed to enable them to undertake complex and uncertain tasks independently. This leads to the view that professionals need the freedom to apply the appropriate skills to any given situation. Managers, however, in exercising their responsibility for the overall performance of their organisation, are required to coordinate, direct and control the professionals who perform the tasks. Ultimately, managers are brought into conflict with 'professional' resistance to control.[20] In order to achieve their goals, professionals tend to focus on their individual clinical contribution and their treatment of the patient, while managers focus on the organisation as a whole and endeavour to ensure that all parts of the organisation are coordinated.

The demand for healthcare and the costs of providing it have increased significantly in Australia over the past decade. Efforts to control the costs, coupled with advances in medical technology, have had an impact on health organisational structures and the organisational subsystems. Advances in medical technology have resulted particularly in increasing diversification, based on intensive training and subspecialisation in all professional disciplines. Such diversity and specialisation of activities necessitate an extensive division of labour, which, coupled with an already complex organisational structure, requires an elaborate system of coordination of tasks, functions and social interactions. Coordination by means of organisational hierarchy (traditional bureaucracy) is difficult. Administrative rules and procedures serve to coordinate routine events; however, for non-routine, complex patient care problems, one of the primary means of integration must be the voluntary coordination and willingness of the participants to work effectively together to deal with unusual events. The value system emphasising patient care is the basic factor influencing voluntary coordination.

In many healthcare systems, this has led to the development of a matrix-type organisation, with both hierarchical (vertical) integration through departmentalisation and formal chain of command, and lateral (horizontal) integration across departments. These complex organisations have, as workers, sophisticated specialists or professionals who are required to combine their efforts in project teams coordinated by mutual adjustment. Here, coordination is achieved by mutual adjustment because line management and staff functions, as well as a number of other distinctions, tend to break down. Some matrix designs express themselves as 'divisionalised' structures with semiautonomous units or sections responsible and accountable for their own budgets. In some matrix organisations, the functional (vertical) divisions retain most of the control so that the teams are set within a bureaucratic structure from which it is often difficult to break free. However, there have been cases where innovation and efficiencies have been achieved.

Public versus Private Hospital Environment

It is important to recognise that the organisational environments outlined above may differ in Australia between the public and private hospital systems. Private organisations have tended to be more traditional in the bureaucratic sense. That is, they are more hierarchical and often have traditional authority positions. This is partly due to the complexities of the relationships and the ownership of some of the organisational issues. In the public sector, most (although not all) medical staff are salaried employees. In the private system, fewer specialist medical practitioners are employed: most work on a private basis, thereby making them a key 'customer' of the organisation which brings in revenue by choosing to admit patients to any one hospital over other potential institutions in the geographical region. As long as access to facilities and equipment is provided by the hospital to enable medical practitioners to complete their required tasks in an efficient and coordinated manner, clinician interest in, and ownership of, the organisational issues can vary considerably. This is often because 'the organisation' is not the only or even the major affiliation they have with healthcare institutions. The medical practitioner's income and livelihood, although connected to the organisation, is basically the relationship with the patient (depending on the specialty) and can be satisfied outside the organisation. However, structural designs in private hospitals are changing. As private hospitals move from being stand-alone cottage industries to networked conglomerates of private businesses, the organisational structures have become more business-like. Private hospitals have become larger, more highly specialised and complex, and offer tertiary services; as such, their organisational structures are beginning to look like those in the public sector.

Boundaries within the Work Environment

No matter how an organisation is structured, the boundaries between work groups reinforce the relationships and accomplishment of the work within groups. They also hinder the development and maintenance of relationships among people and the accomplishment of work that crosses the boundaries of different groups. In complex organisations such as healthcare organisations, there is no perfect structure.[21] As a newly qualified professional functioning in such systems, it is important to understand the complexities of the relationships and work boundaries that will influence the achievement of either your work or your unit's work.

CREATING A LEARNING CULTURE WITHIN A HOSPITAL

While nurses' learning needs are ultimately their own professional responsibility, there are many ways these can be achieved within their employing organisation.

In-service Education

Many health service organisations arrange in-service sessions in wards during the day/evening shift changeover period. These sessions usually last about 30 minutes and nurses attend during their afternoon tea break. In-service sessions are usually prepared by the ward staff and are informal. One or more nurses are usually responsible for organising in-service sessions, and ideally they seek input from the other staff on desirable topics. Some wards expect all staff to give regular in-service sessions, which can provide very good learning opportunities.

Organisation-based Education Courses

Short courses are often made available to nursing staff at no or minimal cost. These courses are an excellent opportunity to access updates on various aspects of clinical practice, and also provide an opportunity for employees to display to the employer their interest in further opportunities and responsibilities. Staff undertaking these short courses should be mindful not to limit themselves to organisation-based courses as, inherently, these are biased to the beliefs and values of the institution. A balanced approach should be made and more formal university- or profession-based qualifications should also be sought.

Support for External Courses

Most hospitals offer financial support for staff members who wish to undertake formal university-based courses. Surprisingly, there are often few applicants for these grants. For those who do apply, emphasising the knowledge and skills that will be acquired as a future resource for the organisation is usually the key to achieving support. Some organisations offer support to staff who undertake courses that the employer considers desirable – for example, graduate qualifications in specialty areas such as mental health, midwifery or critical care.

Developing a Learning Culture

A key element to retaining and recruiting nursing staff is to create a culture that values and empowers nurses to develop professionally and personally. It means creating a culture where learning is valued, and where everyone is making improvements. By creating such a facilitating culture it should be possible to develop a learning organisation.[22]

Learning organisations also promote the notion of lifelong learning among their staff. There are two elements to creating lifelong learning. One is the need for organisations to ensure staff are oriented, have opportunities for professional development, and are adequately prepared to implement and use new equipment and technology. Second, the organisation needs to build the capacity for staff to seek out development opportunities independently throughout their careers. This approach demonstrates an organisation's professional duty to support and nurture new graduates, new staff and undergraduate students. While it is accepted that human capital investment in health or education is the key to future prosperity and economic growth,[23] the final responsibility for learning rests with individuals themselves, a function of their current work needs and interests in their longer-term career aspirations.[24]

Performance Management Systems

The employment of registered nurses is generally governed by a formalised performance planning and review (PPR) system that takes place annually. This PPR system involves registered nurses meeting with their supervisor, identifying and documenting their performance goals, and establishing a plan to achieve those goals. This process should not be seen as a pointless bureaucratic activity, but rather as an opportunity to achieve learning goals. Specific learning goals that may be included in a PPR are presented in Figure 5.1.

Performance plans should be relevant to employer expectations and service focus. Attending a course on diabetes will not be seen as desirable if the ward does not care for such patients. Documentation of learning goals not only makes the employee responsible for achieving the goals but, importantly, also places a responsibility on the supervisor and the organisation to assist the staff member to achieve the goals by providing educational sessions.

In the next 12 months I will fulfil my role as a registered nurse by:

Clinical

Observing cardiac angiography and cardiac angioplasty

Attending the hospital 2-day program 'Managing diabetes'

Education

Giving in-service sessions on angiography, angioplasty and managing diabetes

Acting as preceptor to a new staff member

Management

Discussing 'in charge of shift' role with clinical nurse consultant

Undertaking 'in charge of shift' role 'buddied' with a senior nurse on three shifts

Research

Discussing current ward research with nurse researcher

Reviewing a research article for journal club

Figure 5.1

Performance planning and review (PPR) learning goals

Educators and Other Resource People

Nurse educators are employed in hospitals to facilitate staff education. Registered nurses should approach their nurse educator and supervisor to discuss their learning needs. However, there are many other ways to improve knowledge. There is usually only one educator allocated to several wards and the educator's workload may be largely dictated by broad organisational needs. For example, hospital standards usually require all nurses to undertake a cardiopulmonary resuscitation competency annually, which is a time-consuming responsibility for the educators. Nurse colleagues and other healthcare professionals can be consulted informally as matters arise, although care should be taken to back this up with formal documents such as procedure manuals, resource manuals, online journals and evidence-based practice guidelines published by reputable professional groups; these are usually located at the nurses' station in the ward.

NURSING ORGANISATIONAL ISSUES AND POTENTIAL CONFLICT SITUATIONS

Clinical nurses are concerned mainly with giving care and providing for the needs of their patients. However, nursing executives tend to focus on the overarching organisational issues that involve the governing of the hospital as a whole. There are thus many organisational and administrative issues that have an impact on the everyday working lives of clinical nurses and have the potential to lead to conflict situations. We now look at some examples of these issues.

Balancing the Budget

As healthcare costs continue to rise, government health budgets are increasingly being stretched, and hospital departments and service areas are required to compete among themselves for the limited funding now available; for example, the medical division competes for funds with the surgical division. Clinical departments have budgets for nursing wages, equipment and disposables, and the distribution of funds between various departments and service areas can become a source of much conflict across divisions within hospitals.

Human Resources Management

The processes of employing staff, providing orientation, managing performance and resignations are all regulated by government legislation and organisational bureaucratic structures and systems (e.g. the Nursing Act in the relevant jurisdiction and hospital orientation programs). These requirements may sometimes be seen to conflict with the ability of the organisation to bring about change.

Organisational Performance

Healthcare organisations are required to evaluate the extent to which they deliver quality care. Formalised processes such as quality assurance programs and accreditation exist to fulfil this function. Performance is also measured in terms of the cost of services performed. Clinical staff are expected to collect data on patient/nurse dependency ratios to help justify spending and plan for future services. However, the collection of such data may seem unnecessary or take time away from the delivery of patient care.

Variation of Policies and Procedures

Healthcare organisations have developed a variety of documents to guide staff in their provision of quality, consistency and external justification of care. These documents may be very specific and apply only to one ward, or they may be more generically applicable to the whole hospital. The documents may be clinical in nature (e.g. how to undertake a dressing) or more administrative (e.g. how to apply for annual leave). Because these policies/procedures may be so parochial, there is the potential for dissatisfaction for registered nurses who move around the same or different hospitals. Official hospital policies and procedures should be adhered to in the same manner as a legal guideline.

Unfortunately, policies often become out of date and the informal culture within an organisation may be such that it is acceptable not to follow the official policy for this reason. These situations should be brought to the attention of the clinical nurse consultant (or similar) so that the policy can be reviewed and reissued to reflect current practice and research. It is common for junior nursing staff to assist in the development and review of policies with assistance from their supervisor and this can be an excellent learning opportunity.

Informal and Unofficial Practices

Because hospitals consist of people, the element of informal, unofficial mores and procedures will exist. These can be confusing for a newcomer to the ward or organisation, as these practices are not explicit and are not included in official orientation manuals. Preceptors or co-workers may be helpful in enlightening new colleagues on these matters. However, it is more likely such practices will be learnt through observation at best, and trial and error at worst. Perceptions of competency or seniority among ward staff are often linked to familiarity with the unofficial culture.

CONFLICT MANAGEMENT

Conflict is a natural and unavoidable aspect of any setting of human life. Conflict occurs when individuals have different needs or desires, or when they have different ideas about the best way to meet goals. Conflict can be useful and lead to positive change or, at least, allow discussion of issues so that some sort of resolution can be achieved. Unfortunately, conflict can also be destructive, causing personal anguish as well as decreased productivity.

Types of Conflict

Registered nurses regularly experience conflict during the course of their work, whether it is during their day-to-day work practices or secondary to larger organisational conflict. The three main types of conflict that occur within healthcare organisations are intrapersonal, interpersonal and intergroup conflict.

Intrapersonal conflict occurs within an individual rather than between individuals.

CASE STUDY 5.1

After Phuong had finished her graduate year on an oncology ward, she felt unsure of the next step to take in her career. A lot of her fellow graduates were going overseas on a working holiday – something she had always wanted to do. On the other hand, she felt that perhaps she should consolidate her experience a little more before she went. After all, she had only worked on one ward; she should probably move to another area to increase her confidence and experience. She did like her ward, though, and that was another problem. The nurse educator and charge nurse were really nice and they were strongly encouraging Phuong to take a place in the Graduate Diploma in Oncology. Phuong liked oncology, but she wondered if it was only because she had not tried anything else.

REFLECTIVE QUESTIONS

1. What might happen if Phuong left and then decided she wanted to return?
2. What are some of the intrapersonal conflicts Phuong may be experiencing?

Interpersonal conflict occurs between individuals in the work environment. If two people are on an equivalent power level, interpersonal disagreements may simply cause annoyance. However, if one person has real or perceived authority over the other, the situation has the potential to lead to conflict.

CASE STUDY 5.2

As a new graduate, Helen was assigned a preceptor named David. At first Helen was grateful for his help, but as she grew more confident she started to think that David did not always know as much as he made out. She wanted him to treat her the same as any registered nurse on the ward, but he would not leave her alone and kept giving her long, boring lectures that slowed her up when she was trying to get her work done and made her look silly in front of her patients. Helen was at a loss about how to deal with the problem. She wanted to brush David off, but she worried that he would turn nasty – after all, he was often in charge of the shift. What if he started allocating her the hardest patients or told the charge nurse that she was not performing well? Helen dreaded going to work when she knew that David was also rostered on.

REFLECTIVE QUESTIONS

1. What options might Helen consider to deal with this potential conflict?
2. How might Helen engage David to improve the situation?

Intergroup conflict occurs between professional groups or different departments.

CASE STUDY 5.3

One thing Mark felt quite confident in when he graduated was stoma care. He had undertaken quite a few placements where patients had stomas, but when he got a job in a surgical ward he was surprised to find there was a nurse employed in the very grand-sounding job of stomal therapy consultant. One day, as he was educating a patient about his stoma care, the charge nurse apologised for interrupting but asked him to come to her office straightaway. When he arrived, he found the stomal therapist there also. Mark sat there in disbelief as the two senior nurses told him that he was not to perform stoma care or education with his patients, as it was not his role. When he protested that he felt it was within his abilities, they became quite short with him. Didn't he appreciate how lucky he was to work in a place with such a resource? they said. It was people like him who were jeopardising professional opportunities and specialised nurses, they added. When Mark went home that night, he felt so angry he wanted to resign.

REFLECTIVE QUESTIONS

1. What strategies might Mark use to reduce or defuse the conflict so as to maintain his professional practice?
2. Is there a compromise that would allow Mark to continue to use his skills and feel like he is contributing to the care delivered to his patients?

Conflict Resolution Strategies

Various options exist for conflict resolution:

- *Compromise/collaboration:* the conflicting parties work together to reach a mutually satisfactory outcome.
- *Competition:* one party attempts to defeat any opposition.
- *Cooperation/accommodation:* in this case one party gives in or tries to smooth over the conflict.
- *Avoidance/withdrawal:* the individual avoids any attempts to resolve the conflict or pretends it does not exist.

Deciding which strategy to choose can become a challenge, and depends on the following:

- the urgency with which the conflict must be resolved
- the power/status of the person you are experiencing conflict with
- how important you perceive the issue to be
- previous experience and comfort within conflict situations
- personal factors such as being tired and having other worries on your mind.

Conflict Resolution in the Healthcare Organisation

Conflict may not always be able to be resolved to the satisfaction of all parties; however, if patience and willingness to appreciate another's point of view and a focus on shared goals are present, there is a good chance that at least an acceptable compromise can be reached. Conflict for nurses in the workplace should always be resolved with the emphasis on patient safety and quality care first, followed by what is the best outcome for the majority of staff.

Aiming for a 'win–win' situation is often promoted as the preferred option of conflict management, but this should be considered carefully. In situations where patient care is jeopardised, an urgent and even non-consultative decision must be made. In these situations the authority of the nurse leader/s should be sought. However, more minor grievances should be resolved by those involved.

CONCLUSION

This chapter presents an overview of the traditional bureaucratic organisational structure and examines the way in which professional bureaucratic structures have evolved within health services in Australia, as well as the differences between the public and private hospital environments. Understanding the structure, design and purpose of healthcare organisations gives staff an awareness of how organisations operate and how organisational culture is developed. In addition to providing an understanding of organisational structures, the chapter outlines strategies for improving culture and organisational climate and for dealing with negative cultures in hospitals. The chapter concludes with a discussion on areas of potential conflict in healthcare organisations and strategies for resolving conflict.

CASE STUDY 5.4

After graduation, Fiona worked on a surgical ward in a large city hospital that was committed to evidence-based practice. Policies for wound dressings were updated regularly to reflect the latest research. After a few years, Fiona returned to her hometown and started working at the local hospital. During orientation she was shocked to learn that wound care policies differed for each surgeon. For example, laparotomy wounds were washed in the shower for surgeon A, with antiseptic for surgeon B and with saline for surgeon C. The nurses seemed to have little idea of or interest in what wound research had been done.

Fiona tried to discuss her frustrations with her colleagues but could not convince them to work towards a standardised best-practice approach. 'You'll never get the surgeons to agree' and 'We don't have much infection, so it probably doesn't matter which way we do the dressings' were common statements. After a while, Fiona just gave in and learnt each surgeon's preference. She had succumbed to the ward culture.

REFLECTIVE QUESTIONS

1. Why did Fiona succumb to the ward culture?
2. What approach could Fiona adopt in order to slowly modify the culture and move it towards a best-practice approach?

CASE STUDY 5.5

At a ward meeting, the nursing staff decide they would like to trial 12-hour shifts, which would mean working only 3 days per week. The nurse manager is supportive and agrees to look into the matter. There is excitement in the ward until the nurse manager reports back that the Nurses Act prohibits 12-hour shifts and that the Nursing Union is against any change being made to shift length. The ward staff feel frustration and disbelief that they are unable to do something they all want because of what they see as 'red tape'.

REFLECTIVE QUESTION

Can you think of other examples of human resources management conflict?

EXERCISE 5.1

1. Consider the organisation or organisations you have worked in. How would you describe the culture? What leads you to categorise the culture in this way?
2. Is the culture you are working in (or have worked in) conducive to positive teamwork and good patient outcomes?
3. Consider what actions you can take that would improve the department or organisation you work in. Write a list of the practical steps that you could use to turn the culture around.
4. Write down a list of the things you do that improve culture within your department or work team. Then write a list of the things you do that detract from the work culture of your team or department. What comments would you make about these two lists and your personal responsibility for workplace culture?

RECOMMENDED READING

Daly J, Speedy S, Jackson D, editors. *Nursing leadership.* Sydney: Churchill Livingstone; 2004.

Heifetz R, Grashow A, Linsky M. *The practice of adaptive leadership: tools and tactics for changing your organization and the world.* Boston: Harvard Business Press; 2009.

Malloch K, Porter-O'Grady T. *The quantum leader: applications for the new world of work.* Boston: Jones and Bartlett; 2005.

Mick SS, Wyttenbach ME, editors. *Advances in health care organization theory*. San Francisco: Jossey-Bass; 2003.

Porter-O'Grady T, Malloch K. *Quantum leadership: a textbook of new leadership*. 2nd ed. Boston: Jones and Bartlett; 2007.

REFERENCES

1. Kaufman G, McCaughan D. The effect of organizational culture on patient safety. *Nursing Standard* 2013;**27**(43):50–6.
2. Scott-Findlay S, Estabrook CA. Mapping the organizational culture research in nursing: a literature review. *Journal of Advanced Nursing* 2006;**56**:498–513.
3. Marquis BL, Huston CJ. *Leadership roles and management functions in nursing: theory and application*. 5th ed. Philadelphia: Lippincott; 2006.
4. Hemmelgarn AL, Glisson C, James LR. Organizational culture and climate: implications for services and interventions research. *Clinical Psychology: Science and Practice* 2006;**13**:73–89.
5. Sergeant J, Laws-Chapman C. Creating positive workplace culture. *Nursing Management* 2012;**18**(9):14–19.
6. Laschinger HK, Cummings GG, Wong CA, et al. Resonant leadership and workplace empowerment: the value of positive organizational culture in reducing workplace incivility. *Nursing economics* 2014;**32**(1):5–16.
7. Jacobs R, Mannion R, Davies HTO, et al. The relationship between organizational culture and performance in acute hospitals. *Social Science and Medicine* 2013;**76**:115–25.
8. Tambur M, Vadi M. Workplace bullying and organizational culture in a post-transitional country. *International Journal of Manpower* 2012;**33**(7):754–68.
9. O'Farrell C, Nordstrom CR. Workplace bullying: examining self-monitoring and organizational culture. *Journal of Psychological Issues in Organizational Culture* 2013;**3**(4):6–17.
10. Casali GL, Day GE. Treating an unhealthy organizational culture: the implications of the Bundaberg Hospital inquiry for management ethical decision making. *Australian Health Review* 2010;**34**:73–9.
11. Park JS, Kim TH. Do types of organizational culture matter in nurse job satisfaction and turnover intention? *Leadership in Health Services* 2009;**22**(1):20–38.
12. Manley K, Sanders K, Cardiff S, et al. Effective workplace culture: the attributes, enabling factors and consequences of a new concept. *International Practice Development Journal* 2011;**1**(2):[1]. Online. Available: <www.fons.org/library/journal.aspx>.
13. Brown A. *Organisational culture*. 2nd ed. Harlow, UK: Prentice Hall; 1998.
14. De Bono S, Heling G, Borg MA. Organizational culture and its implications for infection prevention and control in healthcare institutions. *Journal of Hospital Infection* 2014;**86**(1):1–6.
15. Cameron KS, Quinn RE. *Diagnosing and changing organizational culture*. Reading, UK: Addison-Wesley; 1999.
16. Gifford BD, Zammuto RF, Goodman EA, et al. The relationship between hospital unit culture and nurses' quality of work life. *Journal of Healthcare Management* 2002;**47**:13–26.
17. Sovie MD. Hospital culture – why create one? *Nursing Economics* 1993;**11**:69–75.
18. Taylor FW. *The principles of scientific management*. New York: Harper; 1911.
19. Mintzberg H. Organization design: fashion or fit? *Harvard Business Review* 1981;**Jan–Feb**:103–16.
20. Southon G. Health service structures, management and professional practice: beyond clinical management. *Australian Health Review* 1996;**19**:1–5.

21. Charns MP. Changing health care organisations for increased effectiveness. *Australian Health Review* 1984;**7**:98–105.
22. Chapman L, Howkins E. Developing a learning culture. *Nursing Management* 2001;**8**:10–13.
23. Calpin-Davies PJ. Management and leadership: a dual role in nursing education. *Nurse Education Today* 2003;**23**:3–10.
24. Legge D, Stanton P, Smyth A. Learning management (and managing your own learning). In: Harris MG, editor. *Managing health services: concepts and practice.* 2nd ed. Sydney: Elsevier Mosby; 2005.

CHAPTER 6

Preparing for role transition

Jan Sayers and Esther Chang

INTRODUCTION

Transitioning from the graduate role is both exciting and challenging. Exciting because you are finally embarking on your professional career, and challenging because of the high-paced demands of the healthcare environment. You may experience a mix of feelings and emotions – from exhilaration to self-doubt and inadequacy – as you try to meet the requirements of your new role and the expectations of your workplace.[1] As described in Chapter 2, the first step in your career trajectory is that of a novice.[2] Gradually, as you develop confidence in your role and acquire more skills, you will move from being a novice through the stages of being an advanced beginner, a competent nurse, then a proficient one and, ultimately, an expert nurse or midwife.[2] Having an understanding of roles within health settings may enable you to better understand why people behave the way they do in certain situations. Role theory provides students and new graduates with a useful theoretical perspective from which to consider the novice role. In this chapter, we will explore the following aspects of role theory in relation to transition:

- roles and society
- role acquisition – primary, secondary and tertiary
- role stress – incongruity, conflict, ambiguity
- establishing and nurturing role relationships and a positive self-concept.

In your new graduate role, you will find yourself in situations where both your personal and university-acquired values, ideals and behaviours may require some adjustment in order to meet the expectations of the clinical setting.[3–7] Transition from student to graduate is a challenging process that you will find both exciting and rewarding. During this period, you will experience rapid growth as a person and as a professional, and as a result of this process you are likely to experience emotional highs and lows. It is likely that you will feel some anxiety and apprehension about how well you will function in your new role and whether or not you will meet the expectations of the institution, your colleagues and your patients.[8] No amount of prior learning or experience can completely prepare you for role transition, but thoughtful preparation can help to ease the stress and strain.[9] In this chapter, we focus on furthering your understanding of the graduate role and how you can prepare yourself to meet the organisational expectations of your role performance during transition by utilising role theory as the underlying perspective.

ROLES IN SOCIETY

Roles are assigned to individuals and groups in society because they describe predictable and patterned behaviour. In other words, each recognisable role has certain behaviours that are associated with it. This process makes it easier for us to function because we know what to expect from others. Each member of society can hold a myriad of roles at any one time; our immediate role may change from one situation to the next; and we can play numerous roles across the course of our life. Furthermore, the way we regard ourselves is highly dependent on the roles we hold and how they are valued by the people that interact with us. Learning to conform to role expectations starts when we are very young because most people seek the approval and acceptance of others: the approval of others is a strong motivation to conform throughout our lives. The feeling of not fitting in can be uncomfortable and influence us to adapt our behaviour very quickly to be accepted by the group to which we wish to belong.[10] Resisting the pressure to conform can be difficult; however, in some situations if the behaviour change required by the group is so great that we feel our behaviour is no longer acceptable to ourselves, or if it requires more effort to maintain our behaviour than we are willing or able to give, this can prove to be just as uncomfortable. Such feelings may lead to role relinquishment and group abandonment.[10]

One way of looking at your behaviour is to see yourself as an actor playing a part and following scripts that direct your performance. The first notions that led to the development of role theory were generated in this way.[11–13] Our role scripts contain the rules about how others in society expect us to behave. Many of our roles come to us because of our abilities, education and training, and these are more likely to be formal, in that they have an identifying role name and are tightly controlled – that is, they are more tightly scripted by society. The registered nurse role is a good example, as the practice of registered nurses is regulated and subject to codes of conduct, ethics and standards.[14,15] All professional groups experience this type of role control. However, there remain many aspects of a professional role, no matter how formal, that are not always clearly scripted or accessible. These aspects can depend on the situation or the context in which they occur. Expectations of the graduate role differ according to whether the graduate is working in a hospital ward or in the community. Even experienced graduates will talk about the challenge of meeting set expectations when moving from one specialty area to another.[16] Most graduates will never fully understand their professional role until they are experiencing or acting their part. Furthermore, script expectations may not become clear to an actor until the person transgresses the role boundaries or does not fully address what is expected by interdependent others. When expectations are not met, fellow actors exert pressure to control an actor's behaviour in order to bring it into line with expectations. Resisting the pressure to conform takes a good deal of effort and resolve on the part of an actor.

A word of advice: even though acceptance by nursing and midwifery colleagues will be crucial to your professional development and comfort in the clinical setting, it should not come at the cost of losing your personal values or those you developed at university.[3] Furthermore, the responsibility to make role expectations 'right' is not a task for the new graduate alone. The tertiary sector and industry are also responsible and need to work towards removing the incongruity between sector expectations that can make beginning practice for the new graduate more stressful than necessary.[17]

Learning the role of the registered nurse or midwife, like other formal roles in society, involves not only acquiring knowledge about the role and all its dimensions but also an awareness that there are aspects of the role that are only accessible through experience. Careful preparation is essential to a smooth transition, and of equal importance is the acceptance that your conception of the graduate role will be altered to some degree by exposure to the expectations of others in the workplace.

Primary and Secondary Role Acquisition

As mentioned above, role acquisition is a social process. Your decision to become a registered nurse or midwife has evolved over time and can be divided into primary, secondary and tertiary phases.

During the primary phase of socialisation you internalised values, beliefs and behaviours from significant others that motivated you to become a student.[18] This

---

EXERCISE 6.1 Changing Images of the Nursing/Midwifery Role

1. If you had been asked on your first day of university to draw an image of a nurse/midwife, what would you have drawn? How would they have looked? What would they have been doing? In what role situation would you have depicted them?
2. What aspects of the above picture would you like to change? What parts do you feel should stay the same? Consider the ways in which your image of your profession and associated roles has changed over the course of your studies.
3. Discuss these findings with your study group.

motivation is in part related to an internalised set of expectations about your professional role, expectations that have probably been altered in many ways by your education. Exercise 6.1 will allow you to compare your earlier expectations of your professional role with the ones you hold now; it will be interesting to consider how your perceptions have changed over time.

Secondary socialisation has to do with acquiring knowledge, skills and dispositions such as those you have learnt during your university program.[18] Your present image of the graduate role has been shaped by this process, and this is probably evident from your reflection in Exercise 6.1. It is during this phase that your professional values and standards are formed and integrated with a developing understanding of your profession's scope of practice and variety of service. Despite an almost completed undergraduate education, however, you may still feel somewhat unclear about what the graduate role fully encompasses. A good place to begin to increase your understanding is by reviewing the various codes and standards that apply to practice as a registered nurse or registered midwife.

An understanding of the codes and standards that apply to the professional behaviour of registered staff is essential for students who are preparing for transition. Australian undergraduate nursing and midwifery programs aim to address the standards developed by the Australian Nursing and Midwifery Council (ANMC) within its curricula, and this then forms the basis for curriculum approval by the registering authority. In addition, universities and health facilities use these standards for the clinical assessment of students and new graduates.[14] The ANMC has also developed codes of professional[19] and ethical[20] conduct for nurses in Australia. Similar codes and standards developed by the Nursing Council of New Zealand (NCNZ)[21] apply to nurses and midwives in New Zealand.

The competencies address not only the expected standards for registered nurses, but also the competencies related to enrolled nurses.[15] It is important that enrolled nurses who upgrade their qualifications to become registered nurses understand that there are higher expectations of professional behaviour in the new role. As is often the case when you have been successfully working in an associated role, elements such as a sense of responsibility and accountability can be underestimated or discounted in regard to the new and more responsible role and result in increased stress.[7] For graduating students who entered their Bachelor of Nursing with enrolled nurse qualifications it may be beneficial to discuss with registered nurses from similar educational backgrounds the challenging aspects of their transition to the workforce. This process allows graduates to 'reframe their practice' within the realities of the work setting.[8] Simulated learning experiences may also serve to provide a feeling of the responsibility and accountability associated with the new role that is not achievable through clinical practicum in the student role.

As a graduate, you will encounter a variety of other nursing- and midwifery-associated roles within your immediate team in the workplace. These roles may include the assistant in nursing (AIN), mothercraft nurse, enrolled nurse (EN), clinical educator (CNE or CME) and nurse unit manager (NUM). As a graduate, it is imperative to acknowledge that staff occupying these roles will have attained varying levels of education and have differing knowledge and skill sets. Additionally, they are bounded by varying scopes of practice identified in their role descriptions and competencies. It

EXERCISE 6.2 Understanding Role Dimensions through Competency Standards

1. Review the competency standards for registered nurses and enrolled nurses.
2. Identify how the standards differ between these two levels.
3. Discuss the implications of these differences for the registered nurse or the registered midwife role.

EXERCISE 6.3 Exploring How Competency Standards are Integrated in Clinical Practice

1. Interview a second- or third-year graduate.
2. Explore with the graduate the meaning of the relevant competency standards.
3. Ask the graduate how these competency standards are addressed in their present role.
4. Compare the responses of the graduates interviewed.
5. Discuss the factors that promote or hinder integration of the competency standards in practice.

is the responsibility of each staff member occupying these roles to work within the parameters of their role. As a new graduate, an understanding of the assistant in nursing and enrolled nurse roles is important as you will gradually find yourself being responsible for supervising these staff in clinical practice.

Exercise 6.2 suggests that you review your relevant standards (ANMC/NCNZ) and compare these competencies with those that guide the practice of the enrolled nurse. By undertaking this activity you will become clearer about your role in relation to a closely associated role. This activity will provide you with a clearer understanding of the competencies of a group of health workers that you will often supervise in practice and to whom you will delegate responsibilities.

While Exercise 6.2 will broaden your understanding of the registered nurse or registered midwife role, your understanding will be greatly enhanced by exploring with a clinical nurse or midwife the application of these standards in practice. Exercise 6.3 explores how the national competency standards are expressed in the workplace.

Tertiary Role Acquisition

Tertiary socialisation occurs when you enter specific work situations as an employee.[22] At this point, you will be required to demonstrate the expected behaviours associated with your professional role. It is often the case that the beliefs, values and behaviours developed through primary and secondary socialisation do not fit easily or exactly into the institution where you have chosen to work. As role acquisition is a lifelong process,

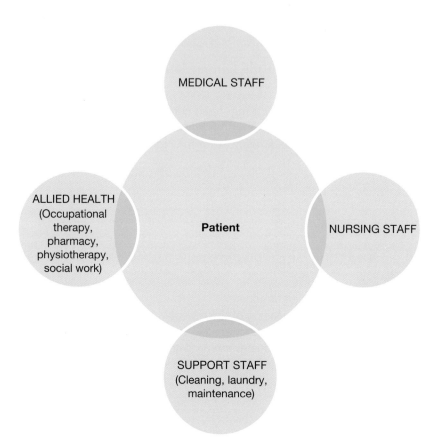

Figure 6.1
Role partners

you have entered a new and important phase of learning that focuses on acquiring the values and norms relevant to the clinical context. Your professional identity is formed during this phase and the values and attitudes learnt in other phases of socialisation may be changed or modified.

Your role set will have a significant influence on your behaviour during your transition. A role set is made up of role partners who have an interdependent role relationship with you – for example, medical staff, your nursing unit manager, other nurses and your patients,[23] as shown in Figure 6.1. It is important that you have a clear idea of who your role partners are and their areas of responsibility and skill. This knowledge will help you to function more effectively as a team member.

Each member of your role set will be affected in some way by what you say or do, and will have attitudes and beliefs about what to expect from you in your new graduate role. Sometimes these attitudes and beliefs will differ from your own expectations of your role and you will experience role conflict. Part of successful preparation for practice should include an exploration of the role of interdependent others in your prospective workplace. Exercise 6.4 assists you in identifying your role set members and what their role responsibilities involve.

EXERCISE 6.4 Identifying and Understanding Your Role Set

1. List the roles in a typical ward situation that are interdependent with nursing or midwifery.
2. Determine the responsibilities and skills associated with each role, and the lines of authority where applicable.
3. Consider the degree of influence these roles can or should potentially exert on your practice.

ROLE STRESS

It is almost impossible for graduates to avoid some level of role stress when you consider the complex socialisation processes involved in learning how to work competently as a graduate.[16] Furthermore, new graduates often report that they feel unprepared for the workload, shift work and managerial responsibilities associated with their role.[8,9,24–27] Many studies also indicate that graduates have difficulty maintaining what they consider to be excellence in nursing care in the face of workload expectations, and that this can result in strong feelings of stress, inadequacy, guilt and disillusionment.[4,9,16,24,27] It appears that the ideals and values new graduates learnt at university can often set them apart from other staff.[9,17,24,28]

The responsibility for determining educational standards and clinical practice requirements for undergraduate nursing and midwifery courses rests with the accrediting body. In Australia this is the Nursing and Midwifery Board of Australia, and in New Zealand either the Nursing Council of New Zealand or the Midwifery Council of New Zealand (MCNZ). While universities focus on educating students in relation to the competencies in their fullest sense, and embrace the theoretical and ideological aspects of nursing or midwifery, the clinical sector continues to expect proficient 'hands-on' practitioners upon graduation.[17,26,28] Students attending clinical practicum as part of their university study are allocated to a mainly supernumerary role where they have time to consider their theoretical knowledge and how this informs their clinical actions. However, as graduates they still need time to adjust these values to the reality of the hospital workplace, which can result in role stress as they attempt to grapple with the level of proficiency needed in the often resource- and staff-constrained clinical settings.[10] Moreover, this high expectation by clinicians in healthcare facilities for all graduates to be competent and accountable for clinical decisions can be even more stressful for those graduates who have an initial qualification.[9] This discontinuity between sectors leads to a general lack of recognition of the graduate as a new clinician and a misunderstanding of the graduate's educational preparation.[26,28] Pressure is often exerted by a graduate's role set to control and regulate the behaviour of novices in line with the traditional norms set by the clinical sector.

It would be a great loss to our professions if frameworks for practice developed at university, such as critical thinking, reflective practice, evidence-based practice and cultural safety, were abandoned by the graduate in order to 'fit in' with a controlling social environment. There is room to move on both sides; that is, for new graduate clinicians, clinical educators and academics to work together to implement innovative programs or strategies to redress the discontinuity. An example of such a strategy can be the design of clinical practicums in the final year of the degree, which provide students with experiences that mirror the reality of the hospital workplace they will encounter on graduation. This can, for example, include the allocation of several patients of different dependency levels so that students can learn to plan and complete their caring practices competently within the expected timeframe. Clinical experiences such as this may offer the best opportunity for maintaining the theoretical frameworks for practice while still achieving the requirements of their professional role, especially if these students are also given adequate support and understanding during this practicum by staff while they learn to cope with the pressures and expectations of the workplace. Role stress can be reduced if tertiary programs endeavour to prepare graduates more realistically for transition, and industry eases the process of transition for new graduates by respecting their achievements and supporting their beginning practice.[9,24,26,28,29]

Types of Role Stress

Four types of role stress have been identified – role incongruity, role conflict, role ambiguity and role overload – and it would be unusual for new graduates not to experience some degree of strain on commencing work. Role strain is the outward expression of stress that can be evident in your behaviour.[30] You may feel frustration, tension or anxiety in response to role stress, which may result in distancing, denial and avoidance.[31] These negative effects can eventually have an impact on your patient care and your relationships with others, and so it is important to try and identify the symptoms when they occur.

Role incongruity

This aspect of role stress is largely cognitive and is related to the dissonance in values or self-concept between the graduate and their workplace.[32] Case study 6.1 illustrates role incongruity where the graduate's personal skills or values about their role may not align with the requirements of the role as expected by the health facility. Role incongruity can be lessened in situations where the work environment and workplace culture encourages open communication and reciprocal exchanges between staff. Your interpersonal skills, respect for others, a willingness to listen and self-reflection are important considerations here.

CASE STUDY 6.1

During the first few weeks working on her new ward, Maria admitted feeling frustrated and stressed because she was not able to provide patient care at the standard she had been educated to provide. She was resentful of the other staff whom she believed did not care that her patient care was being compromised.

REFLECTIVE QUESTIONS

1. Do your values about your caring role differ from those of the other staff working on your ward?
2. What could account for the difference in values between staff?

3. How can Maria resolve this situation and find a way to work with the other staff, while maintaining her own values?
4. What support could Maria access to work through her concerns?

Many nurses resolve their role incongruity by developing a pragmatic and multidimensional understanding of nursing values and their professional self-concept. When this occurs, the nurse is able to integrate the nursing values that incorporate holism and caring for the humanistic needs of the patient with their professional role, while maintaining loyalty to the institution and its work values, rules and regulations.

New graduates are also vulnerable to workplace incivility.[33] Examples of uncivil behaviour include a staff member dismissing your ideas or comments, belittling you or making demeaning remarks to you. This inappropriate behaviour can leave you feeling demoralised and may lead to feelings of not belonging or of anger. An effective strategy to manage change or adapt to difficult situations is to develop resilience.[33] Ensuring you stay connected with people you know and trust, and talking to them about the issues that concern you, is one way of developing resilience as this allows you to gain perspective about the situation and consider strategies that you can use to address it. This also helps you to determine how important the issue is and the degree of influence you may have to change the situation. Another way that resilience is developed is by being patient with yourself as you adapt to your new workplace. If you can do this, then you are accepting that your experiences may be challenging but with time and perseverance you may feel that you are accepted in your new role and workplace. Being positive and trying to view difficult situations as a challenge that you can ultimately overcome also helps to build resilience.[33]

Some graduates, however, are not able to move on and may decide to leave their profession or to capitulate their own values fully to the values of the institution and workplace culture.[34] It is up to each individual to reflect on the continuing expectations of his or her role. Unless graduates are prepared to reflect honestly on their practice, it is difficult to resist task-oriented and ritualised care based on the bureaucratic ideals of efficiency and conformity.

Role conflict

Role conflict involves the recognition of the urge to act in different ways to what one may want, because of different role pressures. Compliance with role pressure from one source will make compliance with another difficult, and may affect both behaviour and feelings. This conflict can occur within the new graduate or between two or more individuals who have different perceptions of the role to be enacted.[30] One example of role conflict can be encountered when graduates feel pressured because of competing priorities in their work role. Conflicting situations can arise during times when the ward may have inadequate or less experienced staff. Case study 6.2 demonstrates the conflict a graduate can experience between work and personal role pressures.

CASE STUDY 6.2

During the night, Roger's 3-year-old daughter, Lindy, was ill with a high fever. By the next morning her temperature had subsided, but she was not well enough to be left at her kindergarten. Roger, a single parent, had no close family support or friends who could help. He was feeling stressed about his conflict, as he would prefer to remain at home and care for Lindy rather than go to work. He was rostered on for the day shift, and he knew that if he did not go to work his nurse unit manager would be upset with him. Roger did not want to let down his manager and the other staff, but he really wanted to stay at home and be with Lindy.

REFLECTIVE QUESTIONS

1. What would you do in this situation?
2. How would you approach the nursing unit manager if you found you were unable to work your shift because of a personal matter?
3. What could Roger do to avoid a similar situation of role conflict arising in the future?

If work role requirements are not completed at the set times expected during the shift, then role conflict may develop between the graduate and any other interdependent role set member or group. One way to avoid this type of role conflict is to organise a plan at the beginning of the shift concerning which aspects of the work role need to be actioned within set periods of time. Staff will be more supportive if they see that there is a determined effort to complete aspects of the role within an expected timeframe. Another example of role conflict can be caused by personal demands that have an impact on the work role.

Because of a general misunderstanding of the nursing and midwifery role, particularly in regard to relatively recent changes in nursing and midwifery education and career development, graduates often face this type of role conflict. It is in the interest of the nursing and midwifery disciplines that these situations are negotiated in a way that promotes the status of nurses and midwives and enlightens the understanding of others.

Role ambiguity

Situations arise for new graduates where expectations by role set members are not clearly expressed, leaving graduates feeling confused and uncertain of their role behaviour.[30] Expectations of the new graduate may be unstated and only found when reflected in the values and behaviour of other staff. These expectations include the impressions that role partners have developed about the position of new staff members, and these may be adapted for each new employee. Exercise 6.5 may be useful in determining the unstated role expectations that exist in your prospective workplace.

Role overload

This type of role stress occurs when graduates are unable to meet all of the expectations of their role.[30] Aspects of their work that new graduates often find difficult include time management, adapting to shift work, lack of managerial abilities, and getting through the volume of work required in times when staff shortages are a

EXERCISE 6.5 Examining the Influence of Role Partners' Expectations

1. Reflect on an incident during one of your clinical placements where you felt your practice was inconsistent with what other staff expected.
2. Describe the people who were in your role set at that time.
3. Write a short summary, or illustrate the experience with a diagram.
4. In retrospect, what do you feel the expectations of your role partners were?
5. Were these expectations stated or unstated norms of the clinical setting?
6. Explore the effect of your role partners' expectations on your nursing practice and self-concept during this incident and since.
7. What did you learn from this experience?

common occurrence in the healthcare sector. Case study 6.3 presents an example of role overload that new nurses may experience in attempting to meet time management commitments on the ward.

CASE STUDY 6.3

Joanne, a new graduate, was not enjoying her role on a busy ward. She said she found caring for her patients very satisfying but explained that sometimes she was not able to complete her work on time. She felt that this affected her relationships with the other staff, who sometimes ignored her when she asked them questions or indicated that she needed help.

REFLECTIVE QUESTIONS

1. If this situation occurred to you, how would you feel?
2. How would you respond in a similar situation?
3. How could you prevent a similar situation from occurring again?

Exercise 6.6 will encourage you to challenge your perceptions and expectations of your clinical role and can be utilised for continuing professional development.

EXERCISE 6.6 Reflection on Time Management

Reflect back on your student role activities during clinical practice.

1. How did you prioritise your work?
2. Were the strategies you used effective?
3. What might you do differently as a new graduate?

To prepare yourself for this particular role stress, it may be helpful for you to experience a facilitated clinical block that includes exposure to shift work and managerial responsibilities similar to those undertaken by new graduates.

It is important that you recognise the symptoms associated with the four types of role stress and seek support to balance their negative effects. One important piece of advice is to find out as much as possible about the institution you are joining, as this may assist in making your transition much smoother. Of particular note is whether or not the facility offers supportive initiatives such as orientation, supervision and preceptor programs.

If you recognise that you are feeling role strain it is your responsibility to develop a number of personal coping strategies. These may include: seeking assistance from other staff, graduate peers and/or family and friends; activating your existing coping mechanisms; or simply having fun and maintaining activities outside the work role.

Maintenance of Role Relationships and Self-concept

Finding support from role models or peers and learning to manage your emotions and relationships more effectively during transition can make a significant difference to your self-concept as a beginning graduate. Your self-concept is the way in which you see yourself: it is related to your emotional and social intelligence and is important because it influences your behaviour towards others. Your beginning professional self-concept, which is your sense of who you are as a professional upon graduation, has developed through your interaction with others, principally your lecturers, clinical facilitators, peer group and patients. Once these reactions are internalised they become part of your image of yourself and set up your self-expectations.[7,24,29,35] In your beginning practice, you will attempt to meet these expectations.

Self-esteem is enhanced by positive feedback from others that supports and aligns with the expectations you hold for yourself in the role of a registered nurse or midwife. If you receive negative responses about your role, your self-concept may be called into question and you may experience a degree of self-doubt. Figure 6.2 presents activities that may assist you in maintaining your self-esteem during times of self-doubt in your role.[35]

A positive self-concept can only be maintained over time if your role partners and peers acknowledge your contribution.[35] A strategy that will help you in this regard is to find a supportive role model. A role model is someone you admire and identify with, someone whose professional characteristics you value.[28,35,36] If you are able to form a

Reflect on positive aspects of your practice as a nurse
Search out other nurses who will provide support and encouragement
Involve yourself in work projects that will offer you a sense of achievement
Develop supportive personal affirmations based on your known strengths
Recognise that it is unrealistic to expect to be liked by all your colleagues or to succeed at everything you do

Figure 6.2
Advice for maintaining positive self-esteem

relationship with this person, you could approach your role model for advice and support in times of stress. Role models can also act as mentors and assist you in achieving your career goals.[32,35,36] This relationship should be positive, constructive, developmental and grounded in reality. It should enhance your self-esteem and make you feel more accepted as a new graduate. A good mentor can contribute to your role satisfaction.[35-38]

A support network made up of your peers can be another useful asset in maintaining a healthy self-concept during transition.[31] In most instances, when you commence employment you will attend an orientation program with other new graduates. This is an opportune time to discuss with these colleagues the notion of forming your own support network. By meeting on a regular basis, either face-to-face or online, this group could help you cope with your new role and the changes you will have to face in adapting your self-concept to the reality of the workplace. Mutual sharing of the highs and lows can be extremely useful in relieving role stress. In addition, forming a new-graduate group can be helpful in raising issues with management and lobbying for changes within the institution that would be of benefit to new graduates.

As you are well aware, how you feel and relate to others is closely aligned to your emotions; and as transition is often a period of heightened emotions, developing your emotional intelligence is another invaluable means of coping and of managing your relationships with members of your role set. Emotional intelligence, as defined by Goleman,[39] is characterised by five attributes: (1) self-awareness; (2) self-regulation; (3) motivation; (4) empathy; and (5) social skills. These attributes allow us to recognise the early signs of emotional stress in ourselves and to control subsequent behaviour with others, and this is particularly useful when our self-concept is under threat. Emotional intelligence helps us to understand the emotions of others and to behave towards them with this understanding in mind.[31] You can become more emotionally intelligent by critically reflecting on your behaviour and focusing on the part your emotional reactions played in motivating that behaviour.[31,40] This reflection, in light of further reading on emotional intelligence, will heighten your self-awareness.

CONCLUSION

This chapter has discussed aspects of role theory that will help you in preparing for transition. The acquisition of the graduate role is a social process that undergoes primary, secondary and tertiary phases. During the primary phase, significant people in your life were influential in shaping the values and beliefs within you that motivated you to study. You are now almost at the end of your secondary phase of socialisation where a university program has provided you with the knowledge, skills and dispositions appropriate for practice as a registered nurse or midwife. During this phase your ideals and values about the nursing role have been enhanced through academic study and clinical exposure. The primary and secondary phases of role acquisition have been synthesised to form your professional role expectations. Your expectations will now undergo another stage of development during transition.

Transition is a period of highs and lows when the realities of the clinical setting and the expectations of your role partners will exert pressure on your present image of yourself as a graduate. Transition is not an easy process, but the role stress that may occur can be moderated by thoughtful preparation, formal and informal support strategies, and developing and maintaining a positive self-concept and personal resources, including emotional intelligence. We hope that this chapter has provided you with useful strategies to improve role stress and strain and smooth your personal experience of transition.

ACKNOWLEDGMENT

The authors would like to thank and acknowledge Katherine Milton-Wildey and Suzanne Rochester for their contributions to this chapter in previous editions of the text.

RECOMMENDED READING

Fox K. Mentor program boosts new nurses' satisfaction and lowers turnover rate. *Journal of Continuing Education in Nursing* 2010;**41**:311–16.

Hart PL, Brannan JD, De Chesney M. Resilience in nurses: an integrative review. *Journal of Nursing Management* Online 2012. doi:10.1111/j.1365-2834.2012.01485.x.

Hayes B, Bonner A, Pryor J. Factors contributing to nurse job satisfaction in the acute hospital setting: a review of recent literature. *Journal of Nursing Management* 2010;**18**:804–14.

Parker V, Giles M, Lantry G, McMillan M. New graduate nurses' experience in their first year of practice. *Nurse Education Today* 2014;**34**:150–6.

Walker A, Earl C, Costa B, Cuddihy L. Graduate nurses' transition and integration in the workplace: a qualitative comparison of graduate nurses' and nurse unit managers' perspectives. *Nurse Education Today* 2013;**33**:291–6.

REFERENCES

1. Anderson P, Edberg AK. The transition from rookie to genuine nurse: narratives form Swedish nurses 1 year after graduation. *Journal of Continuing Education in Nursing* 2010;**41**(4):186–92.

2. Benner P. *From novice to expert: excellence and power in clinical nursing practice.* Menlo Park, CA: Addison-Wesley; 1984.

3. Duchscher J. A process of becoming: the stages of new graduate professional role transition. *Journal of Continuing Education in Nursing* 2008;**39**:441–50.

4. Duchscher J, Myrick F. The prevailing winds of oppression: understanding the new graduate experience in acute care. *Nursing Forum* 2008;**43**:191–206.

5. White J. The client and the healthcare environment. In: Crisp J, Taylor C, editors. *Potter and Perry's fundamentals of nursing.* 3rd ed. Sydney: Mosby/Elsevier; 2009.

6. Beecroft P, Dorey F, Wenten M. Turnover intention in new graduate nurses: a multivariate analysis. *Journal of Advanced Nursing* 2008;**62**:41–52.

7. Mooney M. Facing registration: the expectations and the unexpected. *Nurse Education Today* 2007;**27**:840–7.

8. Hodges H, Keeley A, Troyan P. Professional resilience in baccalaureate-prepared acute care nurses: first steps. *Nursing Education Perspectives* 2008;**29**:80–9.

9. Kelly J, Ahern K. Preparing nurses for practice: a phenomenological study of the new graduate in Australia. *Journal of Clinical Nursing* 2008;**18**:910–18.

10. Milton-Wildey K, O'Brien L. Care of acutely ill older patients in hospital: clinical decision-making. *Journal of Clinical Nursing* 2010;**19**:1252–60.
11. Michener H. *Social psychology*. Toronto: Wadsworth; 2004.
12. Goffman E. *Presentation of self in everyday life*. New York: Anchor Books; 1959.
13. Harre R, Secord P. *The explanation of social behaviour*. Oxford, UK: Blackwell; 1972.
14. Wilson V. Introduction to nursing, midwifery and health. In: Dempsey J, French J, Hillege S, et al., editors. *Fundamentals of nursing and midwifery: a person-centred approach to care*. Sydney: Wolters Kluwer/Lippincott, Williams & Wilkins; 2009.
15. Australian Nursing and Midwifery Council. *ANMC National competency standards for the registered nurse*. Canberra: ANMC; 2006 Online. Available: <www.nursingmidwiferyboard. gov.au/Codes-and-Guidelines.aspx>.
16. Duddle M, Boughton M. Intraprofessional relations in nursing. *Journal of Advanced Nursing* 2007;**59**:29–37.
17. Parry J. Intention to leave the profession: antecedents and role in nurse turnover. *Journal of Advanced Nursing* 2008;**64**:157–67.
18. Poole M. Socialisation and the new genetics. In: Germov J, Poole M, editors. *Public sociology: an introduction to Australian society*. Sydney: Allen & Unwin; 2007.
19. Australian Nursing and Midwifery Council. *ANMC Code of professional conduct for registered nurses*. Revised. Canberra: ANMC; 2006 Online. Available: <www. nursingmidwiferyboard.gov.au/Codes-and-Guidelines.aspx>.
20. Australian Nursing and Midwifery Council. *ANMC Code of ethics for the registered nurses*. Revised. Canberra: ANMC; 2002 Online. Available: <www.nursingmidwiferyboard.gov.au/ Codes-and-Guidelines.aspx>.
21. Nursing Council of New Zealand. *NCNZ Code of conduct for nurses*. Revised. Wellington: NCNZ; 2012 Online. Available: <www.nursingcouncil.org.nz/Nurses/Code-of-Conduct>.
22. Roy C. *Introduction to nursing: an adaptation model*. 2nd ed. Englewood Cliffs, NJ: Prentice Hall; 1984.
23. MacGuire J. The function of the 'set' in hospital controlled schemes of nurse training. In: Smith J, editor. *Sociology and nursing*. Edinburgh: Churchill Livingstone; 1968.
24. Duchscher J. Transition shock: the initial stage of role adaptation for newly graduated registered nurses. *Journal of Advanced Nursing* 2009;**65**:1103–13.
25. Lavoie-Tremblay M, O'Brien-Pallas L, Gelinas C, et al. Addressing the turnover issue among new nurses from a generational viewpoint. *Journal of Nursing Management* 2008;**16**:724–33.
26. Romyn D, Linton N, Giblin C, et al. Successful transition of the new graduate nurse. *International Journal of Nursing Education Scholarship* 2009;**6**:article 34.
27. Newton J, McKenna L. Uncovering knowing in practice during the graduate year: an exploratory study. *Contemporary Nurse* 2009;**31**:153–62.
28. Morrow S. New graduate transitions: leaving the next, joining the flight. *Journal of Nursing Management* 2009;**17**:278–87.
29. Burns P, Poster E. Competency development in new registered nurse graduates: closing the gap between education and practice. *Journal of Continuing Education in Nursing* 2008;**9**:67–73.
30. Hardy M, Conway M. *Role theory*. Norwalk, CT: Appleton & Lange; 1988.
31. Stein-Parbury J. *Patient and person: interpersonal skills in nursing*. 4th ed. Sydney: Elsevier Australia/Churchill Livingstone; 2009.
32. Benner P, Benner R. *The new nurse's work entry: a troubled sponsorship*. New York: Tiresias Press; 1979.
33. Laschinger HK, Wong C. Workplace incivility and new graduate nurses' mental health: the protective role of resiliency. *The Journal of Nursing Administration* 2013;**43**:415–21.
34. Young M, Stuenkel D, Bawel-Brinkley K. Strategies for easing the role transformation of graduate nurses. *Journal for Nurses in Staff Development* 2008;**24**:105–10.

35. Price S. Becoming a nurse: a meta-study of early professional socialization and career choice in nursing. *Journal of Advanced Nursing* 2009;**65**:11–19.

36. Niven N. *The psychology of nursing care.* 2nd ed. New York: Palgrave Macmillan; 2006.

37. Murray T, Crain C, Meyer G, et al. Building bridges: an innovative academic-service partnership. *Nursing Outlook* 2010;**58**:252–60.

38. Weng R, Huang C, Tsai W, et al. Exploring the impact of mentoring functions on job satisfaction and organizational commitment of new staff nurses. *BMC Health Services Research* 2010;**10**:1–9.

39. Goleman D. *Emotional intelligence: why it can matter more than IQ.* London: Bloomsbury; 1996.

40. Akerjordet K, Severinsson E. The state of the science of emotional intelligence related to nursing leadership: an integrative review. *Journal of Nursing Management* 2010;**18**:363–82.

CHAPTER 7

Processes of change in bureaucratic environments

Patrick Crookes, Kenneth Walsh and Steve Outram

LEARNING OBJECTIVES

When you have completed this chapter you will be able to:

- outline a realistic yet constructive explanation of the culture of innovation in contemporary nursing
- understand the imperative of developing effective nursing leaders in the years to come
- reflect upon practical and theoretical knowledge regarding ways in which one can function and actively participate in decision making in rapidly changing environments
- identify ways of dealing with the stresses involved in working in rapidly changing environments
- devote time to thinking now about being a leader of the future.

KEYWORDS: transformational leadership, transactional leadership, oppressed group behaviour, self-empowerment, change management

INTRODUCTION

This chapter discusses the forces that operate within bureaucratic health service environments and the impact upon individuals and groups within them. It also discusses some of the recent positive movements towards assisting innovation and change in these environments.

Change can be likened to a fast-flowing river: it continues remorselessly and it is very easy to get caught up in its currents. Once you are within a context where change is happening all around you, it becomes very difficult to do anything other than work extremely hard to keep your head above water. This is the situation for many nurses when they take up their first position in health services. However, as we shall see, it is not a situation that is peculiar either to nursing or to relatively inexperienced people.

WHAT IS AN ORGANISATIONAL BUREAUCRACY?

This section will discuss briefly the nature of the environment in which most nurses work, before going on to discuss the spirit of innovation that may or may not exist within it. Whatever setting, large or small, urban or bush, nurses work in an organisation. Major theorists and writers on organisations[1,2] agree that, despite differences in perspective, organisations exist in order to fulfil goals and they do so by carrying out defined, consciously coordinated activities. In other words, they exist for specific purposes, such as the provision of healthcare, and are structured to fulfil that purpose.

In an effort to ensure this happens, people working in healthcare organisations are typically managed in relatively systematic ways and their efforts coordinated by fairly formal leadership structures.[3] A major influence on our understanding of the shape and functions of organisations in the 20th century was Max Weber, via his notion of the 'bureaucratic organisation'.[2] In bureaucratic organisations, goals are achieved by grouping together employees who carry out similar work, overseen by individuals who have been placed in positions of authority. Submission to this rule of authority is due to a set of related beliefs. Weber believed that a position of authority should be achieved as a result of individuals acquiring, and being viewed as possessing, specialist technical knowledge. In such a system, obedience is due not to the person who holds the authority but to the impersonal order that has granted the person this position.

BUREAUCRACIES IN HEALTHCARE

Given this description, it can be seen that traditional hospitals consisting of groups of wards and clinical departments, designed for a specific function such as surgical and medical nursing or radiography services, are clear examples of bureaucratic structures. The same can also be said for health services provided in community and other non-institutional settings, in that they are all managed by professionals who possess the relevant qualifications and experience. These managers are attributed with defined levels of authority to enforce the rules and policies of the organisation. In turn, they are themselves expected to abide by the same rules and policies. In terms of change and its management, the main implications of this are that, in such organisations, the impetus for change and its direction are invariably mandated from above; and, due to the fact that the division of labour is based on roles or structures, insufficient action is taken to ensure ownership by the workforce. According to Charles Handy,[4] the chosen route to efficiency via concentration and specialisation in a bureaucratic culture has reached a dead end because it restricts flexibility and runs counter to the cultural preferences of most of the people it needs in order to work. It is interesting, therefore, to note that health services are still managed predominantly through bureaucratic management structures. The management of change is thus affected because, in addition to the above, the multidisciplinarity, mutual respect, trust and sense of self-worth required to allow agreement and cooperation across the whole organisation rarely exist.

Another implication is that newly graduating nurses, as fairly lowly placed members of the organisation, may find themselves feeling relatively powerless and inconsequential. This is reinforced by the processes of line management with its typically 'top-down' approach to running its business (including the management of change) and an emphasis on adherence to policy. In such circumstances in some organisations, there may be little opportunity for staff to participate in change in anything other than a passive role. There is a tendency from the outset, therefore, for newer members of the nursing team to operate with a passivity which over time translates into a state of learned helplessness.[5] This is defined as the 'behavioral state of a person who believes control over the environment has been lost and his or her efforts are ineffectual or futile'.[6] It has been said that professionals such as nurses tend to be socialised into such a mindset.[7–9] Such writers argue that, quite quickly after entering the workforce (within a few months), many nurses can be seen to have adopted a bureaucratic orientation to their work whereby decisions are made very much with the rules and regulations of the employing institution in mind. They do so as a means of minimising the risk of contravening policy or custom and practice. This is opposed to legitimising actions and decisions from a service perspective (where the emphasis is on the dignity and humanity of the patient) or a professional perspective (where the emphasis is on occupational standards, transcending institutional policies and practices). Furthermore, it is these authors' view that nurses adopt this orientation because this appears to help them to avoid conflict with supervisors and peers and so 'fit in'[10] as quickly as possible.

'OPPRESSED GROUP BEHAVIOUR' IN NURSING: ITS IMPLICATIONS FOR INNOVATION

The situation described above can be reinforced even further in nursing by the presence of what has become known as 'oppressed group behaviour'. According to Roberts,[11,12] this model of behaviour reflects literature on colonised Africans, Latin Americans, African Americans, Jews and, more recently, women.[13] These groups are said to have been oppressed by virtue of being controlled and exploited by dominant forces external to themselves.

In his seminal text *The Pedagogy of the Oppressed* (1971), Paolo Freire[14] explains how, over time, the norms and values of the dominant group come to be accepted as the 'right' ones by all concerned. In turn, the leaders of the oppressed group, as they emerge, tend to identify with the characteristics of the dominant group (e.g. white people, landowners, those guarding them, men) as a means of 'fitting in' and being accepted. This typically includes their coming to view those they have 'left behind' with a degree of cynicism and even disdain. Meanwhile, those who have been left behind are said to behave in a submissive–aggressive manner[15] whereby malice, or even aggression, felt towards the oppressor(s) is not expressed towards them but rather at easier targets – others within their group, usually those even lower down the pecking order. Fanon calls this 'horizontal violence'.[16]

Over 30 years on from Roberts' article,[13] horizontal violence as a symptom of oppressed group behaviour is still seen as a major issue in contemporary nursing.[13,17,18] However, the term most widely used today is 'bullying'. Bullying may take the form of personal attacks, erosion of professional competence and reputation, and attack through work roles and tasks;[19] it does not include being asked to undertake legitimate tasks or to take instruction from a legitimate authority. In contemporary nursing there is recognition that such bullying exists, and most organisations have measures in place to deal with it.

The result of all the above is that the leaders emerging from oppressed groups may not value the views of their subordinates, while those same subordinates tend not to make their views known because they see no point in doing so. A catch-22 scenario thus often exists.

While this may seem to be a bleak picture, there are examples of health services trying to utilise the expertise of all their staff to ensure provision of the best possible care via initiatives such as Essentials of Care (EOC)[20] in New South Wales, changes to clinical governance and Magnet Hospitals.[21] However, many newly graduating nurses find themselves working in a bureaucracy where work tends to be guided by adherence to policy and procedure. Changes to those policies will almost inevitably occur as a result of top-down initiatives and will do so via the processes of line management. As such, the socialising tendency will be to adopt a bureaucratic, as opposed to a social or professional, orientation to their work. They will do this along with peers and supervisors who will exhibit, to some degree, oppressed group behaviour, which has been indicated to lead to a tendency to stifle change and innovation from the bottom up.

Some Solutions?

So, given that most nurses work within a bureaucratic structure, how can they position themselves so as to be able to deal constructively with change, participate in it and perhaps even initiate it?

Part of the answer to this question requires change to the nursing profession as a whole. Susan Jo Roberts published her seminal work on the theory of oppressed group behaviour and its application(s) to nursing back in 1983.[11] She and her colleagues[12] updated this work in 2009 through a review of the literature. This work provides a history of the concept, and goes further to provide useful and practical suggestions on how to avoid or diminish the oppressed group behaviour. In essence, this amounts to the need for:

- an acceptance among nurses that oppression and its related behaviour exist within its ranks
- a recognition that such behaviours are not due to the fact that nurses are inherently inferior, but rather that they have come to feel so within a wider culture that does not value them properly
- the development of nursing leaders who do not subscribe to the view that the rank and file are to be viewed with disdain
- the rediscovery, under the guidance of such leadership, of the cultural heritage of nursing.

Together, Roberts believes, such initiatives will lead to a situation where the more powerful players in health service politics (doctors, managers) will come to view nurses and nursing more positively, basically because nurses themselves have a positive view of themselves. Roberts quotes Torres:[22] 'the freedom to develop nursing's own destiny can only come from nursing's own initiative; it will not be freely granted by other groups.'

Nurses, like individuals in all oppressed groups, need to engage in self-empowerment. If this could then be amalgamated with a sense of pride and confidence that what they do is effective and of benefit to society (supported obviously by evidence of their efficacy), the influence that nurses exercise on healthcare and the policy that underpins it will surely come to reflect the proportion of the health services workforce which nurses constitute.

An Alternative to Learned Helplessness

Martin Seligman,[23] who originally studied the detrimental effects of learned helplessness, has in more recent times studied learned optimism. If we can learn to be helpless, we can also learn to be optimistic, he argues. By understanding our individual strengths we can learn to be positive, have realistic goals, make plans to achieve them, and be ready to share them when the opportunity arises. By understanding our strengths and how we make good things happen in our lives, we can use this information to find solutions and buffer us when things do not go as well as we planned.

Another important mechanism for staying positive is to be realistic – a key concept related to reactance theory.[24] Those who succeed at it gain a sense of wellbeing from the perception that they can make a difference, not that they necessarily have already – at least not yet. Thinking through what we would like to change and being realistic about whether it is possible to do so, given our sphere of influence, is a basic tenet of being a change agent.

As well as being realistic, it is helpful to have a support network. Unfortunately, those who have researched this field[25,26] have found that professionals such as nurses are actually quite bad at asking for and/or accepting help and support from others. Instead, they have a tendency to see themselves as strong, and as being seen to be so by others. It is therefore important to develop supports. Some forms of support may be informal, such as debriefing with colleagues, whereas others can be of a more formal nature, such as critical companions[27] or clinical supervision.[28] Many health services now recognise the importance of providing staff with opportunities to reflect upon their practice and provide systems of peer support and, sometimes, counselling services.

Solution-focused Approaches

Another recent positive innovation for solving problems in nursing has been the advent of a solution-focused approach (as opposed to a problem-focused approach) to nursing.[29] This approach also comes out of the positive psychology movement, especially solution-focused counselling. It can be applied to nursing as both an approach to working with clients and an approach to working with each other to find innovative solutions to workplace issues.[29]

The problem focus is so familiar as to be almost invisible. The problem focus on deficits and what is wrong has entered our language. Problems have blame and ownership and negative connotations: 'that's going to be a problem'; 'that's not my problem, that's your problem'; 'who caused the problem in the first place?' Problem-saturated thinking can psychologically disengage the thinker from the issue by mobilising anxiety and putting the thinker into a psychological 'away state'[30] which can rob them of psychological resources required to solve the problem. 'Problems' can trigger stress and confusion, and thinking can be clouded as a result.[31]

In contrast, the solution approach is focused on the positive future goal the change is aimed at achieving. The solution-focused approach looks for what works and what is going well. It endeavours to build on the strengths of individuals and teams, and it uses creativity and imagination to focus on a positive possible future and how to get there.[32] The solution-focused approach assumes that nothing happens by chance. When something bad happens, something made it happen. However, the same is true when things go well; something makes the good things happen. What we need to do is to explore what makes the good things happen and do more of this, and find out what makes the bad things happen and stop doing that. In this way we take a more positive view of ourselves and others, and we build on the strengths that we already possess.[33]

This approach enables the person to think about how they want things to be and the actions to take. It is based, first and foremost, on shared values and shared goals and how to achieve these together. By focusing on these positive shared elements, the evidence for change is seen as less threatening. Solutions to problems are not imposed. Rather, solutions are seen as coming from the engagement with the key stakeholders and are developed together.[31] Solutions developed in this way are more likely to be supported and sustained.

LEADERSHIP AND NURSING'S FUTURE

In all likelihood, the future contribution of the nursing profession will be measured in terms of its ability to influence the delivery of evidence-based, cost-effective care in multidisciplinary, multiagency environments. Success in this will depend on the nursing profession's ability to produce transformational leaders capable of effecting the necessary change.

Transformational leadership means changing the realities of our environment to conform more closely to our values and beliefs. Covey[33] identifies the goal of transformational leadership as being to 'transform' people and organisations in a literal sense – to change them in mind and heart; to enlarge vision, insight and understanding; to clarify purposes; to make behaviour congruent with beliefs, principles and values; and to bring about changes that are permanent, self-perpetuating and momentum building. Kouzes and Posner[34] have written extensively about transformational leadership. Backed by an impressive empirical base, they assert that there are five practices of exemplary leadership – namely: (1) modelling the way; (2) inspiring a shared vision; (3) challenging the process; (4) enabling others to act; and (5) encouraging the heart.

In his book *Creating Culture Change: The Key to Successful Total Quality Management*, Phillip Atkinson differentiates between 'transformational' and 'transactional' leaders.[35] He identifies transformational leaders as being independent, visionary and inspirational, driven by long-term goals, visions and objectives. They are also said to possess a clear vision of what they wish to achieve, expect high standards from others and are little concerned with detail. They are the change makers who provide a mission for others to follow. On the other hand, transactional leaders are good at achieving short-term results, typically by promoting teamwork and working in a practical manner on focused issues. Transformational leaders will often provide the frame of reference and strategic boundaries within which transactions can be conducted. Transformational leaders create new initiatives and stimulate action and loyalty, whereas transactional managers are better at administering systems and making things happen on a daily basis, and have an important role in sustaining change once it has been introduced. Both types of leadership are therefore important, especially in practical fields such as nursing and, while they develop different approaches, successful exponents of both types give direction and motivation, and reward and recognise success. They both also develop and meet the needs of staff. The personal styles that managers adopt are therefore important – research has shown that the leadership style and the use of emotional intelligence have a measurable impact on work atmosphere and the enhancement of team performance.[36]

Davidson and Peck suggest[37] that the key characteristic of good leaders is the ability to tune their responses to the context in which they are working. They assert that what we ideally need are leaders who possess both skill sets, and that one solution may be the acquisition of a repertoire of leadership skills. They propose that leaders should aim to develop skills from a broad range of dimensions, which are summarised as:

- *intellectual* – the theories and concepts available to individuals to inform their personal and intellectual responses
- *psychological* – the understandings and insights that individuals have of their behaviours and relationships with others
- *performative* – the range of behaviours individuals can enact in the leadership role.

Davidson and Peck also suggest mechanisms through which this repertoire can be exercised. In summary, these are the abilities to identify and exercise aspects of self and leadership behaviours which have been learned through experience, while being sensitive to the needs and responses of self and others. The underlying assumption of this model is that the effectiveness of individuals as leaders is determined by the range of dimensions available to them and the ability to exercise the appropriate related mechanisms.

To date, nursing has produced many highly skilled transactional managers, but leaders in possession of transformational skills are still less common in the profession. A strategy that may help in this regard would be for individuals to consider ways in which they might develop transformational leadership skills. Kouzes and Posner[34] have a number of resources in relation to their 'exemplary leadership behaviors' which can be found at www.leadershipchallenge.com.[38]

Evaluation and research to date indicate that transformational leaders in healthcare enhance practice and the patient experience. They may also be pivotal to the implementation of evidence-based practice. Kitson and colleagues[39] highlight that not only is it important for there to be strong evidence to support the change being advocated (along with an environment supportive of that change), but also facilitation of the change by leaders is vital. It seems that high-quality facilitation skills may well be vital to high-quality leadership.

LEADERSHIP AND CHANGE MANAGEMENT

We noted at the outset of this chapter that change is faster and more complex than ever before. It is an inevitable phenomenon, and whether or not we want to accept change we must learn to manage – or at least cope with – it.[40] The need for change emerges when, as a result of pressure from either intrinsic or extrinsic sources, the balance of a system is disturbed.[41] Although change can create anxiety, successful change thrives alongside risk and uncertainty and this can lead to real opportunities for creating a better way forward – innovation.[42]

It is therefore important to understand change processes, and to have insight into why things happen in order to offset feelings of uncertainty and anxiety. Crookes and Froggatt[43] provide useful insights into making a difference in practice. An experienced change manager will encourage participation to engender ownership of change among staff, but having insight into the change process could allow others also to identify how they can play a more active part in the change process. It is interesting to consider how people affected by change react. Rogers and Shoemaker[44] categorise these responses along a continuum: innovators, early adopters, early majority, late majority and laggards. However, many attempts at organisational change are unsuccessful. Moore[45] adapted the continuum developed by Rogers and Shoemaker and suggested that there is a gap between the innovators and early adopters on the one hand and everyone else on the other. This has come to be known as Moore's chasm, and the goal of the change manager is to bridge this chasm. Geoghegan[46] has suggested that this chasm can be explained by exploring the different values that people on each side of the chasm hold. Innovators and early adopters typically favour revolutionary change; they are visionary, project-oriented risk takers; are willing to experiment; and are generally self-sufficient. Conversely, everyone else in an organisation is likely to favour evolutionary change; be pragmatic, process-oriented and risk averse; want proven applications; and may need significant support if they are to change. It is worth noting that Geoghegan's work was based on the difficulty organisations have in introducing new IT systems and it is worth asking the question, 'Does this model, based on different values, work in hospital and other health-related settings?' It is also interesting to identify which side of the chasm you would prefer to be on.

In exploring the different ways in which organisational change has been explained, it is self-evident that this entails an examination of how an organisation moves from one state to another and what it does to get there. One of the earliest approaches, and one that is still popular, is Kurt Lewin's[41] Unfreeze, Move, Refreeze model. This approach focuses on a staged approach to change. The first stage, unfreezing, requires that people in the organisation accept that there is a need for change. This will often entail an inquiry into the 'ways things are done around here' and a challenge to the beliefs, values, attitudes and behaviours that are characteristic of the status quo. This is the most difficult stage and can provoke strong reactions and resistance. It is necessary to create a sense of criticality. To do this, it is helpful to have all the necessary factual information on hand to support the need for change, as well as to prepare a compelling message showing why the status quo needs to be challenged.

A useful tool for exploring 'the way things are done around here' is the 'cultural web' (see Figure 7.1 on p 103).[47] The web is made up of six elements: stories, symbols, power structures, organisational structures, control systems, and rituals and routines. At the centre of this web is the 'paradigm', which refers to the aggregation of all of the narratives that emerge when one analyses each of the elements and their underlying assumptions – the 'big picture'. For example, in any given organisation, what is the acceptable daily behaviour that is valued by management? What stories do people currently tell about the organisation? What do people expect when they walk into the organisation? What are the symbols to be found in the organisation, such as the way people dress? By addressing each of the six elements a picture is created of what it is really like in the organisation. The process is then repeated, but this time thought should be given to how one might like the organisation's culture to look if everything were correctly aligned – the ideal 'big picture'. It is now possible to map the difference between the two. Where are the existing strengths? Where are the weak points, and what needs to be done to change them? What new beliefs and behaviours need to be promoted? What new stories would people ideally like to be telling about the organisation? In this way, it is possible to identify the priorities for achieving strategic change in the organisation – the 'move' element of Lewin's model. Refreezing occurs when people can be seen to have embraced the changes and they have been incorporated into everyday life, such as in job descriptions. Key leadership roles can therefore be seen to support the changes and to ensure that a reward system is in place to support them.

Interestingly, Edgar Schein[48] adopted the unfreezing, move, refreezing model to apply to individual change – what he termed 'cognitive redefinition'. In his view, the motivation to change (unfreezing) has three sub-processes: disconfirmation, survival anxiety and learning anxiety. Disconfirmation occurs when present conditions lead to some form of dissatisfaction, such as when old ways are no longer always successful and start to be seen as invalid. The resulting 'survival anxiety' can stimulate change. However, this stimulus might not be sufficient to bring about change if the individual has created a stronger sense of 'learning anxiety'. Learning anxiety can include a fear of failure and loss of 'face', and may lead to defensiveness and resistance. Once there is sufficient dissatisfaction, successful change (the move stage) can occur provided the individual can identify exactly what needs to change and provide a clear and concise view of what the altered state looks like. This change can be seen to be permanent (refreezing) when the new behaviour becomes habitual. This may be facilitated by imitating role models, as well as by experimenting through trial-and-error for personalised solutions, leading to the creation of a new identity.

In their exploration of the transition from student to professional, Reid and colleagues[49] also stress the significance of identity formation. In their discussion of the Australian Professional Entity Project and the European Journeymen Project they argue that the most successful transitions from 'expert student' to 'novice professional' occur when the student has developed an *intrinsic meaning* in relation to their discipline. That is, unlike the narrower, almost mechanistic engagement with the discipline – an *extrinsic meaning* – the successful student develops a new mindset that centres on a wider understanding of their discipline. By way of explanation, the musician not only knows the right notes to play, but also knows the musical traditions, the possible interpretations, the nuances and subtleties of different techniques, and has a sense of belonging to a musical community of practice. They see themselves as a musician and they 'talk like a musician'. Like the 'move' stage in the work of Lewin and Schein, Reid and colleagues stress the 'trajectory' that a student will follow to accomplish successfully the transition from student to professional.

Another approach to change that continues to find support from change managers is John Kotter's[50] Eight-Step Model. The model comprises the following steps:

1. Create a sense of urgency around the need to change.
2. Form a powerful coalition. This is likely to include a strong leader and other influential people.

3. Create a vision for change. This will give clarity and enables people to make sense of the need for change.
4. Communicate the vision. This is fundamental. Kotter advised that one should identify at least seven different ways of communicating and use each method at least seven times.
5. Remove obstacles. This includes overcoming the resistance of colleagues who object to change, as well as removing systems or processes that get in the way.
6. Create short-term wins. In this way the benefits of the change can be seen, particularly if the early 'quick wins' are inexpensive to achieve.
7. Build on the change. Kotter points out that early successes do not mean the change has become embedded and sustainable. This might entail changing your change team as a way to bring in new ideas, as well as setting goals to build on the early momentum.
8. Anchor the changes in corporate culture. This entails working to ensure that the changes are found at the core of the organisation's work, that leaders continue to endorse the changes, and that any recognition and reward policies support the changes.

The importance of Kotter's work, and possibly why it still receives a lot of support, is that it is not so much a model that explains organisational change as a *checklist* for implementing organisational change. Some critics have argued that his ideas about getting change started are stronger than his ideas about embedding change and making it sustainable. Nonetheless, it is a useful model to consider.

Table 7.1 compares these different change theories in a way that allows us to see the similarities between them; no theory alone is *the* accepted model.

Implications of Change

A common implication of change, whether successful or failed, is the psychological effect on individuals and, indeed, organisations. As an individual and as a member of an organisation, the newly graduating nurse needs to be prepared for these psychological effects because, as has been asserted throughout this chapter, change in healthcare is constant and is often imposed on nursing staff with little or no consultation.

While the above theories of change are overarching in scope, they do little to explain the emotions related to change other than the motivation to adopt or reject it. When situations change and previous understanding does not enable decisions to be made, we are likely to experience a sense of loss.[51] Marris[52] contends that the fundamental crisis of bereavement is due not to the loss of others but to the loss of some aspect of self. Mead and Bryar[53] concur that the grieving process could apply in many contexts that would not normally be thought of as bereavement, and they contend that when we lose objects, or even an activity, we lose a part of ourselves. The same could be said of a job, or a work role within it.

Esty[51] identifies four kinds of loss experienced by employees in the wake of organisational change: (1) loss of the familiar; (2) loss of security; (3) loss of control; and (4) loss of optimism. All of these things, Esty[51] maintains, contribute to our occupational identity, which in turn is a major contributor to our perception of self.

TABLE 7.1

Comparison of change models

Lewin's model: unfreeze	Move	Refreeze
Prepare the organisation and break down the existing status quo. Develop a rationale and compelling message for why things cannot stay the same. Challenge the beliefs, values, attitudes and behaviours.	Resolve uncertainty and find new ways of doing things. People start to behave and act in ways to support the new direction. (Not everyone will act in this way and those people need to be addressed.)	The outward signs of the refreeze are a stable organisation chart, consistent job descriptions, and a demonstrable sense of confidence. New ways of behaving are embedded into everyday policies and practices.
Schein's model: unfreeze	**Move**	**Refreeze**
Dissatisfaction with present conditions such as not meeting personal goals. Previous beliefs now being seen as invalid creates 'survival anxiety'. However, this may not be sufficient to prompt change if learning anxiety is present.	With a real desire to change, it is necessary to identify exactly what needs to change. A concise view of the new state is required to clearly identify the gap between the present state and that being proposed.	Refreezing is the final stage where new behaviour becomes habitual. A new self-identity is established and new interpersonal relationships may be created.
Kotter's eight steps		
1. Create urgency. 2. Form a guiding coalition. 3. Develop a vision for change. 4. Communicate the vision.	5. Empower broad-based action. 6. Generate short-term wins.	7. Consolidate gains and produce more change. 8. Anchor new approaches in the culture.

Source: *Adapted from N Stragalas, Improving change implementation: practical adaptations of Kotter's model.* OD Practitioner *2010;42(1):31–8.*

William Bridges can be seen to be supportive of this view, observing that it is not change per se that people find difficult, but rather the process of adapting: 'It isn't the changes that do you in, it's the transitions. Change is situational; new policy, new boss, new site. Transition is the psychological process people go through to come to terms with the new situation. Change is external; transition is internal.'[54]

Perlman and Takacs[55] expanded on the acclaimed work *On Death and Dying* by Elisabeth Kubler-Ross[56] to describe employees' grief responses to change. The ten steps they described (equilibrium, denial, anger, bargaining, chaos, depression, resignation, openness, readiness and re-emergence) detail the emotional responses of individuals confronted with change. Schoolfield and Orduna[57] identified that the process of unfreezing requires changing the values, attitudes and customs of individuals. During this stage, one might expect to encounter some or all of the Perlman and Takacs phases.[55]

Changes for the Profession as a Whole

While this chapter has discussed change at an individual level, some systematic processes that are being used in nursing bring about change that provides not only for more efficient organisations, but also for better patient outcomes and greater staff satisfaction with their working environment. Probably the most comprehensive approach to this sort of change, which incorporates most of what we have stated thus far about change in bureaucratic environments, is practice development.

Practice development, according to McCormack and colleagues,[58] is:

> ... a continuing process of improvement towards increased effectiveness in person-centred care, through the enabling of nurses and healthcare teams to transform the culture and context of care. It is enabled and supported by facilitators committed to a systematic, rigorous and continuous process of emancipatory change (p 256).

We believe that the single most important element in the definition is also the underlying philosophy: person-centredness. Person-centredness is acknowledging the personhood, or shared humanity, of all people. This is the starting point and shared value of practice development and its guiding principle.

In relation to person-centredness, values are worked out explicitly with all the people involved in practice development. Practice development provides many ways of doing this, but when it is done well it breaks down the barriers between 'them' and 'us' and helps people to see each other as being more similar than different.

It also gives the work a compass bearing, so that each solution and action can be evaluated in the light of shared values that are lived – that is, there are good values–practice interaction and good values congruence.

Practice development is also about evolving cultures of innovation through facilitation in order to bring about emancipatory change – change that frees people to work in ways that support dignity for themselves and others. It is practical in that it works with the people and the context at all levels of healthcare. It is very much about personal leadership, but not just at the level of people with recognised leadership roles: everyone is seen as a leader of something and someone, and everyone can work in ways that facilitate person-centred change, even if they do not have the formal role of facilitator. Most importantly, practice development incorporates the views and knowledge of service users and involves them in the process.

In these ways, practice development builds on the strengths already existing in organisations and further builds the social and intellectual capital so that worker agency, rather than worker resistance, is developed. The collective (including clients) is seen as a rich resource of innovative ideas and, through various processes, solutions to problems are generated by the collective wisdom of the group.

There are many ways of doing this and the strength of practice development is that, in solution generation, as in all other activities, no one process is prescribed. The key is that whatever process we use, person-centred emancipatory change is the goal. It is our underlying shared humanity that counts.

Practice development as a program of practice change is being undertaken more and more in health services in Australia, New Zealand, the United Kingdom and continental Europe. It is beyond the scope of this chapter to detail practice development principles and processes. Manley and colleagues[59] provide a comprehensive overview of the approach.

CONCLUSION

Change is something that has been with us forever. In fact, that is perhaps the only thing that will never change. In this chapter we have attempted to explain and illustrate why bureaucracies operate the way they do, and we present ideas on how nurses may make a difference in these environments. Working through the exercises and undertaking the recommended reading will help to reinforce what we hope is, after the negativity of the earlier part of the chapter, a constructive and optimistic message for the future.

~~~~~~

CASE STUDY 7.1

Charles has begun working on a new ward. The staff say they are involved in practice development and are working to develop a person-centred culture.

REFLECTIVE QUESTIONS

1. What do you understand by the term 'practice development'?
2. What would a person-centred culture mean for both staff and patients?
3. What are the benefits of a person-centred approach to care for the patients and staff?

~~~~~~

CASE STUDY 7.2

Elise works in a unit where the staff seem to be innovative and creative and work together to find solutions to shared problems. They say that part of the reason they work so well together is because of the support they receive from their manager. They describe her as being a transformational leader.

REFLECTIVE QUESTIONS

1. What is transformational leadership? How does it differ from transactional leadership?
2. What does the literature say about the strengths of a transformational leadership style?
3. What does the literature say about the strengths of a transactional leadership style?

~~~~~~

CASE STUDY 7.3

Declan works in a busy surgical ward. He has been asked to join a group of staff who are working together to improve staff access to learning opportunities and staff development. He has been told the group uses a solution-focused approach.

REFLECTIVE QUESTIONS

1. How does a solution-focused approach differ from a problem-based approach to change?
2. As a group using a solution-focused approach, what would you explore together in order to find a solution to the problem?
3. What other learning opportunities can you provide for staff in your environment?

EXERCISE 7.1

1. Review the characteristics of transactional and transformational leaders (see Case Study 7.2). Next, compare these characteristics with four people you know: one in a senior management position, one in middle management, one an experienced registered nurse and, finally, yourself.
   > Do any of these people demonstrate the characteristics of either of these types of leader?
   > Which type do you most easily fit into, and which would you most like to be?
2. As a registered nurse, do you believe that you have a choice about whether or not you occupy a leadership position?
3. Think now about how you might best go about becoming the leader you would like to be and make a plan to help you get there. Ask colleagues and managers to help you do this.

EXERCISE 7.2

1. Reflect on a change you have been involved in, or affected by, and then try to answer the following questions:
   > Was the change planned or unplanned? Was an established model of change used?
   > Can you identify the actions taken to unfreeze, move and refreeze the behaviour of individuals involved?
   > Was the change process, in this instance, successful or not? How could it have been more successful?
   > Did oppressed group behaviour play any role in events?
2. Consider the points put forward about oppressed group behaviour, preferably in light of the recommended reading. What do you think you might do to ensure that you do not suffer from horizontal violence, as well as avoiding treating others in this way?

EXERCISE 7.3

1. Using the 'cultural web' tool shown in Figure 7.1, write down what you would say for each element of your university and create an overall picture of your life as a student.
2. Now repeat the exercise, but this time do it for a hospital or medical setting with which you are familiar.
3. Compare the two narratives. What is the difference between the two? What aspects of university life are missing in the hospital setting, and what new aspects are there that you might look forward to, or be apprehensive about, in the hospital or medical setting?

THE CULTURAL WEB

The 'cultural web' is a tool for mapping the often tacit aspects of organisational culture to identify potential barriers to change and provide a stimulus for action planning. It can be used to examine both existing and desired cultures at the level of the whole institution, or with subsets of the institution such as departments.

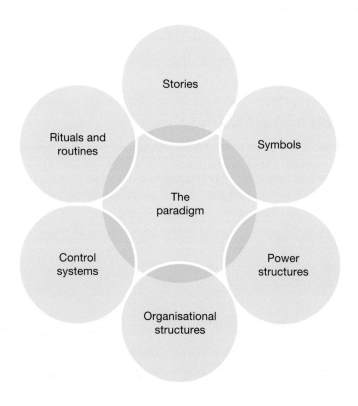

Figure 7.1

The cultural web

Source: *G Johnson, R Whittington, K Scholes*, Fundamentals of strategy. *Pearson Education; 2012.*

Elements of the cultural web

1. **Stories**: the 'mythology' of the organisation – stories of events and people frequently told by members of the organisation to each other, outsiders and new recruits.
2. **Symbols**: the physical, visual and verbal representations of the organisation, including logos, offices, buildings, titles, and commonly used language and terminology.
3. **Power structures**: not just senior management, but also the individuals and groups found throughout the organisation who exercise significant influence on decision making, operations, strategic direction and, most importantly, organisational values and beliefs.
4. **Organisational structures**: the formal power structure (as defined by organisation charts) as well as informal alliances and groupings.
5. **Control systems**: financial systems, quality systems, and reward, promotion and performance management mechanisms.
6. **Routines and rituals**: the daily behaviour and actions that determine what is expected to happen in given situations and what is valued by management.
7. **The paradigm**: created by the preceding six elements, the paradigm is the set of assumptions that is held in common and taken for granted in the organisation. Transformational change often requires a change in the paradigm.

Source: *Adapted from G Johnson, K Scholes*, The cultural web. *www.odhq.net/cultural-web.*

RECOMMENDED READING

Covey SR. *The 7 habits of highly effective people.* 2nd ed. London: Simon & Schuster; 2004.

Crookes PA, Davies S, editors. *Research into practice: essential skills for reading and applying research in nursing and health care.* 2nd ed. London: Harcourt Brace; 2004.

Kouzes J, Posner B. *The leadership challenge: how to get extraordinary things done in organizations.* 5th ed. San Francisco: Jossey-Bass; 2012.

Manley K, McCormack B, Wilson V, editors. *International practice development in nursing and healthcare.* Oxford, UK: Blackwell; 2008.

Walsh K, Crisp J, Moss C. Psychodynamic perspectives on organisational change and their relevance to transformational practice development. *International Journal of Nursing Practice* 2011;**17**(2):205–12.

REFERENCES

1. Handy C. *Understanding organisations.* 4th ed. London: Penguin; 1993.
2. Pugh DS, Hickson DJ. *Writers on organizations.* 5th ed. Thousand Oaks, CA: Sage; 1997.
3. Lippitt R, Watson J, Wesley B. *The dynamics of planned changes.* New York: Harcourt; 1958.
4. Handy C. *Gods of management.* 3rd ed. London: Century Business; 1991.
5. Seligman M. *Authentic happiness: using the new positive psychology to realize your potential for lasting fulfillment.* New York: Free Press; 2002.

6. Anderson KN. *Mosby's medical, nursing and allied health dictionary.* 5th ed. St Louis, MO: Mosby Year Book; 1998.

7. Darbyshire P. Thinly disguised contempt. *Nursing Times* 1988;**84**:42–4.

8. Green GJ. Relationships between role models and role perceptions of new graduate nurses. *Nursing Research* 1988;**37**:245–8.

9. Corwin RG, Taves MJ. Some concomitants of bureaucratic and professional conceptions of the nurse role. *Nursing Research* 1962;**11**:223–7.

10. Melia K. *Learning and working: the occupational socialisation of nurses.* London: Tavistock Publications; 1987.

11. Roberts SJ. Oppressed group behaviour: implications for nursing. *Advances in Nursing Science* 1983;**5**:21–30.

12. Roberts S, Demarco R, Griffen M. The effect of oppressed group behaviours on the culture of the nursing workplace: a review of the evidence and interventions for change. *Journal of Nursing Management* 2009;**17**:288–93.

13. Cleland V. Sex discrimination: nursing's most pervasive problem. *The American Journal of Nursing* 1971;**71**:1542–7.

14. Freire P. *The pedagogy of the oppressed.* New York: Herder & Herder; 1971.

15. Carmichael S, Hamilton C. *Black power.* New York: Random House; 1967.

16. Fanon F. *The wretched of the earth.* New York: Grove Press; 1963.

17. Farrell GA. Aggression in clinical settings: nurses' views. *Journal of Advanced Nursing* 1997;**25**:501–8.

18. Duffy E. Horizontal violence: a conundrum for nursing. *Collegian (Royal College of Nursing, Australia)* 1995;**2**:5–17.

19. Hutchinson M, Vickers M, Wilkes L, et al. A topology of bullying behaviours. The experiences of Australian nurses. *Journal of Clinical Nursing* 2010;**19**:2319–28.

20. NSW Health. *Essentials of Care Project.* Online. Available: www.health.nsw.gov.au/nursing/projects/Pages/eoc.aspx [Viewed 13 December 2014]. (*Note:* This project is based on the UK-based project: Ho D, Craig E. Essence of care: a key approach in improving patient care. *British Journal of Nursing* 2009;18(12):740–4.)

21. Joyce JT, Crookes PA. Developing a tool to measure 'magnetism' in Australian nursing environments. *Australian Journal of Advanced Nursing* 2007;**25**:17–23.

22. Torres G. The nursing education administrator: accountable, vulnerable and oppressed. *Advances in Nursing Science* 1981;**3**:1–16.

23. Seligman MEP. *Learned optimism.* New York: Pocket Books; 1998.

24. Brehm JW. *A theory of psychological reactance.* New York: Academic Press; 1966.

25. Crookes PA. Personal bereavement in registered general nurses. PhD thesis. University of Hull, UK, 1996.

26. Crawley P. Once a nurse always a nurse – unless you are a patient! *International Journal for the Advancement of Counseling* 1984;**7**:261–5.

27. Titchen A. Critical companionship: part 1. *Nursing Standard* 2003;**18**:33–40.

28. Walsh K, Nicholson J, Keough C, et al. The development of a group model of clinical supervision to meet the needs of a community mental health nursing team. *International Journal of Nursing Practice* 2003;**9**:33–9.

29. Walsh K, Moss C, FitzGerald M. Solution focused approaches and their relevance to practice development. *Practice Development in Health Care* 2006;**5**:145–55.

30. Rock D. SCARF: a brain-based model for collaborating with and influencing others. *Neuro Leadership Journal* 2008;**1**:1–7.

31. Walsh K, Crisp J, Moss C. Psychodynamic perspectives on organisational change and their relevance to transformational practice development. *International Journal of Nursing Practice* 2011;**17**(2):205–12.

32. McAllister M, editor. *Solution focused nursing: rethinking practice.* Houndmills, UK: Palgrave Macmillan; 2007.

33. Covey SR. *The 7 habits of highly effective people.* 2nd ed. London: Simon & Schuster; 2004.

34. Kouzes J, Posner B. *The leadership challenge: how to get extraordinary things done in organizations.* 5th ed. San Francisco: Jossey-Bass; 2012.

35. Atkinson PE. *Creating culture change: the key to successful total quality management.* Bedford, UK: IFS Publications; 1990.

36. Goleman D. Leadership that gets results. *Harvard Business Review* 2000;**Mar–Apr**:78–90.

37. Davidson D, Peck E. Organisational development and the 'repertoire' of healthcare leaders. In: Peck E, editor. *Organisational development in healthcare: approaches, innovations, achievements.* Oxford, UK: Radcliffe; 2004.

38. Kouzes and Posner leadership site: <www.leadershipchallenge.com> [Viewed 13 December 2014].

39. Kitson A, Harvey G, McCormack B. Enabling the implementation of evidence-based practice: a conceptual framework. *Quality in Health Care* 1998;**7**:149–58.

40. Zukowski B. Managing change before it manages you. *Medsurg Nursing* 1995;**4**:325–33.

41. Lewin K. *Field theory in social science.* London: Routledge & Kegan Paul; 1951.

42. Poggenpoel M. Managing change. *Nursing RSA Verpleging* 1992;**7**:28–31.

43. Crookes PA, Froggatt T. Techniques and strategies for translating research findings into health care practices. In: Crookes PA, Davies S, editors. *Research into practice: essential skills for reading and applying research in nursing and health care.* 2nd ed. London: Harcourt Brace; 2004.

44. Rogers EM, Shoemaker FF. *Communication of innovations: a cross-cultural approach.* New York: Free Press; 1971.

45. Moore G. *Crossing the chasm: marketing and selling high-tech products to mainstream customers.* New York: Capstone Trade (HarperCollins); 1991, revised 1999 and 2014.

46. Geoghegan WH. Whatever happened to instructional technology? Paper presented at the 22nd Annual Conference of the International Business Schools Computing Association, Baltimore, MD: 17–20 July 1994.

47. Johnson G, Scholes K. *Exploring public sector strategy.* Harlow, UK: Pearson Education; 2001.

48. Schein E. Kurt Lewin's change theory in the field and in the classroom: notes toward a model of managed learning. *Systems Practice* 1996;**9**:27–47.

49. Reid A, Dahlgren MA, Petocz P, Dahlgren LO. *From expert student to novice professional.* New York: Springer; 2011.

50. Kotter JP. Leading change: why transformation efforts fail. *Harvard Business Review* 1995;**73**(2):59–68.

51. Esty K. The management of change. *Employee Assistance Quarterly* 1987;**2**:90–7.

52. Marris P. *Loss and change.* London: Routledge & Kegan Paul; 1985.

53. Mead D, Bryar R. An analysis of the changes involved in the introduction of the nursing process and primary nursing using a framework of loss and attachment. *Journal of Clinical Nursing* 1992;**1**:95–9.

54. Bridges W. *Managing transitions: making the most of change.* 3rd revised ed. London: Nicholas Brealey Publishing; 2011.

55. Perlman D, Takacs GT. The 10 stages of change. *Nursing Management* 1990;**16**:820–4.

56. Kubler-Ross E. *On death and dying.* New York: Macmillan; 1969.

57. Schoolfield M, Orduna A. Understanding staff nurses' responses to change: utilization of a grief-change framework to facilitate innovation. *Clinical Nurse Specialist* 1994;**8**:57–62.

58. McCormack B, Manley K, Titchen A, et al. Towards practice development: a vision in reality or a reality without vision. *Journal of Nursing Management* 1999;**7**:255–64.

59. Manley K, McCormack B, Wilson V, editors. *International practice development in nursing and healthcare.* Oxford, UK: Blackwell; 2008.

SECTION 2
SKILLS FOR DEALING WITH THE WORLD OF WORK

CHAPTER 8

Caring for self: the role of collaboration, healthy lifestyle and balance

Judy Lumby

LEARNING OBJECTIVES

When you have completed this chapter you will be able to:

- be critically aware of the parameters of remaining healthy inside and outside the workplace
- explore the ways in which values, contexts and lifestyle affect health and wellbeing
- build a knowledge of stress, its manifestations and its effects
- understand how to build resilience in self and others
- ensure that a life balance is maintained so that health is central personally and professionally.

KEYWORDS: caring, coping, allostatic load, healthy lifestyle, teamwork, resilience

INTRODUCTION

Nursing is a role similar to medicine, which demands much of an individual both personally and professionally. But it also gives back in ways that can be life enhancing. The two aspects of one's life – work/recreation, or professional/personal – become inextricably linked when undertaking the work known as nursing. To nurse is to become involved. After all, unless another or others are involved, then the act is not nursing. Central to being a nurse is being involved with another person, either caring for them or assisting them in their own care. This can take many forms: chance conversations about health issues; provisional diagnosis of an illness or disease; managing symptoms such as pain or breathlessness; counselling; advising on choices in treatments such as chemotherapy, dialysis or asthma medication; dressing or draining a wound; or assisting someone to die peacefully in the way they desire. All these acts, and many more, are a normal part of everyday nursing and all involve interacting with another person or persons. However, the compassion and empathy required to be so involved in caring for another can lead to work-related stress and its inevitable repercussions.

Over the past two decades, technology has made what was already a demanding job even more demanding, not only in terms of skills development but also in terms of managing time and priorities. While the introduction of new technology is usually made by doctors, it is nurses who are expected to manage and manipulate it, thus adding to their workload of caring. It is interesting to note that, of all industries, healthcare is one where the introduction of technology has meant not the loss of staff but the *addition* of staff – and even specialist staff – to drive the technology. Unlike many industries, most new healthcare technology has not meant simplification of skills or roles, but rather the extension and even sophistication of roles. In many areas, such as intensive care with technology such as ventilators and monitors, central lines and renal dialysis, it has also meant the opening up of new wards or units and the education of specialist nurses and doctors to work in the new areas. In most cases the technology is linked to the patient; however, because of the safety aspects of technological intervention, it is vital that the nurse keeps an ever-watchful eye on the actual machinery as well as its impact on the patient.[1] Nurses now have to divide their time between caring for the patient and caring for the technology. But who cares for the nurse?

In 1996 a report on the workforce in New South Wales mirrored the reduction in retention and recruitment of nurses across the Western world, with an ageing workforce compounding the problem.[2] By 2012, however, this trend appeared to have been reversed. The Australian Institute of Health and Welfare's labour force audit revealed that the total number of nurses and midwives was 334,078, an increase of 6.8% since 2008. Of these people employed in nursing and midwifery, 238,520 were registered nurses (including midwives) and 51,624 were enrolled nurses.

The workforce itself continued to age, with the proportion of nurses aged 50 years or over increasing from 35.1% to 39.1%. Some 62.6% of all employed clinical nurses and midwives worked in hospitals. And, despite efforts to reverse a gender imbalance, the profession continued to be predominantly female.[3]

The challenging nature of our contemporary healthcare systems contributes to the current dilemma of how we retain highly skilled younger nurses in our health workforce, given the changing social norms and values. After all, nurses were once expected – and even drilled – to care for others to the neglect of self. Such values were deeply embedded in nursing's – and indeed women's – history. Nursing is a profession founded in the convent and the army, institutions in which women were expected to be selfless, obedient and silent. Cultural shifts in recent times, including the expanding education of women, have questioned the belief that selfless dedication leads to healthy and caring individuals.[1] Quite the opposite can occur, with individuals feeling resentful, angry and unfulfilled if their own needs are unmet.

Present-day knowledge about self-development shows that, in order to empower and support another, it is important to be aware of who you are and what drives you forward. Caring for others to avoid confronting yourself is not only dangerous, it is unhealthy for those you care for. Often the carer comes from a position of victim or martyr, two very damaging positions for any individual, let alone those with whom they work. Nurses, like doctors, rely on working with many colleagues and sharing the care of individuals. For this to happen in a way that is in the best interests of the patient, we need to explore our personal values and share these with our professional colleagues so that we can work more effectively.

PERSONAL AND SHARED VALUES

The term *values* means different things to different people. It can refer to our social and cultural principles, goals or standards; it may mean the value we place on another person, or the quality of something in terms of its worth, or the extent to which something is desirable or worthy of esteem (pp 621–4).[4] Inherent in any discussion on values is the subject of ethics, which is a system of moral values – values about what it means to be a good person whose actions are based on a moral code of behaviour. There are at least six moral principles in most professional codes of ethics for health professionals. These are: (1) autonomy, (2) beneficence, (3) fidelity, (4) justice, (5) non-malificence, and (6) veracity. It is incumbent on graduates entering the workforce to analyse their specific profession's code of ethics to ensure that their personal values are not in conflict with such a code. This ensures integrity of the personal and professional conduct with which patients come into contact. In addition, it has been shown that individuals gain a sense of worth and connectedness if the values they hold personally are given expression through their professional practices. This requires us to ensure we achieve a balance between our personal and professional lives.

It has become increasingly clear to those who work in systems such as healthcare that the key to good outcomes is effective teamwork, which requires shared values.[4] While our education and healthcare systems educate and employ individual practitioners such as nurses, doctors or therapists, ultimately our diverse skills are complementary. Our boundaries of practice are not nearly as distinct as we would like to believe, and in many cases our work overlaps and interlinks. Nurses in one context may do what doctors do in another, and vice versa. For example, in isolated areas nurses often work alone with no professional support apart from someone at the end of a telephone line (assuming they have a telephone line). Nurses in these contexts triage, diagnose, treat and manage care in the way that a general practitioner in the city might. In the city, general practitioners may dress wounds and give injections which in a hospital would be the work of a nurse. One solution to 'turf battles' of practice is to use models of care that place the patient, rather than any one practitioner, at the centre of care. This focuses the mind on the core of healthcare practice – the patient – and away from vested interests. One such model of care is that used by nurse practitioners working in many primary healthcare contexts alone or in collaboration with other health professionals.

November 1, 2010 saw a move towards acknowledging and valuing the role of nurse practitioners in our workforce through ground-breaking changes to the Medicare legislation.[5] Since then, approved nurse practitioners and midwives working collaboratively with doctors but in private practice have access to a provider number, thus enabling their patients to receive a Medicare rebate for specific itemised services. Nurse practitioners working in the public healthcare system in some states and territories also have access to a Pharmaceutical Benefits Prescriber Number, which enables them to prescribe medications for their patients through this scheme. While these changes have taken two decades to achieve, against much criticism from national medical bodies, they represent one more step towards the roles of nurses and midwives being validated as making a difference in people's lives. In turn, this validates the lives of those nurses and midwives who are dedicated to improving access to quality care.

In this way their sense of worth, and of connectedness, is reinforced, thus leading to emotional wellbeing for the practitioner.

Collaborative multidisciplinary models of practice that fully involve the patient have been shown to be highly satisfactory and empowering for both providers and patients.[6] It could be said that practitioners who are unwilling to work in a team that involves the patient may be violating the ethical principles inherent in any professional code of conduct. Nevertheless, true collaboration in healthcare remains difficult to put into practice for reasons that are mainly to do with enforcing power and control rather than providing best patient care.

To work in a team so that care is not fragmented, individual practitioners need to take time out to consider their values individually and share them in a way that underpins the paradigm of care in which they work. This is rarely done, resulting in severe conflict in some cases because the individual practitioners may have different values concerning who to treat, with what and for how long. While ultimately there may be one decision maker, it is worthwhile for the whole team to take time to discuss the patient's wishes, needs and cultural beliefs, and to include the patient. In such cases the nurse is often privy to information never shared with the doctor/s. This is not necessarily because the doctor is not a good listener, but because the doctor may not be available, whereas the nurse cares for the patient for long periods of time, often in quite an intimate way. Alternatively, the doctor may have very well thought-out arguments for why a treatment should be considered. Unless there is a space for such conversations to happen before the event, decisions will always be made from only one perspective, with critical implications for healthy workplaces.

Toni Sullivan[4] comments on the way in which collaboration requires individuals to change or even reaffirm their values if they are to work in new ways with others (p 622). Collaboration itself can change individuals in many ways because of the experience of being forced to consider others and their ways of thinking and working. For many, the fact that others may have different values and ways of working is extremely confronting, requiring much reflection on personal values as well as a willingness to balance personal values with shared values when working in a team.

THE PERSONAL IN THE PROFESSIONAL: A MATTER OF BALANCE

In a role that demands so much, both personally and professionally, what can a nurse do to maintain a sense of equilibrium, of balance, so that work remains satisfying, indeed rewarding? The mass of material on a healthy, balanced life and health-related issues is complex in terms of what to believe and what to ignore. There are journals, tabloid newspapers, magazines and talk-back shows bombarding us with information about diet, exercise, relationships, cosmetic surgery, alternative therapies and drugs. How does one individual make sense of such a mountain of material? For reasons of space, and because there is so much good research devoted to this area which individuals can access, this chapter does not intend to address such debates. A reliable way of gaining the most up-to-date data is to download the weekly *Health Report* material from the ABC website (www.abc.net.au/health/). Perhaps the most interesting thing to note in all the debate about health, however, is the way in which we have focused on our bodies over the past three decades to the point of obsession, perhaps neglecting other components of wellbeing.

Since the early 1980s particularly, there has been an emphasis on, even a fanaticism over, health and fitness. Health and wellbeing have become big business. Indeed, the reality is that, as a population, the incidence of type 2 diabetes is more prevalent as obesity figures increase. Exercise is now one of our largest industries as joggers pound the streets with the latest equipment, expensive personal trainers become increasingly popular, and gymnasiums promise weight loss, weight gain, weight redistribution and happier, more successful lives, all for an annual fee. Pharmaceutical companies bombard us with new and better vitamin/mineral compounds in which the secret to longevity is supposedly contained. Food is dissected to within an inch of its organic components, categorised and labelled accordingly. We can buy it fat-free, chemical-free, preservative-free, sugar-free, calorie-free and taste-free.

The recent demand for perfect health (and the perfect body) – as opposed to 'being healthy' – has created whole new job categories. Fitness trainers, lifestyle managers, beauty therapists and psychic gurus have capitalised on and helped to manufacture our obsession with our bodies. In the United States this has reached manic proportions, with the restructuring, reorganising and reorientation of people now a huge industry. Bodies are manufactured, manipulated and managed. The ultimate medical manipulation of our bodies is, of course, plastic surgery. Advertising constantly bombards us with messages concerning our ability to reinvent our own bodies through diet, exercise and surgery. As a cultural medium, our bodies are also regulated by norms perpetuated through these media images. The advertising associated with the commodification of our wellbeing has had both positive and negative impacts. While providing a vector for the dissemination of information, it has also increased the anxiety and confusion we have about avoiding illness (and perhaps even death) and having the perfect life and body.

Accordingly, the general public has become much more likely to seek alternatives to those offered by conventional medicine. One of the most significant consequences of the contemporary focus on physical, mental and emotional wellbeing, and the growing disillusionment with the conventional system, has been the increasing rejection of conventional medicine and medical practices in favour of what are termed 'alternative' therapies.[7] These so-called alternatives are in fact traditional therapies, ousted when modern medicine gained its scientific foothold in the mid-1800s. A recent study of parents with children being treated for cancer showed that about 50% had also sought alternative therapy.[8]

Treatments that are becoming increasingly popular include acupuncture, homeopathy, iridology, hypnotherapy, naturopathy, aromatherapy and herbs. These have been incorporated into many people's lives for some time now as daily routines. For patients who are accessing both conventional and alternative medicine, the cost of healthcare is doubled and, nationally, this increases the overall amount spent on health (and illness).[9]

Recognition of traditional Chinese medicine has recently translated into registration of practitioners, and into universities offering undergraduate and postgraduate degrees in this area of knowledge. Patients with illnesses such as autoimmune disorders, irritable bowel syndrome, cancer, arthritis, infertility and even asthma are the most likely to consult such practitioners because they are often unable to gain relief through conventional medicine. There are also those who attend traditional therapists as a preventive measure, and those who simply want to optimise their feeling of wellbeing, of being supremely healthy.

WHAT IS HEALTH AND WHAT IS ILLNESS?

The concepts of health and illness are, of course, not immutable but are constructed culturally and historically. In turn, these constructs structure the way health and illness care are delivered and, therefore, received. For example, whereas most Western countries have traditionally focused their notions of healthcare on illness, specifically acute illnesses, other cultures focus on staying healthy and preventing illness. As a result, the way a society funds its healthcare usually reflects its perceptions of health and illness.

Health is currently defined by the World Health Organization (WHO) in its constitution as 'a state of complete physical, mental and social well being and not merely the absence of disease or infirmity'.[10] This general definition of health reflects current popular notions of health in the West, although this rarely translates into a different funding regime. As advances in science have enabled mass immunity from certain infectious diseases, at the same time as nutrition and sanitation have improved, people in developed economies have broadened their views of illness and health. They are now able to envisage a life longer and healthier than that of their mothers and fathers (unless they are Indigenous Australians) and, as a result, they can rethink the very notion of what constitutes a healthy life. It is a conception of health that moves beyond the mere absence of disease. As a result, the late 20th century witnessed a new focus on mental/emotional health. Indeed, psychological wellbeing is now considered an essential part of being healthy, although it is yet to receive the attention or funding it requires.

The following comments were made by a 60-year-old Australian woman on being discharged from a private hospital after a prolonged illness. Her description of what health means to her sums up the contemporary, popular, Western understanding of health that is prevalent in Australia today:

> I don't see [health] as purely a medical thing. To me, being healthy is how
> I'm perceiving life, how I'm relating to people, how I'm coping with
> day-to-day things. And I guess there are more things that influence that
> than the physical condition of your body (Rae: personal conversation).

The WHO's Global Strategy of Health for All by the Year 2000 states:

> All people in all countries should have at least such a level of health that
> they are capable of working productively and of participating actively in
> the social life in which they live.[10]

DEVELOPING A HEALTHY LIFESTYLE

So, how can we work productively every day yet maintain our health and wellbeing so that we have a well-balanced life?

Historically there has been a sustained interest in the notion of coping, in individual coping mechanisms, in why stress in one individual may not be perceived as stress by another, and why things such as cancer survival are not necessarily scientifically determined. This research into coping has important outcomes for individuals and organisations attempting to ensure safe, healthy and productive working days and workplaces. It also answers some important questions. Does a heavy workload increase your stress? Do those who work longer hours feel more stressed, and are they more unhealthy, than those who work shorter hours? What are the major stressors for employees?

Interestingly, research has confirmed that it is certainly not as simple as hours of work; it is more about control – about control over work. It is what Professor Leonard Syme from the University of Berkeley calls 'cell mastery', which involves 'control over destiny; the ability at work to decide how and at what pace we get the job done, and how to be able to traverse life's difficulties and solve everyday problems so they don't overwhelm us'.[11]

The *British Medical Journal* in 1998 reported the findings of a Harvard study of 21,000 female nurses which showed that having a high-stress job in which one has little job control or support is as damaging to the health as smoking, alcohol or lack of exercise.[12] Those with poor health outcomes in this study continued to deteriorate over a four-year period. The measures of health utilised in the Harvard study were physical functioning, limitations due to physical and emotional problems, pain, vitality, social functioning and mental health. Such outcomes have been replicated in a yet-to-be-completed longitudinal study of women's health which is monitoring 42,000 Australian women over 20 years.[13] The healthiest women are those who are self-employed or in family businesses; that is, they feel more in control of their lives. A more recent study cautioned about the limitations of workplace-health research that does not take into account the broader social environment of workers. When such factors were taken into consideration in Canada's National Population Health Survey,[14] the individual's position at work played a limited role in health and wellbeing when the structures of daily life and the agent's personality were accounted for. Indeed, it was shown that, compared with occupational structures, the structures of daily life play a far more important role in psychological distress.

Of course, aspects of work that may have negative effects on an individual's health include lack of control, such as not being able to be one's own boss, have flexible hours or determine ways of undertaking tasks, and lack of support.[14] This knowledge leads to new ways of understanding what interventions are required in terms of making workplaces more satisfactory for workers. Rather than merely reducing hours of work, interventions should enable individuals to feel more in control of their environment while at work. Flexible rostering for nurses would be one way to enable individuals to regain a sense of control over when they work, and if the rostering was done by team negotiation it would add to such control. Control over the practice environment; clinical autonomy; good nurse–physician relationships; clinically competent peers; supportive supervisors; adequate staffing; support for education; and concern for the patients are all characteristics of what have been identified as 'Magnet Hospitals'[15] – those hospitals which attract and retain staff.

Dr Bruce McEwen, from the Rockefeller University in New York, has made meaning of his neuroendocrinology research into stress by applying it to social policies. According to McEwen, when we are under stress our hormonal response attempts to enable us to re-establish homeostasis through allostasis, which means 'achieving stasis through change'.[16] In this way, we survive our minute-to-minute challenges through what is a perfectly healthy response. Thus, while stress is a challenge to the body biologically because it is reliant on the adrenal glands producing catecholamines and cortisol, it is also a means of achieving resilience as individuals in our daily lives. In turn, however, as with most biological mechanisms, balance is crucial. A healthy response can become unhealthy if the body is unable to turn off hormonal responses once the acute stress has passed. This results in a continual stream of hormones being poured into the bloodstream, which can be quite damaging. Inefficient operation of hormonal response is referred to as our 'allostatic load' – that is, the load from the stress mediators on our body. This may be protective or it may be damaging, depending on our biological response as well as our environment. Both play a part in our allostatic load.

The two forms of stress spoken about here are acute and chronic stress. It is chronic stress that is particularly damaging because of the continual outpouring of the stress hormones, causing damage to organs and tissues. And chronic stress is usually not caused by a sudden incidental event, but by longer-term ongoing events such as a personal or professional environment that is full of conflict, or one in which individuals perceive themselves to be out of control. In such cases, hormonal levels are continually high, which over time results in a stress-related disorder such as post-traumatic or dramatic disorder, a disorder in which an individual's body has been sensitised to overreact to things that would not normally be disturbing to others.

McEwen has also identified certain lifestyle choices as responses to stress – for example, overeating, poor dietary choices and lack of exercise – but the problem is that these all synergise with the effects of increased hormonal levels to speed up bodily changes such as increased weight and its side effects. Genetic influences may also add to an individual's allostatic load – for example, familial hypertension and type 2 diabetes, both of which add to biological stress. According to McEwen, cited in Swan,[17] there is also some evidence that certain physical characteristics, such as excess abdominal fat, are indicators of high allostatic load. These characteristics are found mainly in populations that have poorer environments and reduced personal resources, both economically and psychologically. The individuals in such environments have raised hormonal levels due to chronic stress.

One of the techniques used to reduce stress and thus improve cardiac risk factors in patients with coronary heart disease is Transcendental Meditation (TM). In a randomised trial reported in the *Journal of the American Medical Association* (JAMA), one arm of the study offered participants a 16-week trial of TM while the other study arm offered health education. At the end of the trial, those in the TM arm had significantly reduced blood pressure as well as improved levels of fasting blood glucose and insulin, and more stable functioning of the autonomic nervous system, which is significant in controlling stress responses.[18] Another study involving TM was that carried out by Castillo-Richmond and colleagues from the Centre for Natural Medicine and Prevention in Iowa, in the US. This study investigated the effects of stress reduction on carotid atherosclerosis in hypertensive African Americans using TM as the method of reducing stress.[19] The TM group in the study showed a significant decrease in the intima media thickness (IMT) of the carotid artery following the adoption of two sessions of 20 minutes of TM in their daily life. Carotid IMT is a significant predictor of coronary heart disease, with an increase in thickness predicting an increased risk.

More recently, the research into what makes and maintains healthy individuals has moved into the Science of Happiness initiated by Martin Seligman of *Positive Psychology* fame, who showed that the happiest people are those who have discovered their true strengths and used them for others. The 7 Habits of Happy People are said to be: (1) having close relationships, (2) cultivating kindness, (3) exercising, (4) being challenged with activities, (5) discovering meaning in our lives, (6) using our strengths for others, and (7) having a positive mindset.[20]

A study by Otake and colleagues in Japan, in which participants used a counting kindness intervention, showed that kindness produces subjective happiness.[21] And Fowler and Christakis showed that people's happiness depends on the happiness of others with whom they are connected in some way. In other words, it is a collective phenomenon.[22]

WHAT MAKES US HEALTHY WORKERS?

We certainly know that socioeconomic status has an impact on the risk of disease, with those in lower socioeconomic groups having a higher incidence of disease.[23] Whether this is to do with nutrition or lack of control, or with a factor yet to be uncovered, we can only work with the evidence we have so far. Similarly, the 2006 Gallup World Poll, which studies income, health and wellbeing around the world, showed that life satisfaction was strongly related to per capita national income.[23] While not the same as disease, one's satisfaction with life is a major influence on the quality of day-to-day living and perhaps on an individual's health and wellbeing.

An important factor in lowering people's risk of death is social networks. Having strong social networks and friendships, and being involved in social activities, are all variables that make a difference in terms of feeling better and living longer with a healthier mental state.[23]

The plethora of research on health is consistent in saying that exercise and diet are major variables. While writings on both these factors form anthologies in their own right, and there are conflicting opinions about both diet and exercise, there is also some unequivocal evidence that we need to heed. The first is that the body does need some activity to keep it able to function. Staying in bed and immobile is not good for circulation, respiration or flexibility.[24] Contradictions enter the debate when it comes to how much and what kind of exercise is ideal, and at what time in life.

Trends in exercise each decade are clear evidence of the lack of any one body of research that points the way. Professor Stuart Biddle, head of sports psychology at Loughborough University in the UK, has shown that the increased self-esteem and reduced anxiety observed in those who exercise are due to the biochemical changes that take place as we exercise.[25] This may be a key factor in why exercise has such a positive impact on our health and why some individuals become obsessed with exercise.

The intense high-impact aerobic classes of the 1960s have been gradually replaced by the resistance and strength classes, individual workouts and yoga of our contemporary society. Popular forms of exercise today include boxing, resistance cycling, defencercise and pump classes. Pounding the streets, as many of us did for a while before turning to alternative forms of exercise, has been criticised for causing joint and skeletal damage that may manifest as pain and impaired mobility later in life. The two forms of exercise that have remained consistently popular over the years are walking and swimming. These have been identified as the two ideal forms of exercise for the majority of the population who are able to undertake them as activities. And to gain the most benefit, they should be undertaken regularly – that is, at least three times per week.

For postmenopausal women, walking is preferable because of the positive impact of weight bearing on preventing severe osteoporosis. A study into physical activity in postmenopausal women[26] showed that, in those women who engaged in vigorous activity four times per week compared with women who did not engage in such activity, there was a 43% reduced risk of dying. The risk reduction was also there for women who engaged in moderate activity only once a week. They still had a 24% reduced risk of dying compared with those women who undertook no activity at all. As far as osteoporosis is concerned, genetic predisposition is still a major factor, as is smoking and inadequate calcium intake.

Exercise has also been shown to lower the risk of developing breast cancer. In a 14-year study of 25,000 women aged 20–54, those who exercised had a lower risk of developing breast cancer, with the greatest reduction in those women who were leaner than average and exercised for at least 4 hours a week.[27]

In terms of adequate nutrition, while the literature is extensive and often conflicting, several key factors are central. These are that adequate amounts of protein, carbohydrates and fats, adequate fluids, and adequate vitamins and minerals are essential to a healthy daily diet. The conflict in the evidence comes in terms of amounts and types of each, with some diets even dictating the time of day each should be consumed. Recently, the National Health and Medical Research Council (NHMRC) launched Dietary Guidelines for Older Australians in which it has also been shown that bad diets appear to be related to loneliness, grief and depression.[28]

THE CULTURE OF THE CONTEMPORARY WORKPLACE

So, does following a healthy lifestyle and ensuring that your life is balanced mitigate against the impact of an unhealthy workplace? In answering this question, we need to narrow the workplace down to the healthcare workplace, which is somewhat different from many other workplaces. Deidre Wicks, a researcher from Newcastle University, has undertaken one of the most in-depth and contemporary exposés of the healthcare workplace in terms of nurses and doctors.[29] Her study not only provides insight into the conflict inherent within professional boundaries, but also erects signposts for new graduates entering the workplace.

As Wicks comments, 'Power is ever-present within health settings. It is evident in the way people walk, the way they communicate, in who gets recognised as having a presence and who gets ignored' (p 91).[29] Wicks observed in the five months she was in the workplace that it was rare for doctors and cleaners to interact, and this was also the case for doctors and very junior nurses. She also noted that, at times, both doctors and nurses exhibited behaviours of ownership of the ward and, ipso facto, of the patients.

The exercise of power within the hierarchy of medicine, of medicine over nurses and even patients, surprised Wicks in that it had 'survived the reforms of the "new managerialism" in health care settings' (p 98).[29]

The fact that public healthcare, in particular, is dominated by the technologically driven medical specialties marginalises the discourses, and therefore the practices, of those wishing to work in a more contemporary framework of healing. Wicks notes that nurses facilitate this marginalisation through their apparent willingness to pick up the invisible caring components of patient care while the doctors continue their visible curing component. This division has implications not only for healthcare policies but also for healthy workplaces in which the most effective care can be delivered by a functioning, multidisciplinary team. The research previously outlined in this chapter has emphasised the importance of control over one's role and of support in the workplace. Wicks's study reveals clearly that this is not currently so, and the present difficulty in recruiting and retaining nurses may be a clear indicator of a culture that is outmoded and even disabling for many working in it.

To overcome such a culture, those entering the workplace need to articulate their practice clearly, to be open and assertive in their dialogue, and to engage their fellow practitioners in practising what is a more effective team approach. While Wicks's solution of nurses and doctors undertaking undergraduate degrees together may not be feasible in the short term, her goal is still possible in the workplace. This is to move towards integrating the best of modern medicine with a perspective that emphasises 'holism, illness prevention and the relationships between health, illness, individual life history and social structure' (p 181).[29]

Understanding the workplace and its culture is essential for anyone entering the workforce since it assists the initial assimilation of a new graduate. Entering a new work environment is difficult for even a skilled individual who has been in the workforce before but is now entering a new workplace environment such as healthcare.

Healthcare is a multifaceted system in terms of the contexts, the geographical sites, the personnel, and the level of care. Compounding this is the public/private and the federal/state divides. Contexts include acute hospitals, community centres, nursing homes, rehabilitation centres and people's homes. Geographical sites include city and country, and the areas in between. Personnel include nurses, doctors, therapists, technicians, cleaners, dieticians, pharmacists and social workers. The level of care denotes the acuteness or otherwise of the management required, although this is controversial, depending on how health is defined and measured.

With such complexity in the contexts in which care takes place, it is extremely difficult to identify a single culture, as may be possible in a simpler system.

It is little wonder, therefore, that the healthcare system is a difficult culture to traverse for the 'new kid on the block'. More recent changes brought about by the managerialism that has invaded the public sector have created an environment in which the naive tend to struggle. This is mainly to do with the efficiency imperatives that demand productivity gains in the system. In healthcare, where people rather than whitegoods are involved, the main strategies used to make gains have been to reduce staff, increase workload and increase turnover of patients. Given that we have an increasingly elderly and drug-dependent patient population and more sophisticated technology and pharmacology, we now have an industry in which staff are working harder with fewer resources at a time when patients are more highly dependent and yet are discharged to recover at home.

It is important to note that being in control at work is only one part of the very complex equation that makes up the profile of being healthy – an equation that is in its infancy in terms of being solved. After all, as Michael Marmot, Professor of Epidemiology and Public Health at University College, London, points out, the fact that those in control at work may also be on a higher salary and more educated in nutrition must be factored into the equation.[30] Such individuals are more likely to eat fresh fruit and vegetables, which contain antioxidants and vitamins thought to be protective against certain cancers and other illnesses.

A more recent focus on resilience has shown it to be an important characteristic to have if one is to manage stressors in the workplace. Resilience is identified as an inner resource, but Grafton and colleagues showed that it can be developed in oncology nurses through 'cognitive transformational practices, education and environmental support'.[31]

CONCLUSION

The workplace into which new nursing graduates journey is vastly different to the one in which many of us worked several decades ago. The contemporary emphasis on fiscal restraint, organisational restructuring and measurable outcomes rarely takes account of the cost of caring work mainly undertaken by nurses. A Canadian nurse, Brenda Sabo,[32] investigated the consequences of caring work in her doctoral program and discovered that many nurses who care for patients experiencing trauma, pain and suffering, themselves suffer from compassion fatigue. Certain qualities, however, appear to offer protection against compassion fatigue. These are resiliency, hardiness and social support – qualities it may take time to develop. It is up to each one of us in the nursing profession to support our neophyte nurses in every possible way, not only assisting them in their daily caring work but also ensuring that they are able to pursue healthy, well-balanced lives.

CASE STUDY 8.1

You are working in a palliative care ward and have been there for three years. A newly registered nurse has been appointed to the ward after a rotation in the emergency unit, which he enjoyed. He says he feels out of place in this ward because it is so quiet and the patients need much more personal care. You have been asked to mentor him.

REFLECTIVE QUESTIONS

1. How would you go about forming a relationship with this new RN?
2. What would you do when planning your mentorship of him?
3. How would you know if you were succeeding in ensuring he became competent, caring and fulfilled in his new role?

CASE STUDY 8.2

You have been working double shifts in a ward that is constantly understaffed and chaotic due to an environment where the staff work as individuals rather than as a team. You find yourself waking up after a few hours of sleep and lying there dreading your next shift. You are not eating well and have stopped going to the gym because you are always tired.

REFLECTIVE QUESTIONS

1. Imagine yourself in a different space where you are working in a great team of individuals with similar values of giving high-quality care and supporting each other in doing so. Reflect/meditate on this scenario for several days, then develop a plan of action to make it happen so that you become happy and healthy again. Write your plan in your diary.
2. What is the first step you will take in terms of creating this scenario for yourself?

CASE STUDY 8.3

You are working on a very busy post-operative ward with a team of nurses and doctors who work very well together. An experienced RN arrives from Canada to work on the ward and immediately suggests ways of doing things differently – things that worked well in her previous workplace.

Some of her suggestions sound interesting, but the other members of the team ignore her and are beginning to isolate her from their conversations.

REFLECTIVE QUESTIONS

1. What is going on here socially?
2. How are you going to relate to the newcomer when you are working with her?
3. What are you going to do about it in terms of the team around you?

EXERCISE 8.1

1. List the positive and negative influences in your life (being completely honest).
2. Look at the list and identify how you can remove or reduce the negative influences, whether they be people, food, habits or environments.
3. Take 10 minutes a day to meditate. During your meditation, imagine yourself with only the positive influences building up your resilience and happiness.
4. Three months later, redo the list and see what has changed. Reflect on how far you have come.
5. Now think about how your happiness has affected other people.

EXERCISE 8.2

1. You notice that your best friend has lost her enthusiasm for patient care and complains about work every day. How would you go about initiating a conversation about this with her?
2. What three suggestions might you make to enable your friend to regain her previous positive outlook?
3. How would you best support her during this time?

RECOMMENDED READINGS

Hoeger WK, Hoeger SA. *Fitness and wellness.* 8th ed. Wadsworth, OH: Cengage Learning; 2009.

Lupton D. *Medicine as culture: illness, disease and the body.* Revised 3rd ed. London: Sage; 2012.

Reich JW, Zantra AJ, Hall J, editors. *Handbook of adult resilience: concepts, methods and applications.* New York: Guildford Press; 2012.

Sullivan TJ. Collaboration, a health care imperative: reflection on values. In: Sullivan TJ, editor. *Collaboration: a health care imperative.* New York: McGraw-Hill; 1998. p 622.

Swan N. Mastering the control factor, parts 2 and 4. Radio National's The Health Report, 16 and 30 November 1998. Online. Available: <www.abc.net.au/rn/healthreport/index/date1998.htm#November>.

REFERENCES

1. Lumby J. *Who cares? The changing health care system.* Sydney: Allen & Unwin; 2001.
2. NSW Health Department. *Nursing recruitment and retention taskforce, final report.* Sydney: NSW Health Department; 1996.
3. Australian Institute of Health and Welfare. *National Health Workforce Series No. 6. Nursing and midwifery workforce.* Canberra: AIHW; 2012.
4. Sullivan TJ, editor. *Collaboration: a health care imperative.* New York: McGraw-Hill; 1998.
5. *The Health Legislation Amendment (Midwives and Nurse Practitioners) Act.* Canberra: Department of Health & Ageing; 2010.
6. Rose J, Glass N. Community mental health nurses speak out: the critical relationship between emotional wellbeing and satisfying professional practice. *Collegian (Royal College of Nursing, Australia)* 2006;**13**(4):27–32.
7. Phelan A. Culture, cure: orthodoxy embraces alternative medicine. Health for Life. *Sydney Morning Herald* 1997;H1–4.
8. Sawyer MG, Gannow A, Toogood IR, et al. The use of alternative therapies by children with cancer. *Medical Journal of Australia* 1994;**160**(6):320–2.
9. Editorial. *Health and Development* 1998;**181**:2.
10. World Health Organisations Global Strategy of Health for All by the Year 2000.
11. Swan N. Mastering the control factor, part 4. Radio National's The Health Report, 30 November 1998. Online. Available: <www.abc.net.au/rn/talks/8.30/helthrpt/stories/s17549.htm>.
12. Stock S. Sick of work? Your job could be killing you. *The Weekend Australian* 2000;**3–4**:3.

13. Lee C, Dobson AJ, Brown WJ, et al. Cohort profile: the Australian longitudinal study on women's health. *International Journal of Epidemiology* 2005;**34**:987–91.

14. Marchand A, Demers A, Durand P. Do occupation and work conditions really matter? A longitudinal analysis of psychological distress experiences among Canadian workers. *Sociology of Health & Illness* 2005;**27**:602–27.

15. Aiken LH. Superior outcomes for magnet hospitals: the evidence base, in magnet hospitals revisited: attraction and retention of professional nurses. In: McClure ML, Hinshaw AS, editors. Washington, DC: American Nurses Publishing; 2002.

16. McEwen BS. Protective and damaging effects of stress mediators. *New England Journal of Medicine* 1998;**338**:171–9.

17. Swan N. Good stress and bad stress. Radio National's The Health Report, 13 April 1998. Online. Available: <www.abc.net.au/rn/talks/8.30/helthrpt/stories/s10743.htm>.

18. Paul-Labrador M. Transcendental Meditation may improve cardiac risk factors in patients with coronary heart disease. *Archives of Internal Medicine* 2006;June.

19. Castillo-Richmond A, et al. Effects of stress reduction on carotid atherosclerosis in hypertensive African Americans. *Stroke; a Journal of Cerebral Circulation* 2000;**31**:568–73.

20. Seligman MEP. *Flourish: a visionary new understanding of happiness and wellbeing.* New York: The Free Press; 2012.

21. Otake K, Shimai S, Tanaka-Matsumi J, Otsui K, Fredrickson B. Happy people become happier through kindness: a counting kindness intervention. *Journal of Happiness Studies* 2006;**7**(3):361–75.

22. Fowler JH, Christakis NA. Dynamic spread of happiness in a large social network: a longitudinal analysis over 20 years in the Framingham Heart Study. *British Medical Journal* 2008;**337**:2338.

23. Deaton A. Income, health and wellbeing around the World: Evidence from the Gallup World Poll. *Journal of Economic Perspectives* 2008;**22**(2):53–72.

24. Allen C, Glasziou P, Del Mar C. Bed-rest: a potentially harmful treatment needing more careful evaluation. *Lancet* 1999;**354**:1229–33.

25. Clark A. *Exercise your style. Good medicine.* Sydney: Network Distribution; 1987.

26. Kushi LH, Fee R, Anderson K, et al. Physical activity and mortality in postmenopausal women. *Journal of the American Medical Association* 1997;**227**:1287–92.

27. Thune I, Brenn T, Lund E, et al. Physical activity and the risk of breast cancer. *New England Journal of Medicine* 1997;**336**:1269–75.

28. Reiner V. Senior death by diet avoidable. Health. *The Weekend Australian* 2000;**19–20**:7.

29. Wicks D. *Nurses and doctors at work: rethinking professional boundaries.* Sydney: Allen & Unwin; 1999.

30. Marmot M. Inequalities in death: specific explanations of general patterns. *Lancet* 1984;**323**:1003–6.

31. Grafton E, Gillepsie B, Henderson S. Resilience: the power within. Health & Medicine. *Oncology Nursing Forum* 2010;698–705.

32. Sabo BM. Compassion fatigue and nursing work: can we accurately capture the consequences of caring work? *International Journal of Nursing Practice* 2006;**12**:136–42.

CHAPTER 9

Managing approaches to nursing care delivery

Patricia M Davidson and Bronwyn Everett

LEARNING OBJECTIVES

When you have completed this chapter you will be able to:

▲ identify the importance of tailoring models of nursing care delivery to meet the needs of healthcare environments, patients and their families
▲ recognise key roles and responsibilities for nurses in delivering patient care
▲ describe strategies for managing nursing workload and time management practices
▲ consider the role of the registered nurse in an environment of varying skill mix and diverse scopes of practice
▲ discuss the overarching professional, legal and regulatory frameworks that can influence delivery of nursing care.

KEYWORDS: models of nursing care, mentorship, time management, lifelong learning, setting priorities

INTRODUCTION

Contemporary healthcare systems are defined by their complexity and also by the pressures they experience due to rising demands, increasing technological complexity and fiscal constraints. In addition, there is increasing scrutiny by the public to ensure that healthcare is safe and effective. This pressure has been fuelled by the increased recognition of adverse events that are preventable in healthcare systems.[1]

Nursing is a dynamic profession, delivered in a wide variety of settings, and in a range of models and regulatory frameworks.[2] The role, scope and functions of nursing practice are driven by the social, political and economic contexts in which the care is delivered.[3,4] For example, in countries such as the United States there is a greater emphasis on independent nursing practice, whereas in other countries (such as Australia) there is less of an emphasis on these roles because of the later introduction of advanced practice roles, as well as opposition from some sectors in introducing these roles.[5] It is only in recent years in Australia that the nurse practitioner role has been included in healthcare delivery models.[6] Encouraging a range of policy changes has enabled the enactment of the nurse practitioner role.[7] In recent times, funding and policy changes have seen the rapid development of the nursing role in Australian general practice.[8] This represents an exciting time for the nursing role in primary care.

In spite of the diverse range and scope of practice, nursing is focused on facilitating wellness and caring for the vulnerable and infirm in the primary, secondary and tertiary care sectors. Increasingly, there is an emphasis on nurses providing care to populations as well as individuals and communities.[9]

Nursing practice is constantly evolving and, despite the explosion of new technology and labour-saving devices, nurses have never before been required to deliver high-quality patient care within a context of organisational pressures for efficiencies. Despite these challenges, there is an increasing recognition of the importance of nursing in influencing patient outcomes, and of the importance of monitoring and evaluating workforce characteristics, particularly the numbers and ratios of registered nurses to other health workers.[10]

Significant advances and changes in healthcare have occurred since the Second World War. Escalating technological solutions for healthcare, beginning in the 1960s and 1970s, have driven the development of nursing specialties. An example is the coronary care unit,[11] where changes in care patterns have evolved in line with diagnostic and therapeutic advances, leading to a diversification of nursing roles and the subsequent restructuring of inpatient cardiac services. Primary angioplasty and other innovative procedures mean that lengths of stay in hospital are shorter, leaving less time for secondary prevention.[12] This has placed an increasing importance on transitional care and models that interface with community-based care.[13] In many settings, technological innovation and telemedicine have facilitated the reach of the nursing role to populations with limited access.[14] However, population ageing, the increasing burden of chronic conditions and increasing fiscal constraints are now leading nurses and other health professionals to search for alternative strategies that lie beyond technology for more inclusive and humanistic models of patient care delivery. In particular, the importance of prevention, risk management and patient self-management is an increasing focus of nursing care.[15]

In this chapter we look at models of nursing care, the key roles and responsibilities of nurses, managing workload and time management, setting priorities and planning in clinical practice, mentorship and preceptorship, and measuring the outcomes of nursing care. The discussion relates particularly to moving from senior undergraduate student to newly registered nurse, and the skills required in making this transition.

MODELS OF NURSING CARE

Nursing is a diverse and multifaceted profession, and nursing care is delivered across a range of settings and contexts from primary prevention to palliative care. Nursing care can be independent in nature, such as nurse–practitioner-based models, or dependent, based on delegation, such as in intensive care; other models include substitution, such as with physician assistants, and enhancement, such as in nurse-coordinated models of care.[16,17] A comprehensive understanding of the nature of nursing practice requires careful consideration and examination of the dynamic processes that have an impact on the nursing profession, including regulatory and legal frameworks. Models are conceptual tools or devices that can be used to understand and place complex phenomena in perspective. A model is a standard or an example for imitation or comparison, combining concepts, beliefs and intents that are related in some way.[3] This organisation of concepts, together with a philosophy of care, allows nurses to plan, deliver and evaluate nursing care in a systematic manner based on theoretical propositions.[18] Nursing care is both an independent and interdependent practice initiated on the basis of nursing assessment and actions within an interdisciplinary setting. Therefore, as you develop into the registered nurse role, it is important that you also engage in a process of self-reflection to identify the attitudes, values and beliefs you bring to this encounter.

Novel models of care are usually developed in response to perceived deficits in existing care delivery. An example is the care of patients with chronic heart failure (CHF). This condition is an intricate constellation of pathophysiological processes that results in a syndrome eventuating from inadequate cardiac output and neurohormonal activation.[19] CHF has a significant chronic physical and psychosocial impact on the individual and is responsible for substantial family and societal burden. The unpredictable illness trajectory of CHF and subsequent life-threatening complications dictate ongoing management and frequent hospitalisation. Readmission rates of up to 30% have been shown in both Australian and international contexts, with up to 50% of these readmissions attributable to failure to comply with prescribed treatment regimens rather than treatment failure.[20] Models of care that are evidenced-based, patient-centred and multidisciplinary are needed to support self-management and promote service coordination across care transitions.[21]

The burden of CHF has led to the development of innovative pharmacological and non-pharmacological interventions. Innovative care models have been developed and continue to be developed. Many of these have been collaboratively developed by nurses, focusing on nurse-directed interventions. Many of these approaches to nursing care are based on strategies that promote self-management and treatment adherence.[22]

Changes in the contemporary management of CHF reflect the evolution of nursing care delivery in response to changes in practice patterns, patient needs and demographic profiles, and importantly demonstrate that the profession of nursing is required to be flexible and dynamic in achieving improved health outcomes for patients in a diversity of care settings.[23] Further, models of nursing care in chronic conditions, such as chronic obstructive pulmonary disease and diabetes, place an emphasis on continuity of care rather than a perception of acute and chronic care as distinct and isolated care providers. Many of the current healthcare reforms internationally seek to build a bridge between these distinct care models.[24]

Contemporary models of nursing practice need to be appropriate to the needs of individual patients as well as local policy and funding models. As a consequence, these approaches need to be:

- dynamic – responsive to a changing and diverse environment, subject to social, political, economic and cultural change
- eclectic – looking to other disciplines and philosophies to combine factors to improve and complement nursing practice

- responsive – to the needs of health consumers and fiscal priorities
- multidisciplinary – involving consultation with all healthcare professionals and healthcare providers
- interdisciplinary – where the combination of a range of disciplines is greater than the single application of an intervention of a singular profession.

A range of models of nursing care have been developed since the Nightingale apprenticeship style of task allocation based on seniority and experience. Common models of care include team nursing, patient allocation and primary nursing, which all provide a more holistic and patient-centred approach to individual patient care; primary nursing ensures nurse responsibility and accountability beyond the individual shift timeframe. Some health systems have the registered nurse as the coordinator of care, while second-line nurses (e.g. enrolled nurses, nursing assistants), nursing students or unregistered healthcare workers assist in direct and non-direct patient care activities. Since the introduction of tertiary-based education in Australia, direct hospital-based nursing care has been provided primarily by registered nurses with some support from enrolled nurses. Primarily related to the nursing workforce shortage, this composition has changed in recent times and there is increasingly a diversification in skill mix in the clinical setting. The registered nurse is thus required to function in a more problem-solving, communication and delegation role. Therefore, when planning nursing care the registered nurse has to consider:

- constructing interventions using a framework of evidence and/or theoretical propositions
- planning of care delivery informed by assessment of patient, health provider and health system needs
- evaluating health-related outcomes and intervention outcomes
- consulting with all stakeholders in a participative context
- promoting the safety and wellbeing of nurses
- incorporating a multidisciplinary approach where applicable
- configuring healthcare resources to promote accessibility and optimal utilisation
- promoting equity of access for all members of society
- negotiating interventions that are culturally sensitive and appropriate.

Underpinning nursing models is consideration of the processes of clinical decision making, organising care delivery and planning care outcomes. An important part of developing effective models of nursing care is ensuring that there is assessment of outcomes on an organisation, provider and consumer basis. With the increasing view that multidisciplinary collaboration is important for continuity of care, an emphasis on a specific nursing care plan is increasingly considered 'nurse-centric' and isolated from the team approach to patient care. One solution offered as a ward-based method of managing patients in the acute hospital setting is the model of case management.[25] Case management plans provide guidelines for time-based critical incidents during a patient's hospital stay, including the appropriate length of stay and recommendations for evidence-based treatment. As well, the plans offer collaborative interdisciplinary management strategies for all health professionals providing direct patient care, by standardising appropriate use of resources, promoting collaborative team practice, coordinating continuity of care during the patient's admission period, and improving patient and clinician satisfaction.[26,27]

A critical or clinical pathway is a structured care plan that lists essential steps in the care of patients with a specific clinical problem.[28] The critical path is a multidisciplinary plan of care that provides guidelines on the day-to-day management for a patient type or diagnosis-related group. This approach provides recommendations for interventions and investigations, and allows monitoring of resources.[29] A common criticism of clinical pathways is that they are appropriate to acute procedurally based care but are challenging in chronic and aged care because of multiple comorbid conditions. Numerous clinical paths for specific patient types are in evidence in the literature, and many hospitals in Australia and overseas continue to develop their own pathways for patient care using their local multidisciplinary clinical experts. In some practice areas, case managers (often registered nurses) are used to coordinate and monitor patient care activities according to the critical path. In spite of the challenges and criticisms of clinical pathways, the empirical and systematic process of mapping patient care, ensuring accountability and measurement of outcomes often drives organisational efficiencies and improves quality of care, including reducing in-hospital complications and improving documentation.[28] Other models of care include the use of liaison nurses and other consultancy models.[30]

Regardless of the model of care, it is important that the interventions implemented are socially, economically and politically relevant to the local context and treatment patterns. An example of this is cancer care. Increasing consumer advocacy, treatment innovations and improving patient outcomes in cancer care have led to the restructuring of models of nursing care where there is an increasing emphasis on self-management, care continuity, and the recognition of social and psychological issues that have an impact on health outcomes.[31]

KEY ROLES AND RESPONSIBILITIES OF NURSES

The Nursing and Midwifery Board of Australia (NMBA) has developed competency standards for registered nurses and midwives, nurse practitioners and enrolled nurses. These are useful documents. Other useful resources include the *Code of Professional Conduct for Nurses in Australia* and the *Code of Ethics for Nurses in Australia*, which you can access from the NMBA website (www. nursingmidwiferyboard.gov.au). Key competencies for registered nurses involve integrating activities of clinical practice, coordinating care, counselling, health teaching, client advocacy, clinical teaching, supervising, working in a team, mentoring, monitoring patient outcomes and researching. The proportion of each of these activities performed on a daily basis varies with context, experience and employment position, but it is evident that the role of a registered nurse is always varied, complex and challenging. Although job titles vary between career structures for each state and territory of Australia, registered nurses in the hospital setting engage in activities ranging from ward-based direct patient care (clinical nurse), autonomous clinical practice (nurse practitioner), clinical education and support (educator), unit or ward management (manager), hospital-wide clinical consultation in a specialty field (clinician) to management of a clinical division, stream or functional area within or across an area health service (senior nurse manager). Nurses in the community setting have equally varied activities, often liaising and collaborating with a range of allied health disciplines and managing clients requiring chronic disease and/or health promotion management.[29]

For the newly registered nurse, certain skills have been identified as requiring additional support to improve clinical performance, specifically medication administration, time management, and issues of patient comfort and safety.[32,33] As these issues form part of the everyday work of registered nurses, it is vital that beginning practitioners recognise their personal limitations and seek to improve their performance with experience, reflection and support from colleagues. As newly registered nurses are propelled into the busy and often challenging culture of clinical practice, it is important that they look after their physical and mental health and also take the time to reflect and process events.

WORKLOAD AND TIME MANAGEMENT

Determining the metrics of nursing workload and allocation is a fraught and highly political process, with lower numbers of registered nurses and high workloads linked to adverse patient outcomes.[34] Funding of the acute healthcare sector is based on funding models that may include case-mix information and other funding models.[35] The increasing pressure for financial efficiencies presents significant challenges to the practice of nursing and in recent times there has been a change in the skill mix of nurses, particularly in the acute hospital setting. The strong relationship between nursing care and patient outcomes compels nurses to define, describe, measure and cost the nature of their work and contribution to the healthcare experience.[36]

Measuring nursing activities according to physical needs or the dependency of patients alone can fail to include the assessment and clinical decision-making aspects that lead to the subsequent nursing activity and also the coordination and management of the healthcare team. There is also evidence of poor reliability for a number of common workload measurement methods when compared with observations of actual nursing care.[37] When developing nursing workload measures, tension exists between caring for the patient as an individual and the categorising of patients via mainly physical tasks into dependency (workload) levels. These measures also do not accommodate unanticipated events and the complex psychological and social aspects of nursing care. In spite of these challenges, it is important that nurses work towards developing effective and efficient workload systems, and this is clearly a fertile area for future research.[38]

A number of limitations have been identified when considering the measurement of workload. In particular, the assumption that nursing is a linear activity is incorrect. Nurses commonly perform a number of activities simultaneously and also provide a critical role in the coordination of care. Until recent times, research into the ways in which hospitals work and function has been greatly neglected. One key area of deficit in this knowledge base is the lack of data on the contribution of nursing to patient outcomes as well as measurement of nursing workload. Applying systems developed in non-health-related industries can be challenging due to the unique and dynamic nature of the hospital environment. Monitoring workloads using information systems in conjunction with quality improvement activities may enable the three core elements of quality, skill mix and cost of nursing care to be managed more effectively, and certainly nurses should look to technology and health informatics as enabling features of practice.[39,40]

In recent times the skill mix of staff involved in patient care has been broadened, with increasing numbers of nurse practitioners in extended/advanced nursing practice roles, higher numbers of enrolled nurses (division 2) and assistants in nursing who are unlicensed assistive personnel. Many critical care areas that have been traditionally staffed by registered nurses are now challenged to reconfigure models of nursing care to accommodate this diverse skill mix. An additional challenge facing many clinical areas is an ageing nursing workforce and the increasing need to modify work practices to accommodate these factors.[4,41]

From a beginning practitioner's perspective, managing your workload can be an onerous task, particularly in the early period following registration. Having the ability to determine priorities and to communicate your decisions to patients and your staff colleagues is important, rather than being isolationist in style. Being able to verbalise your rationale for decisions will benefit both you and your team. Never be afraid to seek clarification of or to question clinical treatment plans, and always consider a second opinion if you are not sure about your clinical decision. In addition, be aware of personality issues and your own (mis)perceptions. Sometimes an off-hand remark by a senior member of staff may be related to that individual's own sense of being under pressure and not to your performance. Developing the capacity to perceive, assess and manage the emotions of both yourself and others is useful. The dynamic nature of clinical environments means that your activities and priorities will need to be adaptive and flexible. The next section discusses these issues further.

SETTING PRIORITIES AND PLANNING IN CLINICAL PRACTICE

Effective time management involves prioritising tasks, and this can be a daunting prospect for the novice practitioner dealing with competing demands in a complex environment. Determining priorities should be based on astute clinical assessment of the patient group. It is important to perform this at the beginning of each shift to provide a baseline of patients' clinical progress. This assessment should include a rapid head-to-toe assessment and notation of patients' diagnoses and clinical progress. Continued assessment and subsequent care will be contingent on patient clinical need. Taking time to plan for your shift can increase your efficiency compared with leaping into your work in a reactive way. For example, taking time to assess patency of intravenous lines and chest drains can avoid more dramatic consequences later in the shift. In essence, you need to develop your own risk management plan for your shift. Develop your own system to prioritise your work plan, whether it be a notebook with a checklist or a system as you write your report. Remember that you are part of a team; in spite of your commitment to collegial behaviour, sometimes this may not be evident. For example, a medical practitioner may order a new medication halfway through your shift and neglect to tell you. Regardless of this omission, you as the registered nurse are responsible. Therefore, try to make a point to check with medical staff on changes in care plans, and check at medication times for changes in orders.

To be an effective practitioner it is imperative that you spend some introspective time identifying and evaluating your work style. Are you a person who can deal with multiple and competing tasks simultaneously? Or an individual who needs to identify individual discrete tasks? Recognition of your individual work style is an important strategy in the management of your workload. Identifying time-wasting aspects of your work day is an important component in improving your efficiency. Do you make multiple trips to the treatment room for items? Can you take your time and visualise your equipment needs for clinical activities? Do you attempt to document events in the patient's day directly into the progress notes as they occur? Or do you carry around bits of paper and document events retrospectively at the end of your shift? Observe effective practitioners around you and copy their work styles. Focus on working as a team, rather than as an individual and loose collective of discrete practitioners. Attempt to set goals and priorities for your working day and plan accordingly. At the end of each day, identify the barriers and facilitators to achieving these and modify your work style accordingly. Seek feedback and mentorship from senior colleagues whom you trust. In addition, take the time to quickly look up information related to the pathophysiology and pharmacology of the patients you are caring for. This clinical reflection is not only an important aspect of professional growth but will also rapidly escalate your clinical knowledge and competence.

Many newly graduated nurses need to overcome possible coercion and power relationships that dictate the cultural priorities of showering and bed-making over time taken to assess patients and plan their care for the shift. Despite their best intentions, many new graduates take on existing practices in clinical areas because of power relationships and the potency of the socialisation process. It is important to evaluate all practices critically and strive to ensure that your nursing care meets patient needs rather than individual staff or organisational demands.[42,43]

It is impossible to plan nursing care appropriately without an accurate understanding of patients' diagnoses and management plans, as well as their individual needs for assistance.[44] It is important to ask questions and to look up any unfamiliar diagnoses or related issues. It is fair and reasonable that you demand this time as a beginning-level practitioner. Work more effectively, rather than for longer hours. Refusing to take meal breaks can have counter-effects. Accept help readily, and in turn offer help and assistance to your colleagues.

A review of the Australian healthcare system has identified a need for better coordination of care and the need to monitor patient outcomes.[45] It is essential that these important factors are heeded in order to enable a safe, quality healthcare system. At every level of the organisation, from direct patient caregivers to the director of nursing, there should be identification of your core business as patient care, with a readiness to recognise current practice limitations and seek consultation and assistance for continuously improving clinical practice.

CLINICAL LEARNING AS A LIFELONG PROCESS

As students approach the end of their undergraduate degree and begin their career as a registered nurse, there is often a notion that the learning experience is over. However, this is only a brief interlude in the process of being a lifelong learner.[46] Much of what you will learn about nursing is experiential in the workplace; this learning will differ from your university studies, as it is applied and immediate. The qualities of a lifelong learner include an inquiring mind, a positive self-concept, the ability to establish goals and information literacy. These qualities involve taking in and synthesising information and cues from a variety of sources, including online resources. The internet provides immeasurable opportunities for acquiring information, as well as self-development.

As you enter the workplace, it is important to have a realistic expectation of your abilities, knowledge and limitations. Perhaps the most important lesson for the new graduate is that, despite the fact you are employed as a registered nurse, no one expects you to know everything and therefore you should not expect this of yourself. Become comfortable with asking questions and seeking advice. Embrace all opportunities for learning, including attending multidisciplinary events such as medical grand rounds.

As part of being a nurse professional, there is an expectation that you will strive for self-improvement and enrichment of your nursing knowledge and skills over time and be accountable in your clinical practice and professional development. A considerable amount of information and resources will be supplied in new graduate and preceptorship programs.[47] Yet, as part of professional behaviour, a significant onus remains on the individual to seek out information and knowledge. This is an important behaviour to nurture, not only to increase your competency and proficiency as a nurse clinician, but also to enrich your personal and professional growth.

Therefore, in your beginning years of practice you should take the time to stop and reflect on your day's work and seek clarification of incidents and processes from a senior staff member, your supervisor or mentor. A personal journal is an excellent way to monitor your own progress. It is important not to allow fear and doubt to plague your performance and undermine your confidence. If you feel that your work is dragging you down and you are lacking confidence, seek help from a senior nurse, such as the new graduate program coordinator, earlier rather than later. Like most challenges in life, ignoring these feelings will not make them go away; it is likely they will only get worse and encroach on other dimensions of your life. Also, remember that this is not the first or the last time your senior nurse colleagues will hear this story. It is likely that what you are feeling has been experienced by many before you, even by themselves, and will continue to be experienced by others in the future.

MENTORSHIP AND PRECEPTORSHIP

As well as enhancing their beginning skills through lifelong learning and reflective practice, recent graduates need to engage with effective clinical and professional mentors through their workplace or the various professional colleges or clinical societies. Examples include:

- Australian College of Critical Care Nurses: www.acccn.com.au
- Australian College of Midwives: www.midwives.org.au
- Australasian College of Cardiovascular Nurses: www.acnc.net.au
- Australian Nurse Practitioner Association: www.nursepractitioners.org.au
- Australian Practice Nurses Association: www.apna.asn.au
- Australian and New Zealand College of Mental Health Nurses: www.acmhn.org
- Australian College of Nursing: www.acn.edu.au/
- Sigma Theta Tau International: www.nursingsociety.org

The internet provides an excellent medium for obtaining current information. Many professional organisations have chat rooms and you can subscribe to email updates.

The 'reality shock' experienced by new graduates is well recognised.[48] Models of professional learning support have been incorporated in many institutions to ease this transition process. Professional learning support can be derived in a variety of ways, in both formal and informal contexts. The efficacy of a preceptor–preceptee relationship is largely determined by the calibre and commitment of both parties, enthusiasm, personality, and in particular the motivation of the preceptor in that role. In the clinical setting, conflicting rosters can be a major barrier to communication between the preceptor and preceptee. The role of the preceptor is often envisaged as more of a 'how to' or 'where to find' person. The preceptor generally provides collegial support rather than intense clinical supervision and career direction. In many instances, the new practitioner looks beyond the often prescriptive relationship of preceptorship towards a professional mentor.

As with your university clinical placement, in your role as a registered nurse you will be exposed to a variety of role models, some good, some bad. Reflecting on how people around you manage situations and people can assist you in developing your own practice and management style. Many experienced nurses can identify with a particular mentor who has shaped his or her clinical practice development.[49] Heller and colleagues[50] define the characteristics of a good mentor as an individual who:

■ possesses high integrity, honesty and credibility
■ insists on the highest standards
■ sets an inspirational example
■ insists on getting things done
■ demonstrates the ability to envisage the future
■ shows deep concern for the other's performance.[51]

In many instances you will find your mentor will stay with you in your professional journey. In essence, your mentor should be the person you look at and say, 'that's the type of nurse I want to be'. Importantly, the mentoring relationship will also be a partnership based on collaboration and the development of trust, loyalty and mutual respect. Morton-Cooper and Palmer[52] stress the importance of reciprocity and collaboration in a mentoring relationship and identify the following strategies in attracting a mentor:

■ having a positive attitude to work and career
■ standing out in the crowd
■ being willing to take risks
■ having commitment to your own development
■ being receptive to coaching, advice and support
■ showing initiative and motivation
■ having positive self-esteem
■ demonstrating loyalty to individuals and the organisation.

Not all mentoring relationships are successful, and it is important to recognise early relationships that are disabling and do not promote individual growth (e.g. elitism and mutual seclusion); these can cause the mentee to withdraw from other relationships and become excessively dependent on the mentor.[52] In addition to seeking out a mentor for yourself, you also need to consider how to develop these attributes in yourself as part of your ongoing contribution to the profession of nursing and your personal development. We can guarantee that the years will fly by, and soon you will find yourself in charge of a shift and responsible for the transitional development of newly registered nurses and supervision of enrolled nurses and assistants in nursing.

TAKING CARE OF YOURSELF AND YOUR COLLEAGUES

Stress in the workplace can be distressing for nurses. In order to be an effective role model to our patients and colleagues it is important that we pay attention to the messages we preach and look after our own body and mind. This means taking time to exercise, relax, eat and sleep well, together with ensuring we work in a safe environment. Cognisance of these factors, and looking after ourselves and each other, are important strategies in addressing the nursing shortage[53] and minimising the threat of horizontal violence.[54] In order to ensure that nursing is a dynamic and driving force in health, we need to project, both within and externally to our profession, an image of coherence and solidarity.

MEASURING OUTCOMES OF NURSING CARE

The measurement of nursing interventions and patient outcomes is more relevant than ever; the recent drive for an evidence-based approach to clinical management, and the increased emphasis on nursing as a profession, require a patient-centred focus with an emphasis on improving health outcomes.[55,56] However, it is interesting to note that outcome evaluation was first advocated for nursing as early as the 1860s by Florence Nightingale.[57] Although evaluating care has been integral to nursing practice, contemporary trends in management and evaluation create new dilemmas in the selection of methodological approaches and choice of patient and organisational outcomes.[58] It is often difficult to separate nursing from the inputs of other professional groups, as well as incorporating patients' perspectives. As a result, there is an increasing focus on nurse-sensitive patient outcome indicators and how these contribute to the quality of care.[59]

Measurements assessing both process and outcome measures of nursing care are imperative for the development of nursing practice and justification for the nursing role in an interdisciplinary milieu. The impact of nursing can be evaluated in terms of costs, length of stay, clinical outcomes, and patient and carer satisfaction, although it may be difficult within highly technological environments to measure the separate value of nursing care, particularly using biomedical and economic measures. Thus, mixed-method approaches, using both quantitative and qualitative dimensions, may be useful in determining outcomes.[60]

A mission to ensure the delivery of safe, effective, quality clinical care based on evidence is mandatory in the contemporary clinical environment. Many organisations now focus attention on clinical governance as a means of achieving this aim. Clinical governance is defined as a framework through which health organisations are held accountable for continuously improving the quality of their services and safeguarding high standards of clinical care by creating an environment in which clinical excellence will prosper. Clinical governance refers both to the context and outcomes of clinical activities and, importantly, the involvement of all clinical staff in the monitoring and evaluation process. The necessary framework in which to implement a model of clinical governance comprises three main elements:[61]

- structures to allow monitoring and evaluation
- clear documentation of care processes based on evidence
- organisational support for a culture of evaluation and quality practice.

In such frameworks nursing is considered to be a pivotal element in not only directly facilitating patient care, but also coordinating and monitoring care processes.[62] The importance of interprofessional collaboration and the important role of nurses in directing and coordinating care have led to an increased emphasis on the nursing role.[63] Nurses need to evaluate care, measure patient outcomes, and review their practice within a framework of evidence-based practice.[64,65]

CONCLUSION

Nursing is a complex and multifaceted profession playing a critical role in primary, secondary and tertiary care. Nursing requires engagement not only with the healthcare setting but also often with social and education providers. High-quality nursing care is dependent on fostering a collegial profession based on caring and mentoring of its members as well as an evidence-based approach to providing care. Professional development should be directed to the continual improvement and evaluation of effective clinical practice models, as well as the growth of the nurse as an individual, not only professionally but also personally.

Contemporary healthcare settings present challenges for both recently graduated and experienced nurses in delivering appropriate nursing care in accordance with the best available evidence. This mandate requires the development of flexible, dynamic and eclectic models of care that ensure cost-effective, optimal health–related outcomes for patients. Important in the planning of these services is the implementation of strategies to optimise equity of access for all members of society. Recent graduates need to enhance their beginning skills in lifelong learning and reflective practice, as well as engaging with effective clinical and professional mentors. Additional support for professional growth can be gained through the professional colleges and clinical societies. Taking the time to plan for your professional development and seeking mentorship and support are critical in the period following graduation.

~~~~~~

CASE STUDY 9.1

Robert, who has been a registered nurse for 2 months, has started working the morning shift on a complex medical ward. He has been assigned his patients for the day and is working with another registered nurse, Tiffany. Robert and Tiffany are working as a team, with eight patients allocated to them.

It is morning teatime and Tiffany is taking her break while Robert remains on the ward to care for their patients. Soon after Tiffany leaves, Robert is approached by Dr Scott, who advises him that one of his patients has been prescribed intravenous antibiotics and he wants them administered immediately. Robert commences this task straight away. Just as he does so, he is approached by the daughter of another patient, Mrs Tran. Mrs Tran is an elderly patient who requires assistance with her activities of daily living. Mrs Tran's daughter tells Robert that she has helped her mother to the toilet, and that her mother has had diarrhoea. She needs assistance to clean her mother, she says.

Robert tells Mrs Tran's daughter that he will be able to assist her, once he has completed administering antibiotics to another patient, which is a priority at this point in time, he explains. Robert reassures Mrs Tran's daughter that he will 'clean her [Mrs Tran] up' as soon as he has finished giving the antibiotics.

It is soon apparent to Robert that Mrs Tran's daughter is not satisfied with his response. She insists that her mother needs a shower immediately.

Robert explains again that he will be available as soon as he completes his current task, but the daughter disregards him and commences to shower her mother herself without waiting for Robert's help. She complains loudly, in front of her mother and other patients and visitors, that it is not her job to have to shower her own mother.

Later that day, Mrs Tran's daughter approaches Robert and apologises for her behaviour. She explains that she feels ashamed, as she had embarrassed her mother by her behaviour and humiliated both herself and Robert, which was not her intention. She explains that she acted the way she did out of frustration, as she was going to be late for work if she showered her mother. She is already having difficulties at work due to her frequent absences since her mother became ill, she says.

REFLECTIVE QUESTIONS

1. How should Robert prioritise this situation?
2. How could Robert have managed this situation differently?
3. What other resources could Robert have considered using to support himself and Mrs Tran's daughter?

CASE STUDY 9.2

Today is Louise's fourth day shift of her first rotation as a registered nurse. She has started on a specialised gastroenterology unit. She has been working with the educator and has completed and passed her maths test and been deemed safe to administer medications to patients without supervision.

Following the clinical handover, Louise introduces herself to the four patients she has been allocated. She then commences doing a medication round. Her second patient, Mr Hammond, has a chronic gastrointestinal condition that requires him to have multiple admissions to hospital; he has been a frequent inpatient in this unit in the recent past.

Louise approaches Mr Hammond with his medications. She checks his armband and identifies him as the correct patient. After asking him his name and identifying details, she instructs him to take his medications with a drink.

Mr Hammond asks Louise, 'What are these for?' She feels slightly confronted and fails to respond, as she does not know the answer to the question. Mr Hammond senses Louise's confusion and declines to take his medications.

Louise leaves the patient's bedside and uses a pharmacology text to review the medications Mr Hammond has been prescribed and that she has been instructed to administer. She then returns to Mr Hammond and explains what the medications are for. He says that he feels Louise is not competent enough to give him his medications and continues to refuse them from her.

REFLECTIVE QUESTIONS

1. What should Louise do, and why?
2. What resources may be available to Louise?
3. What are the potential implications if the patient does not take his medications?

CASE STUDY 9.3

Louise speaks to an experienced registered nurse on the ward and Mr Hammond takes his medications from her colleague.

REFLECTIVE QUESTIONS

1. How might Louise approach this situation if it occurred again?
2. What are the rights and responsibilities of the patient?
3. What are the regulatory and legal requirements in this scenario?

RECOMMENDED READING

Aiken LH, Sloane DM, Bruyneel L, Van den Heede K, Sermeus W. Nurses' reports of working conditions and hospital quality of care in 12 countries in Europe. *International Journal of Nursing Studies* 2013;**50**:143–53.

Driscoll A, Currey J, Allen JA, George M, Davidson PM. New cardiac models of care reduce patient access to specialist nurses: a Victorian cross-sectional pilot study. *Australian Critical Care* 2014;**27**:17–27.

Ekström L, Idvall E. Being a team leader: newly registered nurses relate their experiences. *Journal of Nursing Management* 2013; first published online:4 July 2013.

Luckett T, Phillips J, Agar M, Virdun C, Green A, Davidson PM. Elements of effective palliative care models: a rapid review. *BMC Health Services Research* 2014;**14**:1–22.

Sundin K, Fahlen U, Lundgren M, Jacobsson C. Registered nurses' experiences of priorities in surgery care. *Clinical Nursing Research* 2014;**23**:153–70.

REFERENCES

1. Austin JM, D'Andrea G, Birkmeyer JD, Leape LL, Milstein A, Pronovost PJ, et al. Safety in numbers: the development of Leapfrog's composite patient safety score for US Hospitals. *Journal of Patient Safety* 2014;**10**:64–71.
2. Bartz CC. Conceptual explorations on person-centered medicine 2010: International Council of Nurses and person-centered care. *International Journal of Integrated Care* 2010;**10**(Suppl.).
3. Davidson P, Halcomb E, Hickman L, Phillips J, Graham B. Beyond the rhetoric: what do we mean by a 'model of care'? *Australian Journal of Advanced Nursing* 2006;**23**:47–55.
4. Duffield C, Roche M, Diers D, Catling-Paull C, Blay N. Staffing, skill mix and the model of care. *Journal of Clinical Nursing* 2010;**19**:2242–51.

5. Pulcini J, Jelic M, Gul R, Loke AY. An international survey on advanced practice nursing education, practice, and regulation. *Journal of Nursing Scholarship* 2010;**42**:31–9.

6. Middleton S, Gardner G, Gardner A, Della P, Gibb M, Millar L. The first Australian nurse practitioner census: a protocol to guide standardized collection of information about an emergent professional group. *International Journal of Nursing Practice* 2010;**16**:517–24.

7. Considine J, Fielding K. Sustainable workforce reform: case study of Victorian nurse practitioner roles. *Australian Health Review* 2010;**34**:297–303.

8. Halcomb EJ, Davidson PM, Brown N. Uptake of Medicare chronic disease items in Australia by general practice nurses and Aboriginal health workers. *Collegian (Royal College of Nursing, Australia)* 2010;**17**:57–61.

9. George VM, Shocksnider J. Leaders: are you ready for change? The clinical nurse as care coordinator in the new health care system. *Nursing Administration Quarterly* 2014;**38**:78–85.

10. Chan TC, Killeen JP, Vilke GM, Marshall JB, Castillo EM. Effect of mandated nurse–patient ratios on patient wait time and care time in the emergency department. *Academic Emergency Medicine* 2010;**17**:545–52.

11. Sloman JG, Julian D. History of the coronary (cardiac) care unit. In: Thompson PL, editor. *Coronary Care Manual.* 2nd ed. Sydney: Elsevier Australia; 2011.

12. Everett B, Salamonson Y, Rolley JX, Davidson PM. Underestimation of risk perception in patients at risk of heart disease. *European Journal of Cardiovascular Nursing* 2014; published online before print 21 October 2014. doi:10.1177/1474515114556712.

13. Naylor MD, Brooten DA, Campbell RL, Maislin G, McCauley KM, Schwartz JS. Transitional care of older adults hospitalized with heart failure: a randomized, controlled trial. *Journal of the American Geriatrics Society* 2004;**52**:675–84.

14. Rabinowitz T, Murphy KM, Amour JL, Ricci MA, Caputo MP, Newhouse PA. Benefits of a telepsychiatry consultation service for rural nursing home residents. *Telemedicine and e-Health* 2010;**16**:34–40.

15. Rolley JX, Davidson PM, Salamonson Y, Fernandez R, Dennison CR. Review of nursing care for patients undergoing percutaneous coronary intervention: a patient journey approach. *Journal of Clinical Nursing* 2009;**18**:2394–405.

16. Halcomb EJ. Expansion of nursing role in general practice: studies suggest patients think that nurses can manage simple conditions but have some concerns about knowledge and competence in some areas. *Evidence-Based Nursing* 2011;**14**:28–9.

17. Shigaki CL, Moore C, Wakefield B, Campbell J, LeMaster J. Nurse partners in chronic illness care: patients' perceptions and their implications for nursing leadership. *Nursing Administration Quarterly* 2010;**34**:130–40.

18. Meleis AI. *Transitions theory: middle-range and situation-specific theories in nursing research and practice.* New York: Springer Publishing Company; 2010.

19. Krum H, Jelinek M, Stewart S, Sindone A, Atherton J, Hawkes A. Guidelines for the prevention, detection and management of people with chronic heart failure in Australia 2006. *The Medical Journal of Australia* 2006;**185**:549–57.

20. Muzzarelli S, Leibundgut G, Maeder MT, Rickli H, Handschin R, Gutmann M, et al. Predictors of early readmission or death in elderly patients with heart failure. *American Heart Journal* 2010;**160**:308–14.

21. Page K, Marwick TH, Lee R, Grenfell R, Abhayaratna WP, Aggarwal A, et al. A systematic approach to chronic heart failure care: a consensus statement. *The Medical Journal of Australia* 2014;**201**:146–50.

22. Riegel B, Moser DK, Anker SD, Appel LJ, Dunbar SB, Grady KL, et al. State of the science: promoting self-care in persons with heart failure: a scientific statement from the American Heart Association. *Circulation* 2009;**120**:1141–63.

23. Davidson PM, Stewart S. Heart failure nursing in Australia: past, present and future. *Australian Critical Care* 2009;**22**:108–10.

24. Wagner EH, Austin BT, Von Korff M. Organizing care for patients with chronic illness. *The Milbank Quarterly* 1996;511–44.

25. Burton CR, Fisher A, Green TL. The organisational context of nursing care in stroke units: a case study approach. *International Journal of Nursing Studies* 2009;**46**:86–95.

26. Oeseburg B, Wynia K, Middel B, Reijneveld SA. Effects of case management for frail older people or those with chronic illness: a systematic review. *Nursing Research* 2009;**58**:201–10.

27. Sochalski J, Jaarsma T, Krumholz HM, Laramee A, McMurray JJ, Naylor MD, et al. What works in chronic care management: the case of heart failure. *Health Affairs* 2009;**28**:179–89.

28. Rotter T, Kinsman L, James E, Machotta A, Gothe H, Willis J, et al. Clinical pathways: effects on professional practice, patient outcomes, length of stay and hospital costs. *Cochrane Database Systematic Reviews* 2010;**3**.

29. Loeb M, Carusone SC, Goeree R, Walter SD, Brazil K, Krueger P, et al. Effect of a clinical pathway to reduce hospitalizations in nursing home residents with pneumonia: a randomized controlled trial. *Journal of American Medical Association* 2006;**295**:2503–10.

30. Wand T, D'Abrew N, Barnett C, Acret L, White K. Evaluation of a nurse practitioner-led extended hours mental health liaison nurse service based in the emergency department. *Australian Health Review* 2014; published online: 13 November 2014.

31. Beaver K, Williamson S, Chalmers K. Telephone follow-up after treatment for breast cancer: views and experiences of patients and specialist breast care nurses. *Journal of Clinical Nursing* 2010;**19**:2916.

32. Dyess SM, Sherman RO. The first year of practice: new graduate nurses' transition and learning needs. *Journal of Continuing Education in Nursing* 2009;**40**:403–10.

33. Fero LJ, Witsberger CM, Wesmiller SW, Zullo TG, Hoffman LA. Critical thinking ability of new graduate and experienced nurses. *Journal of Advanced Nursing* 2009;**65**:139–48.

34. Aiken LH, Sloane DM, Bruyneel L, Van den Heede K, Griffiths P, Busse R, et al. Nurse staffing and education and hospital mortality in nine European countries: a retrospective observational study. *The Lancet* 2014;**383**:1824–30.

35. Goldfield N. The evolution of diagnosis-related groups (DRGs): from its beginnings in case-mix and resource use theory, to its implementation for payment and now for its current utilization for quality within and outside the hospital. *Quality Management in Healthcare* 2010;**19**:3–16.

36. Lucero RJ, Lake ET, Aiken LH. Nursing care quality and adverse events in US hospitals. *Journal of Clinical Nursing* 2010;**19**:2185–95.

37. De Cordova PB, Lucero RJ, Hyun S, Patricia Quinlan M, Price K, Stone PW. Using the Nursing Interventions Classification as a potential measure of nurse workload. *Journal of Nursing Care Quality* 2010;**25**:39–45.

38. Hoi SY, Ismail N, Ong LC, Kang J. Determining nurse staffing needs: the workload intensity measurement system. *Journal of Nursing Management* 2010;**18**:44–53.

39. Mickan S, Tilson JK, Atherton H, Roberts NW, Heneghan C. Evidence of effectiveness of health care professionals using handheld computers: a scoping review of systematic reviews. *Journal of Medical Internet Research* 2013;**15**.

40. Stevenson JE, Nilsson GC, Petersson GI, Johansson PE. Nurses' experience of using electronic patient records in everyday practice in acute/inpatient ward settings: a literature review. *Health Informatics Journal* 2010;**16**:63–72.

41. Fairbrother G, Jones A, Rivas K. Changing model of nursing care from individual patient allocation to team nursing in the acute inpatient environment. *Contemporary Nurse* 2010;**35**:202–20.

42. Laschinger HKS, Grau AL, Finegan J, Wilk P. New graduate nurses' experiences of bullying and burnout in hospital settings. *Journal of Advanced Nursing* 2010;**66**:2732–42.

43. Rudman A, Gustavsson JP. Early-career burnout among new graduate nurses: a prospective observational study of intra-individual change trajectories. *International Journal of Nursing Studies* 2011;**48**:292–306.

44. Kitson A, Marshall A, Bassett K, Zeitz K. What are the core elements of patient-centred care? A narrative review and synthesis of the literature from health policy, medicine and nursing. *Journal of Advanced Nursing* 2013;**69**:4–15.

45. FitzGerald G, Ashby R. National health and hospital network for Australia's future: implications for emergency medicine. *Emergency Medicine Australasia* 2010;**22**:384–90.

46. Barnard AG, Nash RE, O'Brien M. Information literacy: developing life long skills through nursing education. *Journal of Nursing Education* 2005;**44**:505–10.

47. Whitehead B, Owen P, Holmes D, Beddingham E, Simmons M, Henshaw L, et al. Supporting newly qualified nurses in the UK: a systematic literature review. *Nurse Education Today* 2013;**33**:370–7.

48. Parker V, Giles M, Lantry G, McMillan M. New graduate nurses' experiences in their first year of practice. *Nurse Education Today* 2014;**34**:150–6.

49. McCloughen A, O'Brien L, Jackson D. Esteemed connection: creating a mentoring relationship for nurse leadership. *Nursing Inquiry* 2009;**16**:326–36.

50. Heller R, Eaton JP, Johnson R. *Achieving excellence*. London: DK Publishing (Dorling Kindersley); 1999.

51. Davidson P. Becoming a nurse leader. *Contexts of nursing* 2009;258.

52. Morton-Cooper A, Palmer A. *Mentoring, preceptorship, and clinical supervision: a guide to professional roles in clinical practice*. Oxford, UK: Wiley-Blackwell; 2000.

53. Twigg D, Duffield C, Thompson PL, Rapley P. The impact of nurses on patient morbidity and mortality – the need for a policy change in response to the nursing shortage. *Australian Health Review* 2010;**34**:312–16.

54. Chaboyer W, Najman J, Dunn S. Cohesion among nurses: a comparison of bedside vs. charge nurses' perceptions in Australian hospitals. *Journal of Advanced Nursing* 2001;**35**:526–32.

55. Nakrem S, Vinsnes AG, Harkless GE, Paulsen B, Seim A. Nursing sensitive quality indicators for nursing home care: international review of literature, policy and practice. *International Journal of Nursing Studies* 2009;**46**:848–57.

56. Radwin LE, Cabral HJ, Wilkes G. Relationships between patient-centered cancer nursing interventions and desired health outcomes in the context of the health care system. *Research in Nursing & Health* 2009;**32**:4–17.

57. Munro CL. The 'Lady With the Lamp' illuminates critical care today. *American Journal of Critical Care* 2010;**19**(4):315–17.

58. Griffiths P. RN + RN = better care? What do we know about the association between the number of nurses and patient outcomes? *International Journal of Nursing Studies* 2009;**20**.

59. O'Brien-Pallas L, Li XM, Wang S, Meyer RM, Thomson D. Evaluation of a patient care delivery model: system outcomes in acute cardiac care. *Canadian Journal of Nursing Research* 2010;**42**:98–120.

60. Curry LA, Nembhard IM, Bradley EH. Qualitative and mixed methods provide unique contributions to outcomes research. *Circulation* 2009;**119**:1442–52.

61. McSherry R, Pearce P. *Clinical governance*. Oxford, UK: Wiley-Blackwell; 2010.

62. Sullivan E, Francis K, Hegney D. Review of small rural health services in Victoria: how does the nursing-medical division of labour affect access to emergency care? *Journal of Clinical Nursing* 2008;**17**:1543–52.

63. Jennings N, Clifford S, Fox AR, O'Connell J, Gardner G. The impact of nurse practitioner services on cost, quality of care, satisfaction and waiting times in the emergency department – a systematic review. *International Journal of Nursing Studies* 2014; in press, corrected proof.

64. Considine J, McGillivray B. An evidence-based practice approach to improving nursing care of acute stroke in an Australian Emergency Department. *Journal of Clinical Nursing* 2010;**19**:138–44.

65. Stokke K, Olsen N, Espehaug B, Nortvedt M. Evidence based practice beliefs and implementation among nurses: a cross-sectional study. *BMC Nursing* 2014;**13**:8.

CHAPTER 10

Dealing with ethical issues in nursing practice

Megan-Jane Johnstone and Elizabeth Crock

LEARNING OBJECTIVES

When you have completed this chapter you will be able to:

- distinguish between an ethical issue, a legal issue and a clinical issue
- understand what might count as a moral reason for taking action in work-related settings
- explore the function of a nursing code of ethics
- understand the application of ethical principles and moral rights to and in nursing practice
- appreciate the role and responsibility of nurses in promoting and protecting the significant moral interests of patients in healthcare contexts.

KEYWORDS: ethics, moral rights, moral duties, moral decision making, nursing codes of ethics

INTRODUCTION

Nurses in all areas and levels of practice have to deal with ethical issues every day. Sometimes, the issues encountered are relatively straightforward and easy to deal with. At other times, however, the issues may be extremely complex, perplexing and difficult to resolve. In either case, there is always a risk that an ethical issue may not be handled well and a good moral outcome not achieved. Because of this risk (in addition to other considerations such as the demands of ethical professional conduct generally), it is imperative that all nurses – regardless of their years of experience and areas of practice – are well informed about the kinds of ethical issues that may arise in nursing practice. It is also imperative that nurses have the knowledge, skills and 'right attitude' necessary to be able to respond to the issues at hand in an appropriate, ethically warranted and just manner. These imperatives derive from the agreed professional and ethical standards of conduct of the nursing profession in Australia and New Zealand, which make explicit the requirements that all registered nurses must:

- demonstrate satisfactory knowledge of the ethical responsibilities of nurses as morally accountable practitioners
- practise in accordance with the nursing profession's codes of ethics and conduct
- fulfil their ethical responsibilities in all aspects of nursing practice (including identifying and adhering to strategies that recognise, promote and protect the rights of individuals/groups, and advocating for individuals/groups when their rights are overlooked and/or compromised).[1,2]

The ability of nurses to fulfil their ethical responsibilities as morally accountable practitioners, and to respond effectively and appropriately to ethical issues arising in nursing domains, depends on a number of processes, including the ability of nurses to:

- distinguish between ethical, legal and clinical issues
- discern when it is appropriate and also morally imperative to take action to address an ethical issue encountered in a work-related setting
- respond decisively and in an informed and morally wise way to the question: 'What should I do?'
- justify, in moral terms, the stance and action they ultimately take.

Here a number of questions can be raised:

- What is an ethical issue, and how does an ethical issue differ from a legal issue or clinical issue?
- When is it 'right' – and even morally imperative – for nurses to take action in response to an ethical issue they have encountered?
- What (moral) reasons might nurses provide to justify the decisions they make and the actions they ultimately take in response to the ethical issues they encounter?

Before proceeding, a note of clarification is required on the use of the terms *ethics* and *morality*. Contrary to popular opinion among some nurses, there is no philosophically significant difference between these two terms. As Johnstone[3] has noted, if a distinction is to be drawn between them, it is one that is based on *etymological* grounds (i.e. the study of the origin of words), with 'ethics' coming from the ancient Greek *ethikos* and 'morality' from the Latin *moralitas*. This means that the terms have the same meaning, and thus may be used interchangeably, as they are in this chapter and in the literature on moral philosophy generally. With respect to deciding whether to use 'ethics' or 'morality' when discussing ethical issues in nursing, this is a matter of writing style and personal preference, rather than one of philosophical debate.[3] (For a more in-depth discussion on the nature and meaning of these terms, see Johnstone.[3])

DISTINGUISHING BETWEEN ETHICAL, LEGAL AND CLINICAL ISSUES

When practising in a professional capacity, nurses will encounter a variety of problems and associated issues (such as those described in the case studies presented in this chapter). And while many of these problems and issues may have an ethical dimension, it is not always the case that they are ethical issues per se, requiring a moral solution. In many instances, the problems at hand are principally of a clinical or practical nature, requiring a clinical or practical response. In other instances, they may be of a legal nature, for which a response based on legal considerations is required. Although the ethical, legal and clinical dimensions of nursing practice may, and do, overlap, they are nonetheless grounded in and governed by different concerns. In the interests of promoting accountable and responsible professional nursing practice, care must be taken to distinguish between these dimensions and related concerns.[3] To illustrate this, consider the following three scenarios involving the prescription of analgesia for a patient with an end-stage illness.

SCENARIO 10.1

A nurse discovers that an excessively large intravenous dose of an opiate analgesic has been prescribed by an attending doctor. Based on her knowledge of pain management regimens and a clinical assessment of the patient, the nurse is concerned that if the prescribed dosage is administered as ordered, the consequences to the patient could be dire. (Specifically, it could result in the patient's premature death.) She checks with the prescribing doctor, who confirms, with alarm, that he has made 'a terrible mistake' and corrects the error, thanking the nurse for her vigilance. The nurse subsequently administers the revised dose of analgesia to the patient with no ill effects.

SCENARIO 10.2

A nurse discovers that a large intravenous dose of midazolam (a benzodiazepine) has been prescribed by an attending doctor. Based on her knowledge of pain management regimens and a clinical assessment of the patient, the nurse is concerned that if the prescribed dosage is administered as ordered, the consequences to the patient could be dire. (Specifically, it would result in the patient becoming deeply comatose, possibly risking premature death.) She checks with the prescribing doctor, who acknowledges her concern. He advises her that the medication order 'is correct', that it complies with the accepted standards of palliative sedation, and that the drug is to be given 'as prescribed'. The nurse again questions the drug prescription and indicates she is not willing to administer it. The doctor clarifies that the treatment plan has been 'openly discussed with the patient – who initiated discussion about the plan – and totally accords with both the patient's and her family's expressed wishes'. He reiterates that the prescribed regimen accords with the agreed standards of palliative sedation and then advises the nurse that should she fail to administer the drug as prescribed, he will regard this as being tantamount to her interfering with his treatment plan for the patient.

SCENARIO 10.3

A nurse discovers that an excessively large intravenous dose of an opiate analgesic has been prescribed by an attending doctor. Based on her knowledge of pain management regimens and a clinical assessment of the patient, the nurse is concerned that if the prescribed dosage is administered as ordered, the consequences to the patient could be dire. (Specifically, it would, in all probability, hasten the patient's death.) She checks with the prescribing doctor, who confirms that the medication is to be administered as prescribed and that, even though its administration will probably result in hastening the patient's death, this is not the intended outcome. He explains that the dose prescribed is 'in the best interests of the patient' and is 'necessary to alleviate the patient's pain and suffering'. He further states that the prescription in question is simply 'good medical practice'. The doctor upholds this view despite knowing that the patient has requested 'everything possible be done' to prolong her life and has expressed a preference not to be medicated in a manner that would render her unconscious.

~~~~~~

Here the question can be asked: in which of these three scenarios does the medication order constitute an ethical issue, as opposed to, say, a clinical (practical) issue or a legal issue? In order to answer this question, it is necessary to have some understanding of what an ethical issue looks like. In other words, the characteristics of what constitutes a moral/ethical issue need to be clarified.

The Nature of Ethical Issues

It is generally accepted that a situation involves an ethical issue where it has as its central concern:

- the promotion and protection of people's genuine wellbeing and welfare (including their interest in not suffering unnecessarily)
- responding justly to the genuine needs and significant moral interests of different people
- determining and justifying what constitutes 'right' and 'wrong' conduct in a given situation.[3]

Justifying a moral decision or action, in turn, involves providing the strongest moral reasons behind it. Thus, as Beauchamp and Childress[4] explain, merely providing a list of reasons will not suffice to justify a decision. This is because 'not all reasons are good reasons, and not all good reasons are sufficient for justification'[4] (p 390). For example, a majority public opinion supporting the legalisation of euthanasia may constitute a good reason for decriminalising euthanasia yet stop short of providing a *sufficient* reason for doing so. Other 'good and sufficient' reasons will need to be put forward, including moral arguments both for and against the permissibility of euthanasia and why public opinion per se is not relevant or adequate to justify its legalisation.[3]

Reasons or grounds for justifying a person's moral decisions and actions are generally thought to derive from three key sources: (1) moral rules, principles and theories; (2) lived experience and individual personal judgments; or (3) a synthesis of both these theoretical and experiential approaches.[3] In the case of nursing, reasons may be provided by appealing to: (1) nursing codes of ethics; (2) ethical principles; (3) moral rights; and (4) nurses' lived experiences.[3]

Given the above, it can be seen that where a patient's genuine wellbeing and welfare are at risk, where the significant moral interests of different people (e.g. patients, nurses, doctors) are in competition with each other, and where assistance is required to answer the question 'What should I do?' (i.e. what is the morally right thing to do?), a moral problem/ethical issue exists. This is in contradistinction to, say, a legal problem/issue, where what is at stake is upholding the principles and standards of law and 'doing that which is required by law'. It is also in contradistinction to a clinical (or technical) problem/issue, where what is at stake is upholding agreed clinical principles and standards of practice (e.g. upholding the principles of asepsis and the related standards of aseptic wound care). Some problems/issues may, of course, involve all three of these dimensions – that is, involve a combination of ethical, legal and clinical questions and considerations that, in turn, require a multifaceted response guided by an appeal to the principles and standards pertinent to each of these three dimensions. The outcome of deliberations in these instances will ultimately depend on which of the three domains has the weightier claim.

In all three scenarios above, the consequences to the patient of administering the prescribed medication are potentially dire. In the first scenario, however, although the dire consequences stand to be morally and legally significant in that the patient's genuine welfare and wellbeing are at risk of being adversely affected, the problem of the incorrect dose of medication being prescribed is not an ethical issue as such. A clue to why this is so can be found in the consideration that remedying the problem requires little more than correcting the prescription error and enabling the prescribing doctor to account for his mistake. The need to correct the medication error is beyond dispute; correcting the medication error does not compromise anybody's significant moral interests; and little, if any, assistance is required in deciding whether it is right, all things considered, to correct the incorrect dose that has been prescribed or to justify the ultimate action that is taken to correct the error. In short, the problem requires a practical/technical solution, not a moral one. Thus, in scenario 1, there is no need for the nurse to engage in a robust ethical debate about 'What should I do?'.

In the case of the second scenario, a slightly different situation is involved. The consequences of either administering or not administering the prescribed benzodiazepine to the patient are morally and legally significant in that they stand to make a material difference to the life and wellbeing of the patient. What may be at issue here, however, is the nurse's lack of clinical knowledge about palliative sedation and the accepted standards which must be upheld when prescribing and administering a palliative sedation regimen.[3] In this case, the doctor's prescription complies with the accepted standards of palliative sedation, has been openly discussed with the patient, and accords with both the patient's and her family's expressed wishes. Palliative sedation is increasingly recognised internationally as an 'important therapeutic intervention'[5] and an 'integral part of a medical palliative care approach'.[6] While it would be appropriate for the nurse to make further inquiry and address her qualms about the legality and ethics of palliative sedation, in this instance what is primarily required is for her to update her clinical knowledge about the practice and the accepted standards governing it.

In the case of the third scenario, however, a very different situation is involved. The consequences of administering the prescribed analgesia to the patient are morally and legally significant in that they stand to make a material difference to the life and wellbeing of the patient. Moreover, the medication order in this case is problematic on all legal, moral and clinical grounds.

In relation to the legal considerations, the primary question that needs to be answered is: Is what has been prescribed lawful? In order to answer this question an appeal will need to be made to legal (as opposed to ethical) principles, rules and standards.[3]

In regard to the moral considerations, although the doctor's order, decision and intervention are based on benevolent concerns, he has nonetheless failed to give due consideration to the perspective and expressed wishes of the patient. He has also failed to provide a sound and convincing *moral* justification for his actions.

Finally, regarding the clinical dimension of the case, the doctor's actions are not compliant with agreed clinical standards for end-of-life care – including palliative sedation.

The nurse's responsibility to question the medication orders in each of the cases given is unequivocal: in keeping with the competency standards expected of a registered nurse, the attending nurses in these scenarios have a professional, ethical and legal responsibility to identify and question any order, decision and intervention that they judge, on reasonable grounds, to be questionable or inappropriate. In terms of identifying and responding to the possible ethical problem(s) discerned, the nurses in each of these cases must appeal to ethical principles and standards of practice to justify their actions. In sum, the key to identifying and distinguishing an ethical issue/moral problem, as distinct from a legal or clinical issue/problem, lies in recognising that the situation at hand involves a threat to human welfare and wellbeing (including the interest of persons in not suffering unnecessarily), competing and possibly conflicting interests between different people, and the need for assistance in working through what constitutes the 'right' (good) thing to do in the case at hand. Whereas a legal problem/issue is best resolved by appealing to legal principles, rules and standards of conduct, and a clinical problem by appealing to clinical principles and standards of conduct, ethical problems/issues are primarily resolved by appealing to ethical principles and standards of conduct. Upon identifying a given ethical issue, the task remains of deciding how best to respond to it and, more specifically, to justify the responses made. The remainder of this chapter now turns to consideration of this issue.

TAKING ACTION TO DEAL WITH ETHICAL ISSUES

Are nurses obliged to take action in response to ethical issues encountered during the course of their professional practice? If so, under what conditions might this be so? The short answer to the first question is: yes. Nurses are not only morally obliged to take action in such circumstances, but have a special professional responsibility to do so.[3]

The moral imperative to take action in order to address and remedy a moral problem or ethical issue can derive from a number of sources, including a strong intellectual commitment to upholding given moral standards of conduct and to 'doing one's duty' in the moral sense of the term. However, moral imperatives to act can also derive from moral feelings aroused by such things as a pang of conscience, a sense of justice, the sight of vulnerable people suffering unnecessarily and an associated altruistic desire to prevent or alleviate that suffering.[3,7] For example, a nurse might feel and state: 'I couldn't live with myself if I did nothing to help patient X. Things were going very badly for him; I just couldn't stand by and do nothing. I felt I had to intervene to alleviate his suffering. It would have been wrong not to.' Nevertheless, justifying moral decisions and conduct requires more than an appeal to feelings. Nurses also need to be able to articulate good and sufficient reasons to justify their actions; as noted earlier, this is because 'not all reasons are good reasons, and not all good reasons are sufficient for justification'.[4] What kind of reasons, then, are sufficient for justifying a nurse's moral decisions and actions? What (moral) reasons might nurses provide to justify the moral decisions they make and the actions they ultimately take?

Reasons or justifications for a nurse's actions can be found by appealing to the following: nursing codes of ethics, ethical principles, and moral rights theory. Although there are several other sources that can be appealed to in order to justify moral conduct (see, for example, Johnstone[3]), the sources considered in this chapter are the most common.

Nursing Codes of Ethics

Nursing codes of ethics are regarded as important guides to ethical professional conduct in nursing. Like other codes of professional ethics, a nursing code of ethics may be described as a conventionalised set of moral rules and/or expectations devised for the purpose of guiding ethical professional conduct. Although codes of ethics are not fully developed systematic theories of ethics, they nevertheless tend to reflect a rich set of moral values that have been articulated through a process of extensive consultation, debate, refinement, evaluation and review by practitioners over time.[3,8]

Codes can be either prescriptive or aspirational in nature. In the case of prescriptive codes, provisions are 'duty-directed, stating specific duties of members'.[9] In contrast, aspirational codes are 'virtue-directed, stating desirable aims while acknowledging that in some circumstances conduct short of the ideal may be justified'.[10] Either way, codes of ethics have as their principal concern directing

> ... what professionals ought and ought not to do, how they ought to comport themselves, what they, or the profession as a whole, ought to aim at.[11]

For example, the *Code of Ethics for Nurses in Australia*[12] and the *Code of Conduct for Nurses in Australia*[13] both make explicit:

- the ethical standards that Australian nurses are expected to uphold in the interests of promoting and protecting the moral interests and welfare of patients
- the actions that nurses can expect to be taken against them if they breach the agreed standards.

The Nursing Council of New Zealand's *Code of Conduct*[14] and the New Zealand Nurses Organisation *Code of Ethics*[15] likewise make explicit:

- the ethical values and principles that New Zealand nurses are expected to uphold in the interests of promoting and protecting the moral interests and welfare of health consumers
- the actions that nurses can expect to be taken against them if they breach the agreed standards.

If a nurse breaches the values and standards explicated in the code, this is generally regarded as sufficient grounds for censuring the nurse's conduct such as by formal disciplinary action.[3]

EXERCISE 10.1 Nursing Code of Ethics

This exercise can be carried out either alone or in a group.

1. Depending on your jurisdiction, visit the home page of either the Australian Health Practitioner Regulation Agency (AHPRA), <https://www.ahpra.gov.au/>, and access a copy of the *Code of Ethics for Nurses* (2008) or the home page of the New Zealand Nurses Organisation (NZNO), <www.nzno.org.nz>, and access a copy of the *Code of Ethics* (2010).
2. Discuss the content of the code you have accessed and whether you think it is a 'prescriptive' or an 'aspirational' code.
3. Either way (i.e. whether the code is a prescriptive or aspirational code), discuss how you would apply it in practice.
4. What factors might inhibit applying the code in healthcare domains?
5. What would you do to ensure the code is applied in practice?

Ethical Princiivilism

Ethical princiivilism is the view that the best way of dealing with ethical problems is by appealing to sound moral principles.[3,4] The principles most widely used are those of autonomy, non-maleficence, beneficence and justice, which are commonly discussed and applied in the healthcare professional and bioethics literature.

Autonomy

The principle of autonomy prescribes that people ought to be respected as self-determining choosers and that it is wrong to violate a person's autonomous choices.[3,4] This is so even if we do not agree with another's choices and regard them as foolish, provided they do not interfere with the significant moral interests of others. Accepting this principle imposes on nurses a moral duty to respect patients' choices regarding recommended medical treatment, nursing and other associated care.[16] Further, this duty is binding even if nurses and other attending healthcare professionals do not agree with the choices that patients may and do make.

Non-maleficence

The principle of non-maleficence prescribes: 'Do no harm.'[3,4] Accepting this principle imposes on nurses a stringent duty not to injure patients and to avoid causing them to suffer any otherwise avoidable harm. Harm, in this instance, may be broadly taken as involving the invasion, violation, thwarting or setting back of a person's significant welfare interests to the detriment of that person's wellbeing.[17]

Beneficence

The principle of beneficence entails a positive obligation to 'act for the benefit of others' – that is, to promote their welfare and wellbeing.[3,4] In sum, it prescribes: 'Do good.' Beneficent acts can include such virtuous actions as care, compassion, empathy, sympathy, altruism, kindness, mercy, love, friendship and charity – all of which stand to find ready application in nursing and healthcare contexts.

Justice

The principle of justice can be conceptualised in a variety of ways.[3] However, for the purposes of this discussion it is sufficient to conceptualise justice in the following ways: as fairness (an intuitive sense of justice) and as an equal distribution of benefits and burdens (a rational sense of justice). For example, it might be concluded on the basis of both an intuitive and rational appeal to the principle of justice that it is manifestly unfair and disproportionately (unequally) burdensome to withhold care and treatment from a patient simply because he is over 65 years of age. In this instance, people over the age of 65 years would be arbitrarily forced to carry a burden of suffering associated with the non-treatment of their medical condition that others under 65 years of age with the same medical condition are not forced to bear.

Although ethical principlism is not without its difficulties (e.g. in instances where the respective demands of the different principles conflict, there may be no easy solution), it has increasingly come to replace more classical theoretical approaches to identifying and responding to moral problems in healthcare contexts. Ethical principlism can be especially helpful in providing reasonable standards against which a nurse's conduct can be measured and judged as 'ethically wrong'. For example, if a nurse's conduct fails to respect a patient as an autonomous chooser or results in a patient suffering otherwise avoidable moral harm, on the basis of the principles just described, that nurse's conduct could be judged with justification as being in breach of the standards prescribed by the principles in question (e.g. autonomy and non-maleficence) and therefore as 'morally wrong', all things considered.

Moral Rights Theory

Moral rights theory is also widely regarded as an important guide to ethical professional conduct. A moral right is a special interest that a person may have and which ought to be protected and upheld for moral reasons. Moral rights claims are generally taken as involving correlative duties on the part of others to respect the claims made.[3,4] For example, if a patient makes a genuine rights claim in a given healthcare context (such as the right to be treated with respect), then a nurse – or any other attending healthcare professional – has a corresponding moral duty to act in ways that uphold that right – he or she must act respectfully towards that patient.

Rights claims can be either positive or negative. Positive rights claims generally entail a correlative duty to act or do something. Negative rights claims, in contrast, generally entail a correlative duty to omit or refrain from doing something. For example, if a patient claims a right to be kept free of harm, this imposes a correlative duty on an attending nurse to omit or refrain from behaving in a harmful way towards that patient. Likewise, if a patient claims a right to make informed decisions about his or her care and treatment, this imposes on an attending nurse a positive duty to ensure that the patient receives sufficient information to enable him or her to make an intelligent and prudent choice about recommended nursing care and treatment. This may include facilitating consultations with other members of the healthcare team involved in the overall healthcare of the patient.

Rights that are commonly claimed in healthcare include the rights to healthcare, informed consent, privacy and confidentiality, being treated with respect, cultural liberty, and dignity. (For an in-depth examination of these rights from a nursing perspective, see Johnstone.[3]) These rights are also commonly represented in nursing codes of ethics and codes of professional conduct and are often accompanied by explicit statements emphasising that nurses have both a role and a responsibility in promoting and protecting them.

Although moral rights theory is not without its difficulties (e.g. in instances where equally deserving rights claims might conflict, it may not be possible to satisfy all the claims made), it nevertheless has significant currency in contemporary discussions and debates on ethical issues in healthcare. Furthermore, there is room to suggest that the language of rights has perhaps done more to protect the genuine interests (welfare and wellbeing) of patients in healthcare than any other part of the moral vocabulary at our disposal. An important example of this can be found in the World Health Organization's publication series on health and human rights.[18–21]

Moral rights theory can be especially helpful in providing reliable standards against which a nurse's conduct can be measured and judged as morally right or wrong. For example, if a nurse's conduct violates a patient's moral rights (i.e. a set of special interests which ought to be respected and protected for moral reasons), on the basis of an appeal to moral rights theory, that nurse's conduct could be judged with justification as being unethical ('morally wrong'). In keeping with the agreed nursing standards of ethical professional conduct, the nurse's conduct in this situation would deserve being censured. Conversely, if the nurse's conduct upholds a patient's moral rights, his or her conduct could be systematically appraised as being ethical ('morally right') and, thus, meeting the agreed nursing standards of ethical professional conduct.

EXERCISE 10.2 Considering Other Moral Points of View

Pair with another person to complete this exercise.

1. Person A will tell person B about a moral right that he or she believes is at risk of being violated in healthcare domains. Person A should try to give strongly warranted reasons why the moral right identified should be upheld and protected by nurses. Person B should try to make a considered and non-judgmental response opposing the views person A is expressing. That is, person B should mount a 'counter-argument' to the views expressed by person A.
2. Discuss how you felt about presenting and considering the opposing points of view put forward – especially if you did not agree with them.
3. Person B will then tell person A about a moral right that he or she believes is at risk of being violated in healthcare domains. (This must be a different moral right to the one identified by person A in the first part of the exercise.) Person B should try to give strongly warranted reasons why the moral right identified should be upheld and protected by nurses. Person A should try to make a considered and non-judgmental response opposing the views person B is expressing. That is, person A should mount a 'counter-argument' to the views expressed by person B.
4. Share the differences and similarities between these two experiences (i.e. what it was like considering and countering opposing points of view) and discuss the relevance these may have in terms of informing your capacity to deal with perceived risks to or actual violations of moral rights in healthcare when working within a team.

REVIEW OF SCENARIOS

In light of the discussion so far, it can be seen that all of the clinical scenarios presented in this chapter involve ethical issues. Moreover, each of the cases underscores the importance of moral preparedness and the kind of moral capabilities (knowledge, skills and right attitude) that nurses need to develop if they are to be effective in:

■ promoting and protecting people's significant moral interests (including their interests in not suffering unnecessarily)
■ responding justly to the genuine needs and significant moral interests of different people
■ contributing to the positive project of achieving morally just outcomes in morally problematic situations.

The cases also demonstrate how complex and delicate some ethical issues can be and how achieving a morally just outcome can, at times, be a difficult task. The question of how best to achieve morally just outcomes in the additional case studies presented below is one that you might now like to discuss with others.

CONCLUSION

All nurses in all areas and levels of practice have an obligation to conduct their nursing practice ethically. This includes being morally vigilant with respect to their own nursing practice, and also being alert to the practice of others that may undermine and even violate the significant moral interests of patients. Nurses have a responsibility to ensure that they are educationally prepared to be able to recognise ethical issues in the workplace and to take appropriate action in response to them. Taking appropriate action need not always involve some grandiose plan, however. Appropriate action may involve little more than behaving well towards patients, families and co-workers and reminding others of their role and responsibilities (inherent in the profession's agreed ethical standards of conduct) 'to provide just, compassionate, culturally competent, culturally safe and culturally responsive care to the populations they serve'.[12] This, in turn, includes ensuring that people are not disadvantaged or harmed by being treated differently because of their appearance, language, culture, religion, thinking, beliefs, values, perceptions, age (children and the elderly), sex and gender roles, sexual orientation, national or social origin, economic or political status, physical or mental disability, health status (including HIV status, for example), or other characteristics that may be used by others to nullify or impair the equal enjoyment or exercise of the right to health.[3,18–22]

~~~~~~

CASE STUDY 10.1

Molly is a 29-year-old with advanced cancer. She has decided, in consultation with close family members and friends, that, despite the severity of her illness and its symptoms, she does not want any treatment. To ensure that her wishes are respected if she loses the capacity to make choices and consent to recommended treatments and care, Molly has prepared an advance directive. In her advance directive, she has outlined a comprehensive list of medical treatments and nursing care that she does not want and, if she were competent to decide, would refuse. The healthcare team involved in her care is unanimous that, at the time of preparing her advance directive, Molly was competent to make decisions and 'knew what she was doing'.

You are a community nurse visiting Molly at home and notice with concern the progressive deterioration of her condition. She has noticeable difficulty walking and is at risk of falls. You arrange for her to have a personal alarm system in place, but she refuses any additional support services. She also refuses a range of essential nursing interventions that would help to make her more comfortable, including mouth care for a mouth infection, bowel care for constipation, and wound care for various superficial cuts and abrasions that she sustained following a recent fall and that have become infected. Workers from other services who come in to assist Molly are also becoming increasingly concerned about her condition, and report this to your team.

REFLECTIVE QUESTIONS

1. What are the key ethical issues raised by this case?
2. Should you and the team override or respect Molly's wishes?
3. In either case, what moral reasons would you use to justify your decision?

CASE STUDY 10.2

A newly qualified registered nurse is caring for a young man with a severe infection. Staff are aware that he has a history of injecting drug use, although he seems to be actively trying to address his health problems and has recently made some progress. One afternoon, during visiting hours, the new graduate nurse happens to walk past the young man's room and notices that he and his wife are both injecting drugs in the presence of their 4-year-old child. She discusses reporting them to the local child protection authority but the other nursing and medical staff on the ward are strongly against this on the grounds that the patient is 'a delightful young man' and 'seems to have been doing so well'. Moreover, they do not want him to lose trust in the healthcare system and disengage from health services.

The new graduate nurse anonymously reports the couple to the local child protection agency, without telling any other hospital staff apart from a social worker. Although knowing that her report would probably make the young man's life harder in the short term, she believes strongly that she has an obligation to protect his child from possible harm. She knows that, as a registered nurse, she is required by law to report suspected cases of child abuse or neglect to a child protection authority, but still wonders if she has done the right thing.

REFLECTIVE QUESTIONS

1. Did the new graduate do the 'right thing' in this case?
2. Upon what basis have you made your judgment?
3. Do you think the graduate nurse's action will achieve a morally desirable outcome in this situation?

CASE STUDY 10.3

A white Australian man who had been a soldier and served in Vietnam during the Vietnam War is being cared for on a ward where two nurses from Asian backgrounds are employed. Every time one of the nurses comes into his room, the man becomes very agitated and refuses to have them care for him. On one occasion you overhear the man shout at one of the nurses:

'So, you're my nurse? Well, I don't want you. Don't come near me. Don't come near me. I only want an Australian nurse to take care of me.' On another occasion, you see the man suddenly tip a hot cup of tea over one of the nurses when her back is turned to him.

The nurses confide in you that they 'don't want to make any trouble' and that because of this they have agreed not to report the incident to the nurse unit manager. They further confide in you that they are very upset about the man's behaviour, that it has made them feel 'very bad', and that it is not the first time that a patient has treated them in this manner. They also tell you that some staff have 'laughed about it' and told them: 'If you can't take it, then go back to where you came from.'

REFLECTIVE QUESTIONS

1. What, if any, are the moral issues raised by this case?
2. How would you respond to the issues identified?
3. What are the moral obligations of co-workers in this case?

RECOMMENDED READING

Fry ST, Veatch R, Taylor C. *Case studies in nursing ethics.* 4th ed. Sudbury, MA: Jones and Bartlett Learning; 2011.

Johnstone MJ. *Bioethics: a nursing perspective.* 6th ed. Sydney: Elsevier Australia; 2016.

Kerridge I, Lowe M, Stewart C. *Ethics and law for the health professions.* Annandale, NSW: Federation Press; 2013.

Nursing Ethics: an International Journal for Health Care Professionals (Sage Publications).

Staunton PJ, Chiarella M. *Law for nurses and midwives.* 7th ed. Sydney: Elsevier Australia; 2013.

REFERENCES

1. Nursing and Midwifery Board of Australia (NMBA). *National competency standards for the registered nurse.* Canberra: Nursing and Midwifery Board of Australia; 2006. Online. Available: <www.nursingmidwiferyboard.gov.au/Codes-Guidelines-Statements/Codes-Guidelines.aspx> [Viewed 8 July 2014].
2. Nursing Council of New Zealand. *Competencies for registered nurses.* Wellington: Nursing Council of New Zealand; 2012. Online. Available: <www.nursingcouncil.org.nz/Publications/Standards-and-guidelines-for-nurses> [Viewed 8 July 2014].
3. Johnstone MJ. *Bioethics: a nursing perspective.* 6th ed. Sydney: Elsevier Australia; 2016.
4. Beauchamp TL, Childress JF. *Principles of biomedical ethics.* 7th ed. New York: Oxford University Press; 2013.
5. Bruera E. Palliative sedation: when and how? *Journal of Clinical Oncology* 2012;**30**(12):1258–9.
6. Maltoni M, Scarpi E, Nanni O. Palliative sedation in end-of-life care. *Current Opinion in Oncology* 2013;**25**(4):360–7.
7. Staunton PJ, Chiarella M. *Law for nurses and midwives.* 7th ed. Sydney: Elsevier Australia; 2013.
8. Johnstone MJ, editor. Nursing ethics. In: *Developing theoretical foundations for modern nursing ethics,* vol. I. Oxford, UK: Sage Publications; 2016.

9. Skene L. A legal perspective on codes of ethics. In: Coady M, Bloch S, editors. *Codes of ethics and the professions.* Melbourne: Melbourne University Press; 1996.

10. Johnstone MJ. A reappraisal of everyday nursing ethics: new directions for the 21st century. In: Daly J, Speedy S, Jackson D, editors. *Contexts of nursing: an introduction.* 4th ed. Sydney: Elsevier; 2014. pp 157–66.

11. Lichtenberg J. What are codes of ethics for? In: Coady M, Bloch S, editors. *Codes of ethics and the professions.* Melbourne: Melbourne University Press; 1996.

12. Nursing and Midwifery Board of Australia (NMBA). *Code of ethics for nurses in Australia.* Canberra: Nursing and Midwifery Board of Australia; 2008. Online. Available: <www.nursingmidwiferyboard.gov.au/Codes-Guidelines-Statements/Codes-Guidelines.aspx> [Viewed 8 July 2014].

13. Nursing and Midwifery Board of Australia (NMBA). *Code of conduct for nurses in Australia.* Canberra: Nursing and Midwifery Board of Australia; 2008. Online. Available: <www.nursingmidwiferyboard.gov.au/Codes-Guidelines-Statements/Codes-Guidelines.aspx> [Viewed 8 July 2014].

14. Nursing Council of New Zealand. *Code of conduct for nurses.* Wellington: Nursing Council of New Zealand; 2012. Online. Available: <www.nursingcouncil.org.nz/Publications/Standards-and-guidelines-for-nurses> [Viewed 8 July 2014].

15. New Zealand Nurses Organisation. *Code of ethics.* Auckland: NZNO; 2010. Online. Available: <https://www.google.com.au/?gws_rd=ssl#q=New+Zealand+Nurses+Organisation+(2010)%2C+Code+of+Ethics> [Viewed 8 July 2014].

16. Case study: competent refusal of nursing care (with commentaries by Dudzinski & Shannon 2006; Tong 2006). *Hastings Center Report* 2006;**36**:14–15.

17. Feinberg J. *Harm to others: the moral limits of the criminal law.* New York: Oxford University Press; 1984.

18. World Health Organization (WHO). *25 questions and answers on health and human rights.* Health & Human Rights Publication Series, Issue No. 1. Geneva: WHO Press; 2002.

19. World Health Organization (WHO). *WHO's contribution to the world conference against racism, racial discrimination, xenophobia and related intolerance.* Health & Human Rights Publication Series, Issue No. 2. Geneva: WHO Press; 2001.

20. World Health Organization (WHO). *International migration, health and human rights.* Health & Human Rights Publication Series, Issue No. 4. Geneva: WHO Press; 2003.

21. World Health Organization (WHO). *Human rights, health and poverty reduction strategies.* Health & Human Rights Publication Series, Issue No. 5. Geneva: WHO Press; 2005.

22. United Nations Development Programme (UNDP). *Human Development Report 2004: Cultural diversity in today's diverse world.* New York: UNDP; 2004.

CHAPTER 11

Communication for effective nursing

Jane Stein-Parbury

LEARNING OBJECTIVES

When you have completed this chapter you will be able to:

- appreciate the importance of nurse–patient communication in establishing therapeutic relationships with patients
- relate the principles of patient-centred communication to therapeutic interactions
- appreciate that communication competence involves both assertive and responsive skills
- understand key factors that affect communication in nursing practice, especially in relation to cultural competence
- differentiate between the intentions of facilitative and authoritative communication.

KEYWORDS: patient-centred communication, therapeutic nurse–patient communication, communication competence, facilitative communication, authoritative communication, communication in nursing practice

INTRODUCTION

Human communication is a complex process that involves the exchange of ideas, thoughts and feelings, and people communicate continuously through verbal, non-verbal and behavioural means. It is important that nurses appreciate the importance of effective communication in nursing practice, especially in relation to its purpose and function in their interactions with patients.

Effective communication in nursing practice involves an ability to understand patients' personal and idiosyncratic experiences of health and illness, to relay meaningful information to patients that promotes their wellbeing, and to provide patients with an opportunity to participate in their care to the extent that they desire. That is, communication with patients is always focused on the patient. This is a feature that distinguishes effective communication with patients from everyday conversational communication in which the needs of both parties are being met. The needs and desires of patients are what drive nursing communication.

COMMUNICATION IN NURSING PRACTICE

The purpose and function of patient communication in nursing centre on the need to establish therapeutic relationships. An effective therapeutic relationship is characteristically caring, supportive and accepting, and offers reassurance to patients that they are safe.[1] These types of relationships are ones that are helpful in meeting the needs of the patient. Communication in nursing practice serves a vital function in the building of therapeutic relationships with patients. Taking time to listen to and understand patients' experiences conveys a message that the patient matters as a person. This, in turn, results in patients feeling cared for and respected – essential aspects of a helping relationship. Such a relationship is one in which the intent of one person, the nurse, is to assist the other, the patient, by promoting that individual's growth, wellbeing and more functional use of his or her own resources.[2]

It is often assumed that therapeutic relationships need a great deal of time in order to develop in a deep and meaningful way: this is not the case. The relationship can develop with few patient–nurse interactions and in a short period of time.[3] This is because it is the level of vulnerability and dependency of the patient that determines the depth of interpersonal involvement between patient and nurse, not the amount of time spent together.[4-6] The nurse's response to reduce this vulnerability by meeting the patient's needs and providing helpful resources will determine whether a meaningful interpersonal connection is established.

Patients do express a desire to connect interpersonally with nurses, but they are often reluctant to do so because nurses seem too busy and patients do not want to bother them.[7-9] Patients' experiences with nurses' communication reveals that nurses focus more on tasks than on communicating with them.[9] This suggests that not much has changed since Menzies[10] first described how a task-oriented approach to care functioned to protect nurses from the anxiety they might experience when dealing with patient distress. In other words, the needs of the nurse (e.g. completing tasks in a timely fashion), not the patient (e.g. wanting to discuss their concerns with the nurse), remain at the centre of care. It seems that healthcare institutions still do not have systems and practices that demonstrate the core values of patient-centred care.

This may be due to a lack of recognition that the effort involved in relating to patients goes largely unrecognised in current healthcare.[11] Simply put, establishing and maintaining therapeutic relationships with patients is not seen as work. However, knowledge gained about the patient through interpersonal communication and relationship building is central to nursing work because 'knowing the patient' is necessary for patient safety and quality care.[12,13]

Because the interpersonal relational aspects of nursing practice help to construct a professional identity[14] and relational work is grounded in a moral commitment to patients,[15] there is good reason to uphold the value of therapeutic relationships as beginning nurses struggle to adapt to healthcare systems. The development of these relationships is best promoted through the use of patient-centred communication, which is the foundation of patient-centred care.

EXERCISE 11.1 Patient-centred Care

This exercise can be carried out alone but is better done in a discussion group.

1. What is your understanding of patient-centred care?
2. What factors in your workplace facilitate this type of care? What factors are barriers?
3. What can you do to foster the facilitating factors and lessen the barriers?

Patient-centred Communication and Care

Patient-centred communication allows patients to have influence over and input into their healthcare.[16] This involves true dialogue and give and take between nurse and patient, in contrast to telling the patient what to do and expecting compliance or obedience. Patient-centred communication is at the heart of patient-centred care, which is a widely used concept in contemporary healthcare.[17]

The essence of patient-centred care is the recognition of patients as unique beings and requires the nurse to listen to and get to know the patient as a person and to work in a collaborative way with them.[18] A common misconception is that patient-centred care is simply individualised care. While the concept of being patient-centred does involve care that is tailored to the patient, it also includes the promotion of active patient participation[19] and the formation of a therapeutic relationship.[20] Each of these components involves interpersonal communication between nurse and patient. A patient-centred approach to care focuses nurses away from a task orientation and turns their attention to the values and needs of individual patients. A nursing interpretation of patient-centred care includes encouraging patient autonomy, having a caring attitude and individualising care; more importantly, it involves communicating with the patient as a person with unique perspectives and respecting their values.[21] Patient-centred care places communicating with and relating to patients at the heart of nursing practice.

As you enter into professional nursing practice your biggest challenge in communicating with patients may be working in a system that is not patient-centred. Consider the following scenario.

SCENARIO 11.1

Maria was almost as frightened as her 17-year-old son, Steve, when she walked into the emergency department (ED) with him. Steve was suffering from delusional thinking, sleep deprivation and extreme anxiety as a result of drugs he had taken at a party. In the car on the way to the hospital Maria promised Steve that she would stay with him at the hospital, as he was extremely fearful. Because she had called the nurse practitioner in the ED prior to their arrival, Maria was not prepared for the 'red tape' they encountered on arriving in the ED.

When they entered, the triage nurse informed Maria that she must see the clerk first and instructed her to go through a door to her left. She directed Steve down the hall. He looked very anxious, and Maria told the nurse that she would not leave her son, who was very sick and scared, she said. The triage nurse insisted that Maria would need to see the clerk to initiate the paperwork required to process Steve through the ED. When Maria insisted on staying with her son, she could see that the nurse was perturbed.

~~~~~~

This is a rather extreme example of communication that is systems-focused instead of patient-focused. The triage nurse in this scenario may not have even realised this, as she thought she was offering a service to this mother and son. She may not have intended to focus on the task rather than the patient, but this is exactly what happened.

Had Maria followed the nurse's instructions, in all likelihood her son would have become more frightened, even panicked. The nurse's action distanced her from Maria by focusing on making the system work, rather than considering the needs of the individual patient.

It may be challenging for nurses who are new to healthcare systems to stay focused on the patient, rather than on the requirements of the system – for example, to complete tasks at a specified time. The demands of contemporary healthcare systems can distract nurses from interacting with patients.[22,23] Sadly, the work of the nurse is often carried out in a routine and bureaucratic manner that is at odds with a patient-centred approach.[24]

Maintaining a calm demeanour communicates to patients that there is time to communicate. When nurses appear rushed, patients are reluctant to communicate. In these instances, it is the nurses' needs, not the patients', which are being met. Being patient-centred when communicating with patients means that the personal experiences of patients, their desires, values and lifestyle, are the focus of interpersonal interactions.

What difference does a patient-centred approach make for patients? Research demonstrates that when nurses are not rushed and make the time to get to know patients through communicating and relating, patients are more satisfied with their healthcare.[13,25] Once believed to be a proxy measure of quality healthcare, there is now evidence that patient satisfaction – that is, a constructive experience with a healthcare system – is positively associated with both patient safety and clinical quality.[13] Included in the patient experience are functional elements in relation to physical care, timeliness of care, and coordination and continuity of care. In addition, there are relational elements such as participation in decision making, involving families, and providing information that is tailored to the patients' needs. Therefore, attending to both the relational elements through good communication and functional elements through the provision of direct care is what is meant by patient-centred care. It is not just patient satisfaction that is enhanced with the use of patient-centred communication and care. There is evidence to suggest that it reduces patient vulnerability, and improves illness self-management, treatment adherence and health outcomes.[18,21,22,26,27]

EXERCISE 11.2 Becoming Patient-centred

The next time you conduct an initial assessment with a patient, try having the patient take the lead by letting her tell her story before you ask any questions. Save any questions until after the patient has finished with their story. Follow the lead of the patient and make sure that you clarify what they say.

1. How long did the assessment take?
2. What kind of information did you gather? Was it different from typical patient assessments that you have conducted in the past? How so?
3. What difference does it make to let the patient take the lead in an interview?

COMMUNICATION COMPETENCE

By now you will have had some experience of communicating with and relating to patients, but you may not yet feel competent in doing so. You may feel inadequate and poorly prepared for the challenges of communication. You are not alone. In a study focused on difficult communication,[28] nurses spontaneously revealed that they felt their educational program did not adequately prepare them in relation to communication challenges such as dealing with angry patients. Through experience gained in interacting with patients you will have many opportunities to develop into a competent communicator.

Competent communicators are skilled at listening to other people with understanding (i.e. they are responsive) and able to express their own ideas clearly (i.e. they are assertive). Research has demonstrated that nurses are often passive, compromising and accommodating of others, rather than being assertive.[29,30] Most likely this is due to their education, which focuses on understanding and meeting the needs of patients. In addition, it could be that nurses do not perceive being assertive as compatible with being a caring person. Another study[31] concluded that caring behaviour and assertiveness are not incompatible. For example, when advocating for patients – a caring behaviour – nurses need to be able to articulate their views clearly and assertively.

Communication competence is not an end-point but rather a continuous process of reflection and deepening self-awareness. Competent communicators may make mistakes in their interactions with patients, but the difference between them and those nurses who are not competent is that competent communicators recognise errors and contemplate how to address similar situations in the future. Reflecting on experiences with patients is necessary because developing communication skills in nursing involves continuous learning throughout your career.

FACTORS THAT IMPACT ON COMMUNICATION EFFECTIVENESS

The most important contribution you can make to the development of professional communication strategies is to improve self-awareness and practise communication approaches that are known to be effective. To improve communication with patients, you should consider the following issues: cultural competence/understanding; clinical context; dealing with emotions; and metacommunication.

Cultural Competence

Most people hold preconceptions about others: sometimes these are positive and sometimes they are negative. Many people have beliefs about nurses: who they are, what they do, what they should be like. Nurses are likely to hold preconceptions about some types of patients. Categorising people in this way leads to the formation of stereotypes in which all members of a particular group are perceived to possess the same personal characteristics. Common stereotypes are associated with gender, apparent ethnicity, socioeconomic class and sexual orientation. In fact, patients may hold a stereotype that all nurses are kind, caring and compassionate.

All too often, stereotypes are based on the ethnicity of a particular group of people, assuming that all people of a particular ethnic background share the same values, beliefs and cultural mores. Stereotyping is based on a superficial understanding of another's culture. This can be dangerous for effective communication because stereotypes lead to assumptions about people that are often misguided. When acted upon, stereotypes interfere with culturally competent communication and may even be harmful to both the patient and the relationship.

Culturally competent care involves an understanding that people come from diverse backgrounds and may not share the same value and belief systems. It also includes an appreciation of an individual patient's cultural belief systems and values and awareness that there is much diversity within a cultural group.[32] An essential aspect of cultural competence also includes communication and care that is 'safe' in a cultural sense. The concept of 'cultural safety' has been developed from a nursing perspective because patient safety is always at the forefront of practice.[33] Culturally safe practice includes both sensitivity to patient values and beliefs, and an appreciation that social structures, such as healthcare institutions, are disempowering to certain cultural groups, thus creating disadvantage to these groups.[34-36]

Cultural competence essentially relates to the ability to respect other people's way of being and their personal value systems. In this sense, cultural competence is embedded in professional codes of conduct. But there is a danger in thinking that it means that all patients are treated the same. This 'one size fits all' approach to cultural care can be detrimental to good patient care. For example, when considering what a patient desires in the way of healthcare, nurses might consult with just the patient as a singular identity. This is based on the notion that adults are autonomous individuals who can make decisions on their own behalf. However, there are cultures in which individuality is not stressed and identity is collective; that is, decisions are based on what is best for a community of people as the individual is not the most important social unit. This might be difficult for nurses to understand if they have been imbued with the Western notion of personal autonomy.

So, how do nurses become more culturally competent? First, it is important that nurses recognise that *culture* is not the same as *ethnicity*. Ethnicity is biologically determined, while 'culture' refers to a shared worldview, expressed through values, beliefs and customs that are learnt through interaction within a social group. Individual families have a culture, as do schools of nursing and healthcare institutions. 'Culture' refers to values, beliefs and ways of behaving that are shared among a group of people.

The next step in becoming culturally competent is for nurses to understand their own values and beliefs, and this is accomplished through the process of reflection. Not only do individual nurses have their own culture, but there is also a culture within healthcare systems. For example, within the Western world the dominant view of health and illness is through a biomedical lens. This view may not accommodate other ways of knowing and being. For example, many Indigenous Australians hold the belief that illness is the expression of a lack of harmony and continuity, and that healing occurs through social and environmental integration.[37] Understanding cultural systems is achieved by listening and learning about patients' values and beliefs by communicating with them, and by remaining open to views that are different from the nurse's own values. Allowing patients to define who they are and to speak for themselves is part of the communication process involved in becoming culturally competent.

Another approach is to study and learn about the social mores, behavioural patterns and beliefs of other cultures. This is especially needed when nurses are consistently working with people from cultures other than their own. For example, looking someone in the eye, considered to be a sign of honesty in Anglo culture, is considered rude in some other cultures, especially if there is a social status difference between people. Learning the specifics of certain cultures carries a risk, because this approach can lead to superficial understanding based on cultural stereotypes and ignores the reality that there can be as much diversity within a given cultural group as there is between cultural groups. For these reasons, this approach is considered problematic and old-fashioned.[35]

A better approach to achieving cultural competence is through the development of what is termed 'cultural humility'.[38] Cultural humility in healthcare involves nurses understanding not only their own cultural system, but also that of the healthcare system in which they work. In doing so, they will come to appreciate that patients should not be judged in relation to these systems. Rather, they will communicate with patients in order to understand the patients' cultural interpretations and belief systems.[39]

The Importance of Clinical Context

Different clinical contexts will demand different types of interpersonal skills, and competent communication in one clinical context may not translate to competence in another. For example, patients in emergency departments have heightened needs for information and explanations about what is happening to them, while people in a palliative care unit may have higher needs for comfort and understanding, rather than information. Nurses working in mental health settings need advanced skills in counselling and psychotherapeutic techniques, while nurses in intensive care units are served well if they know how to ask specific closed questions of patients (i.e. questions that require 'yes/no' answers), as communication may be limited to that style of interaction when patients are mechanically ventilated. It is useful to contemplate the specific types of communication that are most frequently called for in your chosen clinical context.

Dealing with Emotions

One ongoing challenge for nurses is a commitment to broaden and deepen their communication repertoire. Students enter nursing courses with communicative abilities that are likely to mirror those of the public at large. In his focus on the significance of emotion in human communication, Goleman[40] outlines three prevalent non-productive communication styles: (1) ignoring or trivialising another person's feelings; (2) noticing feelings of distress, but aiming to soothe, placate or cover them over; and (3) recognising feelings, but putting down or disapproving of the person due to the belief that certain emotions are unacceptable. If these styles of interaction are retained in nursing practice, then some patients will not be treated with the respect and dignity demanded by professional codes of conduct. In other words, such commonplace approaches demean the patient's feelings, constitute a barrier to effective communication and are unprofessional.

As well as stereotyping, ignoring or trivialising feelings and expressing disapproval, there are other messages that nurses may convey that are incongruent with holistic patient care which values people's social, spiritual, cultural and emotional concerns. Such possibilities include the use of clichés, false reassurance and suddenly changing the subject.[41] Clichés punctuate everyday conversation, but statements like 'Keep your chin up' are unhelpful in most health settings. Similarly, ritual statements of reassurance such as 'You'll be OK', regardless of pain or prognosis, also are not helpful or therapeutic. Abruptly changing the subject from a patient-initiated concern to something nurse-centred or technical is frequently experienced by the patient as belittling or dismissive.

Metacommunication

Metacommunication relates to any factors that affect one person's interpretation of another person's communication. The context of the message, as well as verbal and non-verbal actions, impinges on the content and potential meaning in the message and on the listener's understanding of what has been heard.

Effective communicators have qualities in common that distinguish them from less successful communicators. These include a high degree of self-awareness, an appreciation for the views of other people, congruence between what they say and what they do, the use of clear messages, and an ability to evaluate the other person's needs and to grasp the main points. These are all essential aspects of a nurse's professional communication responsibilities.

The language spoken, the patient's state of illness/health, expectations, gender and age are factors that affect the sending of messages and their interpretation. Timing is another crucial ingredient. In professional relationships the nurse must assess the patient for readiness to understand information provided or to answer probing questions.[42] Patients who are disoriented, in the recovery room, in pain, have just received a terminal diagnosis or are in an emergency are not candidates for communicating much beyond support and essential information. As nurses often work with patients in these circumstances, the nurse must judge what information has to be conveyed immediately and what should remain for discussion when the patient is in less pain or is more fully alert after surgery or an emergency.

Non-verbal communication is often called body language. Body language relates to the messages that individuals convey by the way their whole body moves, and includes posture, movements, gestures and facial expressions. Assessment of patients' non-verbal communication is often central to recovery. Nurses can observe and recognise patient actions, facial expressions or topic avoidance that indicate they have unspoken health concerns. Patients also assess nurses' non-verbal communications by picking up on incongruities between what the nurse says and how it is being said. Interpretation of non-verbal communication has the potential to be wrong, so it is essential that nurses reflect on their observations and clarify their concerns with the patient.

THERAPEUTIC NURSE–PATIENT COMMUNICATION

Therapeutic communication is oriented towards the patient and his or her healing needs. John Heron[43] provides a useful schema for understanding therapeutic communication techniques. The schema is based on therapeutic intention and has two main categories: facilitative and authoritative. Facilitative interventions build relationships and encourage patients to express themselves, while authoritative interventions are instrumental, such as offering explanations, advice and information.

Facilitative Communication

Facilitative communication is helpful in and of itself, and constitutes the building blocks for a helping relationship between the nurse and the patient. In this type of communication, process is as important as content. This means that *how* you go about speaking and listening is crucial for the patient's recovery and wellbeing. Process relates more closely to non-verbal communication.[41] Some of the main elements of facilitative communication are active listening, sharing observations, questioning (open-ended, closed and focused), clarifying, paraphrasing and the use of silence.

Active listening

In the everyday world, many people only partially listen to others, and they may not notice non-verbal indicators of discomfort, distress or distance. Nurses are therefore professionally obliged to continue to improve both listening and observation capabilities. Within most complex nurse–patient interactions, listening is more powerful than speaking, and the non-verbal behaviours of listening, showing interest and conveying warmth are positively associated with patient satisfaction.[44] Listening actively is 'listening for understanding' and requires that the nurse be fully present and attentive to the patient.[36] Listening is characteristically associated with silence, concentration and astute observation, especially of non-verbal communication.[45] The nurse listens not only for facts, but also for the attached values, attitudes and feelings. Enhancement of these skills requires ongoing commitment, practice, reflection, perseverance and self-teaching.

One of the most important aspects of listening involves the observation of patient cues, which are indirect messages that express a need, desire or feeling. They often take the form of an implied question, or a hint or suggestion. They are important in relation to communication because patients often convey their concerns indirectly, especially in relation to their emotional needs.[46] The most helpful response to a patient cue is active exploration of what it means and an open invitation for the patient to say more. The evidence indicates that nurses are more likely to respond to patient cues with distancing and avoiding rather than acknowledging and exploring the cues.[46,47] While cues can be explored through direct questioning, it is also helpful to share what you have observed with the patient.

EXERCISE 11.3 Listening

Pair with another person to complete the exercise.

1. Person A will tell person B about his or her most memorable recent experience. Person B should try to think about a personal problem, or a workplace issue, while person A is speaking.
2. Discuss how you felt about both roles and experiences, with person A speaking first.
3. Person A then tells the same story again, taking about the same length of time. This time person B will concentrate as much as possible on person A and on what person A is saying.
4. Share the differences between these two experiences and discuss the relevance this may have when person A is a patient and person B is a nurse.

Sharing observations

Reflecting back what the nurse observes is a communication response to a patient who has provided information with unclear emotional or social connotations. The nurse first creates a trusting connection with the person that enables that individual to express his or her feelings[42] by making an observational comment such as: 'It seems like you've had a difficult time ...' Such a statement shows an interest in and understanding of the patient's situation. At other times a patient might imply the presence of strong feelings; in this instance the nurse might respond by saying, 'Many people would be angry if that happened to them.' This is not easy and requires the nurse to concentrate on the patient and gain some certainty about the nature of the feeling being conveyed before naming it. The naming of feelings often normalises them – that is, it allows the patient to know that others are also upset by such experiences. The apt and well-timed naming of feelings can create a sense of relief and understanding about what has been bothering the patient.

Open-ended questioning

Once rapport with a patient is developed, open questions are the most effective way of gaining information to complete ongoing holistic nursing assessment. Open-ended questions begin with phrases like: 'Can you tell me about ...?', 'Would you try to explain ...?', 'How do you feel about ...?' These questions give patients permission to talk about what is bothering them and to speak of anything that they consider important. A good example of an open-ended question that can be used to start a conversation is: 'Would you like to tell me more about yourself?' Open-ended questions are well suited to exploring emotional cues or unexpressed healing or health concerns.

Closed questioning

A closed question is one that requires a short answer, often just 'yes' or 'no'. This style of asking questions is best suited to situations where you need to gain a simple, straightforward answer. For example, asking a patient: 'Are you allergic to any medication?' is an appropriate use of closed questioning. This type of questioning is instrumental and time-saving. If used inappropriately, it is likely to bring a conversation to a sudden halt.

Focused questioning

This type of questioning focuses on a specific topic on which the nurse wants more information. The topic is focused or narrow, but the response is intended to elaborate on something and is therefore longer than one word. Nursing examples of this type of questioning include: 'Will you describe the pain to me?' and 'What drew your attention to this problem?'

Clarifying

It is important that nurses clarify a patient's vague or implied communication, a cue, as failure to do so may result in lack of important information being conveyed. If a patient speaks of pain, for example, it is essential for nursing assessment purposes that the patient describes the pain location and qualities in detail. When listening to a patient it is important that the nurse clarifies the main points that the patient is trying to convey. To ensure that this is so, the nurse can use questioning to request that the patient expand or explain the message. Alternatively, the nurse can use restatement to clarify meaning. Clarification can also be sought through the use of a statement such as: 'I'm not sure I follow you' or 'That's not clear to me.'[42] Most importantly, it is dangerous to pretend that you understand and not to seek clarification.

Paraphrasing

Paraphrasing is often used to confirm with patients the meaning of their message, before the exchange goes much further. It involves using your own words to pull together the key points the patient has made. Paraphrasing often begins with something like, 'Tell me if I've got this right' and continues with a short restatement of what you have understood the patient has said. 'Simple, precise, and culturally relevant terms' are used.[41] Paraphrasing is a very important communication technique for use face-to-face and on the telephone to ensure that you have understood what the person is saying and to give the respondent the opportunity to alter your interpretation if it is not what that person meant.

Silence

Many patients feel scared and alone in hospital, as it is an alien environment for them and they inevitably have concerns and worries about their diagnosis, treatment or future health.

When the nurse is attending a patient in hospital, the experience of the patient can suddenly change from boredom, sleep or pain to multiple actions and words. Hence, it is unusual from a patient's perspective to have a nurse just sit with the patient, a nurse who is not carrying out any procedure, and who is not giving instructions or asking questions. Silence can emphasise a particular point that either the patient or the nurse has made, or convey its seriousness. Some silences are better left as they begin – without words. If the patient is trying to talk about complex matters and is searching for words, silence on the nurse's part shows respect and the recognition that this is not an everyday conversation topic. Sitting quietly with a patient, even for a brief period, shows concern, caring and empathy. Such a silence is accepting, validating and therapeutic.

AUTHORITATIVE COMMUNICATION

Much communication between nurses and patients in busy hospital settings is not therapeutic in its own right. Some communication with patients is primarily social rather than facilitative, in that it is spontaneous and not goal-directed. Other communication is instrumental; that is, the communication aims to get something done. Instrumental communication is authoritative in the sense that the nurse takes the lead. In this type of communication the clarity and content of your words are at least as important as the process involved in imparting that information.

Offering Accessible and Relevant Information

It is important not to confuse information provision with effective communication or with knowledge. For most patients, nurses are a valuable source of information. It is important to remember that even as new graduates your knowledge of the body and its workings is greater than that of many patients. The goal is to provide information that will improve patients' ability to understand what is happening or enable them to improve their own self-care activities.

There are a number of ways in which information can be shared with patients. The following general guidelines ensure that the sharing of information is helpful:[42]

- Share information when the patient has indicated a need for it and is ready to hear the information.
- Find out first what the patient already knows and what he or she wants to know.
- Limit the amount of information given at any one time.
- Use language that is appropriate to the patient and tailored to that person – that is, consider the patient's background and educational level.
- Reinforce spoken information – for example, through the use of written material.
- Frequently check if the patient understands the information.
- Make sure of your own knowledge base.

Summarising

Summarising is similar to paraphrasing in that it focuses on conversation content, but it occurs near the end of the time that you spend with the patient and aims to summarise the important points you have discussed. Nurses can use summarising as an aid to go over information that has been provided, to show the patient what has been achieved, or to create a break before moving on to the next topic. It is a useful technique as it brings a sense of closure to your interaction, provides the patient with an overview of the issues you have discussed and allows for any last-minute clarification.

EMPATHY

Empathy, the ability to put yourself in the patient's shoes, is an essential aspect of all therapeutic communication and underpins both facilitative and authoritative communication. Egan[48] defines empathy as 'listening carefully to the client and then communicating understanding of what the client is feeling and of the experiences and behaviours underlying those feelings'. Before empathy is possible, you need to put your own interests, concerns and needs aside and concentrate on some as-yet-unknown patient concerns – that is, empathy is altruistic.[40,49] Openness without judgment is the beginning of the possibility of empathy, as any perception of disapproval will encourage patients to hide their worries. Empathy is complex and includes active listening, recognising covert communication, validating feelings and responses, understanding ambiguous cues and validating the 'normality' of strong emotions. There is a twofold process inherent in empathy, involving stepping into another person's emotional shoes, then stepping out of them to use cognitive analytical skills and draw on experience with other patients in similar situations.

Considered by nurses to be essential to caring practices, empathy has been shown to decrease in nurses as their clinical experience increases.[50] This decline has been attributed to lack of time, lack of support from colleagues and the increasing emphasis on technical skills. Therefore, as a beginning nurse it is imperative that you remain cognisant of the ongoing need to feel with and understand patients, otherwise your practice will be impoverished.

CONCLUSION

This chapter aims to increase awareness of communication responsibilities for ethical and holistic nursing practice. The focus of communication in nursing practice is placed in the context of relationship building. The concepts of person-centred care and patient-centred communication are reviewed along with solution-focused communication. Communication competence is discussed in relation to the need for both assertive and responsive communication skills. Factors such as cultural differences and stereotyping are outlined, in addition to clinical context and dealing with emotions. A significant part of the discussion focuses on key strategies to improve therapeutic communication, both facilitative and authoritative communication.

CASE STUDY 11.1

In her first year of practice, Jenny was having a great deal of difficulty handling her emotions when caring for patients who were dying. She felt unsure about how to communicate with them and was afraid of becoming too emotional when interacting with them. She was especially fearful of 'saying the wrong thing' and upsetting patients who were dying.

REFLECTIVE QUESTIONS

1. How can Jenny learn more about how to interact with patients who are dying?
2. With whom should she talk about this?
3. How can she learn not to be so emotional when dealing with clinical situations that are potentially emotionally charged?

CASE STUDY 11.2

Laura has completed her first year as a registered nurse in a busy metropolitan hospital. Having rotated through a few clinical specialties, she was thrilled when she was offered full-time employment in a palliative care unit as this was her favourite rotation. She knew that she was able to be sensitive and empathic towards people who were dying and felt she had a lot to offer these patients. However, her work colleagues did not seem to share the same passion and warned her against becoming emotionally involved with patients, saying she would 'burn out'. As a consequence, Laura could feel her compassion and empathy waning. She became fearful that she was becoming 'hardened', as many of her colleagues seemed to be.

REFLECTIVE QUESTIONS

1. What can Laura do to maintain what she knows to be her compassionate and empathic nature?
2. What are some approaches and strategies that she can attempt?
3. To whom should she speak about this?

CASE STUDY 11.3

After completing his new graduate program, Mark decided that he would like to work in a remote area of Australia. Shortly after he began working on an acute medical surgical ward at a hospital in the Northern Territory, he came to the realisation that he had little understanding of the cultures of Indigenous Australians in the area. He was aware that his knowledge was limited by stereotypes and prejudices, and he was careful not to act on this type of information. However, he was having difficulty understanding the sensibilities of the Indigenous Australian patients for whom he cared.

REFLECTIVE QUESTIONS

1. What kinds of strategies should Mark undertake in order to become more knowledgeable, understanding and sensitive when caring for patients who are Indigenous Australians?
2. Where should Mark go to find the information that he realises he needs?
3. How should he handle what he recognises in himself as stereotypes and prejudices that come from his childhood?

RECOMMENDED READING

Doyle C, Lennox L, Bell D. A systematic review of evidence on the links between patient experience and clinical safety and effectiveness. *BMJ Open* 2013;3:e001570.

Lusk JM, Fater K. A concept analysis of patient-centered care. *Nursing Forum* 2013;**48**(2): 89–98.

Stein-Parbury J. *Patient and person: interpersonal skills in nursing.* 5th ed. Sydney: Elsevier Australia; 2014.

Street RL, Makoul G, Arora NK, Epstein RM. How does communication heal? Pathways linking clinician–patient communication to health outcomes. *Patient Education and Counseling* 2009;**74**:295–301.

Zolnierek CD. An integrative review of knowing the patient. *Journal of Nursing Scholarship* 2014;**46**(1):3–10.

REFERENCES

1. Mottram A. Therapeutic relationships in day surgery: a grounded theory study. *Journal of Clinical Nursing* 2009;**18**:2830–7.
2. Rogers C. *On becoming a person.* Boston: Houghton Mifflin; 1961.
3. Shattell M. Nurse–patient interaction: a review of the literature. *Journal of Clinical Nursing* 2004;**13**:714–22.
4. Morse JM. Negotiating commitment and involvement in the nurse–patient relationship. *Journal of Advanced Nursing* 1991;**16**:455–68.
5. Ramos MC. The nurse–patient relationship: theme and variations. *Journal of Advanced Nursing* 1992;**17**:496–506.
6. Graber DR, Mitcham MD. Compassionate clinicians: taking patient care beyond the ordinary. *Holistic Nursing Practice* 2004;**18**:87–94.
7. Papastavrou E, Efstathiou G, Charalambous A. Nurses' and patients' perceptions of caring behaviours: quantitative systematic review of comparative studies. *Journal of Advanced Nursing* 2011;**67**(6):1191–205.
8. Shattell M. Nurse bait: strategies hospitalized patients use to entice nurses within the context of the interpersonal relationship. *Issues in Mental Health Nursing* 2005;**26**:205–23.
9. McCabe C. Nurse–patient communication: an exploration of patients' experiences. *Journal of Clinical Nursing* 2004;**13**:41–9.
10. Menzies I. A case study of the functioning of social systems as a defence against anxiety. *Human Relations* 1961;**13**:95–123.
11. DeFrino DT. A theory of the relational work of nurses. *Research and Theory for Nursing Practice* 2009;**23**:294–311.
12. Zolnierek CD. An integrative review of knowing the patient. *Journal of Nursing Scholarship* 2014;**46**(1):3–10.
13. Doyle C, Lennox L, Bell D. A systematic review of evidence on the links between patient experience and clinical safety and effectiveness. *BMJ Open* 2013;**3**:e001570. doi:10.1136/bmjopen-2012-001570.
14. Deppoliti D. Exploring how new registered nurses construct professional identity in hospital settings. *Journal of Continuing Education in Nursing* 2008;**39**:255–62.
15. Doane GH, Varcoe C. Relational practice and nursing obligations. *Advances in Nursing Science* 2007;**20**:192–205.
16. Epstein RM, Franks P, Fiscella K, et al. Measuring patient-centered communication in patient–physician consultations: theoretical and practical issues. *Social Science and Medicine* 2005;**61**:1516–28.
17. McMillan SS, Kendall E, Sav A, et al. Patient-centered approaches to health care: a systematic review of randomized controlled trials. *Medical Care Research and Review* 2013;**70**(6):567–96.
18. Johnson R. Shifting patterns of practice: nurse practitioners in a managed care environment. *Research and Theory for Nursing Practice* 2005;**19**:323–40.
19. Sidani S. Effects of patient-centered care on patient outcomes: an evaluation. *Research and Theory for Nursing Practice* 2008;**22**:24–37.
20. Hobbs JL. A dimensional analysis of patient-centered care. *Nursing Research* 2009;**58**:52–62.
21. Lusk JM, Fater K. A concept analysis of patient-centered care. *Nursing Forum* 2013;**48**(2):89–98.

22. Papastavrou E, Efstathiou G, Tsangari H, et al. Patients' and nurses' perceptions of respect and human presence through caring behaviours: a comparative study. *Nursing Ethics* 2012;**19**(3):369–79.

23. Corbin J. Is caring a lost art in nursing? *International Journal of Nursing Studies* 2008;**45**:163–5.

24. Jones A. Admitting hospital patients: a qualitative study of an everyday nursing task. *Nursing Inquiry* 2007;**14**:212–23.

25. Haskard KB, DiMattero MR, Heritage J. Affective and instrumental communication in primary care interactions: predicting the satisfaction of nursing staff and patients. *Health Communication* 2009;**24**:21–32.

26. Robinson JH, Callister LC, Berry JA, et al. Patient-centered care and adherence: definitions and applications to improve outcomes. *Journal of the American Academy of Nurse Practitioners* 2008;**20**:600–7.

27. Charlton CR, Dearing KS, Berry JA, et al. Nurse practitioners' communication styles and their impact on patient outcomes: an integrated literature review. *Journal of the American Academy of Nurse Practitioners* 2008;**20**:382–8.

28. Sheldon LK, Barrett R, Ellington L. Difficult communication in nursing. *Journal of Nursing Scholarship* 2006;**38**:141–7.

29. Timmins F, McCabe C. Nurses' and midwives' assertive behaviour in the workplace. *Journal of Advanced Nursing* 2005;**51**:38–45.

30. Iglesias ME, Becerro R, Vallejo B. Conflict resolution styles in the nursing profession. *Contemporary Nurse* 2012;**43**(1):73–80.

31. McCartan PJ, Hargie ODW. Assertiveness and caring: are they compatible? *Journal of Clinical Nursing* 2004;**13**:707–13.

32. Schim SM, Doorenbos A, Benkert R, et al. Culturally congruent care: putting the puzzle together. *Journal of Transcultural Nursing* 2007;**18**:103–10.

33. Ramsden I. Kawa Whakaruruhau: cultural safety in nursing education in Aotearoa (New Zealand). *Nursing Praxis* 1993;**8**:4–10.

34. Doutrich D, Arcus K, Dekker L, et al. Cultural safety in New Zealand and the United States: looking at a way forward together. *Journal of Transcultural Nursing* 2012;**23**(2):143–50.

35. Kirmayer LJ. Rethinking cultural competence. *Transcultural Psychiatry* 2012;**49**(2):149–64.

36. Richardson S. Aotearoa/NewZealand nursing: from eugenics to cultural safety. *Nursing Inquiry* 2004;**11**:35–42.

37. van Schaik KD, Thompson SC. Indigenous beliefs about biomedical and bush treatment efficacy for indigenous cancer patients: a review of the literature. *Internal Medicine Journal* 2011;**42**(2):184–91.

38. Fuller J. Intercultural health care as reflective negotiated practice. *Western Journal of Nursing Research* 2003;**25**(7):781–97.

39. Kleiman S. Discovering cultural aspects of nurse–patient relationships. *Journal of Cultural Diversity* 2006;**13**(2):83–6.

40. Goleman D. *Emotional intelligence. Why it can matter more than IQ.* London: Bloomsbury; 1996.

41. Varcarolis E. Communication and the clinical interview. In: Varcarolis E, editor. *Foundations of psychiatric mental health nursing.* 7th ed. St Louis, MO: Elsevier; 2014.

42. Stein-Parbury J. *Patient and person: interpersonal skills in nursing.* 5th ed. Sydney: Elsevier Australia; 2014.

43. Heron J. *Helping the client: a creative and practical guide.* 5th ed. London: Sage; 2001.

44. Henry SG, Fuhrel-Forbis A, Rogers MAM, et al. Association between nonverbal communication during clinical interactions and outcomes: a systematic review and meta-analysis. *Patient Education and Counseling* 2012;**86**:297–315.

45. Shipley SD. Listening: a concept analysis. *Nursing Forum* 2010;**45**:125–34.

46. Uitterhoeve R, Bensing J, Dilven E, et al. Nurse–patient communication in cancer care: does responding to patients' cues predict patient satisfaction with communication? *Psycho-Oncology* 2009;**18**:1060–8.
47. Chan EA. Cue-responding during simulated routine nursing care: a mixed method study. *Nurse Education Today* 2014;**34**:1057–61.
48. Egan G. *The skilled helper.* 10th ed. Pacific Grove, CA: Brooks/Cole; 2012.
49. Yegdich T. On the phenomenology of empathy in nursing: empathy or sympathy? *Journal of Advanced Nursing* 1999;**30**:83–93.
50. Ward J, Cody J, Schaal M, Hojat M. The loss of empathy in nursing education. *Journal of Professional Nursing* 2012;**28**:34–40.

CHAPTER 12

Evidence-based practice/ knowledge translation: a practical guide

Rick Wiechula, Tiffany Conroy and Paul McLiesh

LEARNING OBJECTIVES

When you have completed this chapter you will be able to:

- describe the key stages of transforming clinical practice using an evidence-based approach
- identify the stakeholders who should be involved and describe their role in evidence-based practice
- discuss the mechanisms that would highlight areas of practice that require improvement
- identify tools and processes for measuring clinical practice
- discuss the implementation strategies used to enact appropriate changes to practice.

KEYWORDS: evidence-based practice, knowledge translation, clinical audit, feedback, implementation

INTRODUCTION

Historically the delivery of nursing care was often based on traditional methods and precedents.[1] The knowledge that nurses used to deliver care was passed from nurse to nurse and may not have changed significantly over time. Over the past two decades there has been a move to incorporate evidence-based practice into healthcare and nursing care delivery. The contemporary healthcare system now demands an increased focus on improving healthcare outcomes using evidence-based research that identifies significant implications for clinical practice.[2] Ensuring positive outcomes for patients such as limited adverse events, lowered length of stay, reduced complication rates and reduced re-admission rates is a high priority in today's healthcare setting.

The term *evidence-based practice* would be familiar to both students and nurses in practice. The term *knowledge translation* may be less familiar. There are many definitions of evidence-based practice.

> Evidence-based practice (EBP) requires that decisions about health care are based on the best available, current, valid and relevant evidence. These decisions should be made by those receiving care, informed by the tacit and explicit knowledge of those providing care, within the context of available resources.[3]

This statement was devised in 2003 in response to a concern that previous definitions placed too much emphasis on the evidence and too little on the decision-making part of the process.[3]

Knowledge translation is defined as:

> ... a dynamic and iterative process that includes the synthesis, dissemination, exchange and ethically sound application of knowledge to improve health, provide more effective health services and products, and strengthen the health care system.[4]

This definition from the Canadian Institutes of Health Research aims also to bring emphasis to the outcome of improving health.[4]

Both terms have become an integral part of contemporary nursing practice, referring to the principal of engaging with the best available evidence to support decision making in practice. There is, however, a subtle difference between them. Evidence-based practice is a broad term that has an emphasis on engaging with the evidence. It encompasses a cycle of activity from producing evidence by conducting primary research, synthesising the evidence by way of systematic reviews, transferring the evidence in the form of guidelines, and using processes to implement the evidence in practice.[5] Knowledge translation also considers evidence to inform practice but is arguably more focused on the pragmatic aspects of achieving changes in practice and improving patient outcomes.[6]

Clinicians will make decisions about the conduct of their practice frequently and within quite different contexts. In day-to-day practice, decisions will often need to be made very rapidly.[7] Faced with a patient whose condition is deteriorating, the nurse will need to consider the available evidence and make an immediate decision about how to proceed. At the other end of the spectrum, it may be apparent that 'usual' practice is not achieving the required outcomes for patients and, as a team, nurses will consider systematically what changes need to occur. For example, if there is an increase in nosocomial infections within a ward, a structured process of the review of practice and the appropriate evidence to inform that practice should occur. The timeframes for these two examples are vastly different, but the principals of evidence-based practice should still apply in both cases.

For the student nurse or new graduate, it may be obvious what role they would play in the day-to-day situation of making immediate decisions about care. If they are unsure of how to proceed, they will generally seek an experienced clinician to help with making a decision.[7] The role that the junior nurse plays in reviewing practice at a ward, or even an organisational, level may not be so overt, but there is an important role to play.

This chapter will consider both engagement with evidence and the practical application of evidence to change practice and improve patient outcomes from the perspective of a clinician. Throughout this chapter we will consider an area of practice that is common to all nurses, hand hygiene, and explore how the principles of evidence-based practice and the processes of knowledge translation can be used to improve this fundamental element of healthcare.

IDENTIFYING PRACTICE THAT REQUIRES IMPROVEMENT

There are many situations that may draw nurses to consider that some aspect of practice requires improvement. The stimulus for considering which aspects of practice are to be reviewed may be internal, instigated by the clinicians at a local level, or external, where a directive comes from an organisational or even regional level.

Clinicians who practise in a reflective manner may simply identify something that occurs in their practice that just does not 'seem quite right' or may not be working. There may be a specific occasion where the outcome for the patient was very poor, potentially resulting in serious injury or even death. This is known as a sentinel event, and the gravity of the situation obviously requires that practice be reviewed.[8,9] Repeated poor patient outcomes for a specific type of practice are an obvious indicator that action is required. You may feel that, as a less experienced nurse, you are not in a position to question current practice in your organisation. However, it is often those with 'fresh eyes', such as new staff and nursing students, who notice these issues and it is important that they are empowered to ask about them. When you become aware of a practice issue, you need to know where to go and what to do with this information.

EXERCISE 12.1

Consider an example of some aspect of your practice that seems like it does not work very effectively. Is there a particular example where things have gone wrong or the outcome for the patient/s has been poor? Talk about that issue with your colleagues. Have they noticed similar things?

There may also be more formal processes to review the quality of care being provided. Most organisations have clinical audit programs in place to monitor the nursing care being provided. This may be at a unit or organisational level. The results of these clinical audit programs should guide the review of current practice.[10] There is a risk, however, that routine collection of audit data becomes just that – data collection without active consideration of the results.

EXERCISE 12.2

It may be noted that the hospital-acquired infection rates in your unit have increased over the past 12 months. The nursing director has asked your unit to consider the role of hand hygiene in this increase.

1. Talk to the senior nurses on the unit where you work about how they monitor and ensure that their practice is best practice.
2. What structures and strategies are currently used at a unit and organisational level?

The impetus to change practice may also come from outside of the organisation. The national in-patient medication chart was endorsed by all Australian state health ministers in 2004 after evidence suggested that the lack of standardisation of medication charts was resulting in unnecessary medication errors. The introduction of the chart followed an extensive pilot study that demonstrated a reduction in overall prescribing errors of nearly one-third.[11] As a result, health departments throughout Australia instructed organisations that they were required to implement the new chart. Organisations then undertook strategies to ensure that this occurred in all units. Less experienced nurses would not be expected to be leading this type of change, but all staff would be expected to conform.

The opportunity to reflect on and engage in a process of using knowledge to change practice can also arise out of knowledge translation research. Researchers building the science around knowledge translation often partner with clinicians on projects with two essential aims. The clinicians involved participate with the objective of improving care for their patients. Their aim is pragmatic. The researchers wish to know more about what processes and strategies work best in implementing changes in practice. Their aim is essentially theoretical. An example of this is The Older Person and Improving Care TOPIC 7 project, where seven groups of clinicians met and were facilitated to each review a different aspect of the care of the elderly patient.[12] Each group identified the best practice in the literature, then moved to measure the current practice in the local setting with a view to implementing best practice in those areas where it was lacking. The researchers were experienced facilitators and were able to guide the clinicians with their individual projects.[12]

Once a problem or gap in practice has been identified, action must be taken. Nurses tend to be problem solvers and face multiple problems each day of their practice. There is a tendency for nurses to want to jump to the solution. Some of the more significant problems that nurses identify in practice require a more detailed and measured approach to assessment, planning and management. Junior and senior nurses alike may be unsure of how to proceed. Ideally, the first step is to identify an individual or a group of people who you can discuss the issue with.[10] The following questions may be helpful in understanding the problem in more detail and may form some of your discussions:

- Is this an issue that others have noted in their practice?
- How serious is the problem? Does it need to be prioritised?
- Are there measurable outcomes that can demonstrate the extent of the problem (e.g. infection rates)?
- Is there a different way of practising already identified that may solve the problem?
- What are the possible cause/s of the problem?
- What are some potential solutions? (Do not rush to implement these just yet, however.)
- Importantly, who else should be involved or be advised of this problem?

No matter what the trigger, once a problem has been identified the process of considering what is best practice and managing the problem should be similar. The remaining sections of this chapter will identify the actions that are involved in this process.

EVIDENCE TO INFORM PRACTICE

Once it has been identified that some aspect of practice requires improvement, the logical next step is to confirm what should be happening – that is, what will be the expected standard of care. In keeping with the principles of evidence-based practice, there should be some form of guidance that makes it clear to clinicians how practice should be undertaken.[5,13,14] Evidence to inform practice can be derived from different sources and may come in many different forms. The evidence-based approach has been criticised for placing too strong an emphasis on evidence from research without considering local context, clinical experience and the specific needs of individual patients. Rycroft-Malone and colleagues (2004) argue that all these evidence types are necessary to guide our practice.[14]

External Evidence

During their education, undergraduate student nurses will have been introduced to the notion of using healthcare research as evidence to inform practice. This may have been part of a problem/case-based learning exercise.[15] Typically, students will work through a case identifying the needs of the patient and then engaging with the evidence to inform decisions about what care should be provided and how that care should be delivered. The process of constructing a clinical question using the PICO mnemonic will be familiar to most student nurses and new graduates.[16] The P is used to define the population of interest, the I indicates the intervention that may be used, the C can be any comparative treatments or strategies, and the O is to indicate what outcomes are expected to be achieved.[16] Searching for research evidence embodied in peer-reviewed journal articles is considered a fundamental skill and would be taught in all contemporary nursing undergraduate programs. Undergraduates are also expected to judge the quality of the evidence they have identified and may have been encouraged to use critical appraisal tools.[17] In clinical practice, however, using primary research reports to inform practice has some significant practical problems. For any given practice area there may be a great many relevant research reports. The expression 'drowning in information, thirsting for evidence' is often used to describe the sometimes overwhelming amount of information available.[18] The results of these reports may differ in their conclusions and the quality of the evidence is not guaranteed. Systematic reviews are a structured and effective way of dealing with this problem.

As their name suggests, systematic reviews are a mechanism of establishing the best available evidence for a given area of practice that is systematic using rigorous methods to identify, appraise and synthesise relevant evidence.[19] Although some clinicians are involved in the conduct of systematic reviews, it is impractical to embark upon a systematic review as part of routine practice. Systematic reviews are conducted by reviewers usually within organisations such as the Cochrane Collaboration and the Joanna Briggs Institute.[20] Systematic review reports summarise all the best available evidence and, where appropriate, provide recommendations for practice and for further research. Although the recommendations can be useful in clinical decision making, systematic review reports often lack contextual information to assist with the process of improving practice.

Of more practical use to clinicians are evidence-based clinical practice guidelines. A good example of such a guideline is the *Prevention and Treatment of Pressure Ulcers: Clinical Practice Guideline*.[21] This guideline was developed using evidence derived from a systematic review. It gives a comprehensive guide to assessment and prevention strategies. Each recommendation is given a rating that indicates the strength of the evidence available. Importantly, the guideline recognises that not all recommendations will be supported by strong evidence; in those cases, an expert panel used a consensus process to derive the recommendations. This guideline is abstracted further to a quick reference guide.[22] Although it may seem confusing to have so many variants of what is essentially the same information, it recognises that busy clinicians will not necessarily have the time to access and read extensive systematic review reports. Evidence is therefore often provided in different forms and formats to meet specific needs. It is important, though, that clinicians consider how the guidance they are accessing is derived. Not all guidelines are evidence-based and their quality will vary.[23] Quality guidelines will detail the processes of identifying and critiquing the evidence they use for recommendations. There should be an overt trail from the recommendation back to the source of evidence.

EXERCISE 12.3

Access the World Health Organization (WHO) *Guidelines on Hand Hygiene in Health Care*.[24] These guidelines are available electronically from the WHO website. Consider the structure and content of the guidelines.

The 'Hand Hygiene' guideline is a large document. Along with significant background information on how the guideline was developed, it details the scientific data in regard to hand hygiene, indicating the guideline is evidence-based. The second part of the guideline provides explicit and detailed recommendations for practice. Part three addresses measurement of hand hygiene practices and outcomes. The information provided can be used to improve hand hygiene practices at a unit, organisational and even national level. Importantly, the guideline has been developed so that it can be applied in as many different contexts and settings as possible, even considering the religious and cultural issues that may be relevant. Although the guideline contains all the evidence around hand hygiene that an organisation would require, at more than 250 pages it is not a document that would be accessed daily. More likely, clinicians will be accessing locally developed guidance.

Local Evidence

Local evidence to inform practice also comes in many guises. In keeping with the principles of evidence-based practice, local evidence can be adapted from external sources, can be knowledge based on clinical experience, and may be the views and preferences of patients.

Research indicates consistently that nurses, particularly students and new graduates, will seek guidance about practice from those they are working with in the first instance.[7,25–27] The advantage of sourcing the knowledge of other clinicians is that it is immediate and contextual. Nurses place a very high value on clinical experience, so it is not unexpected that this would be a focus of their information gathering in the practice setting, particularly when the need to use that information relates to a specific episode of patient care.[7] The potential disadvantage is that it may not be the best evidence for a given clinical decision. While experienced nurses often feel confident about their own practice, they may not be aware of the latest research that could be used to optimise their care delivery.[28] In keeping with the principles of evidence-based practice, we need to critique the evidence regardless of the source.

Routinely, organisations will have documented instructions about the care required. These instructions may be paper-based or electronic. They may be in the form of standard statements, policy or procedure statements.[7] They may be organisation-wide or unit-specific instructions. The instruction can be delivered via various electronic clinical decision support systems,[29] or may simply be sitting on a shelf in a folder.

Regardless of the form of the local guidance, where possible it should be evidence-based. Graham and Harrison (2005) provide a step-by-step users' guide for organisations to incorporate external evidence into local guidance.[23] If an organisation is reviewing an area of practice, it needs first to identify the most appropriate source of external evidence; ideally, an evidence-based clinical practice guideline. The external guidance should be subject to a process of critique, and Graham and Harrison recommend the use of the AGREE tool.[23] This tool is a structured approach using specific criteria to judge the quality of clinical practice guidelines.[30] It is also important that the external guideline is considered in terms of currency and, importantly, content to ensure best fit with the area of practice under review. Many guidelines are focused to a certain area of practice and the scope of the guideline is determined by the developers. For example, in a knowledge translation project conducted in a large tertiary hospital there was a need to access a guideline on the acute pain management of older adults. Although the organisation had existing local guidelines, they were not specific to the elderly.[31] The project team was able to identify high-quality guidelines with a focus on older adults.[32,33] Once an appropriate guideline has been identified, the decision needs to be made as to whether it should be adopted in its entirety or adapted to meet the local contextual needs. Graham and Harrison (2005) recognise that some recommendations from guidelines may not be practical or feasible but caution against altering recommendations that are well supported by evidence. If modifications need to be made, then the rationale should be documented.[23] The WHO 'Hand Hygiene' guidelines were developed with this issue in mind and aimed to provide guidance for both developed and developing countries in all practice settings.[24]

EXERCISE 12.4

Identify your own organisation's guidance for hand hygiene. Determine if the local guidelines are derived from external evidence. Consider the recommendations in the local guidelines and whether there are any significant differences to the WHO's *Guidelines on Hand Hygiene in Health Care*.

MEASURING PRACTICE

The aim of any knowledge translation project is to improve clinical practice based on new evidence or where an existing aspect of care may not be in line with the best available evidence. In both cases an important aspect of determining success is to be able to measure current practice and the outcomes of providing care. This process of measuring is called clinical audit. The clinical audit process can help nurses to:

- use evidence about best practice as a basis for measuring nursing practice
- understand that effective processes of care and patient outcomes depend on consistent best practice
- be actively involved in the change process
- include the patient's perspective in audit activities.[34]

A clinical audit is the systematic and critical analysis of the quality of clinical care. This includes the procedures used for diagnosis, treatment and care of patients, the associated use of resources, and the effect of care on the outcome and quality of life for the patient.[10,35,36] It is also a means by which comparison of actual practice to a practice standard can be made and, through the results of this comparison, any deficiencies in actual practice may be identified and change undertaken to rectify the deficiencies. Clinical audit is a clinically led initiative.[37] It is important that clinicians lead and have ownership of any clinical audit process, as it is their performance which will be judged.

The main reason to audit practice is to improve both the quality of patient care and patient outcomes. The Healthcare Quality Improvement Partnership has identified 11 criteria for best practice in clinical audit:[38]

1. The topic for the clinical audit should be a clinical priority. Both clinical and non-clinical stakeholders must agree to the selection of the audit topic.
2. The clinical audit must measure against standards that are based on the best available evidence.
3. The organisation will enable the conduct of the audit and ensure that the necessary structures and processes are in place to support it. This includes time for staff to participate, as well as administrative and practical support.
4. The clinical audit engages all relevant stakeholders, including those from the multidisciplinary clinical team and non-clinical representatives.
5. The patient group to whom the standards apply is clearly defined, and they and/or their representatives are involved in the clinical audit. If patients are participating in the audit they should be provided with full information about the expectations of them and be given training in audit processes if required.
6. A written protocol describes the clinical audit methodology, timescale and data collection process in detail. This will enable re-audit to be undertaken later in the audit cycle.
7. The audit sample should be sufficient to generate meaningful results. The method of sampling should be specified and reliable.
8. The data collection tools and processes should be robust and valid. Data collection should endeavour to capture all relevant data.
9. Collected data are analysed, and the subsequent results are presented and reported in an appropriate manner that maximises the impact of the audit. Audit results are

delivered effectively to all relevant stakeholders in a way that supports action planning.

10. Action plans are created and implemented. These should identify areas of practice requiring attention, indicate where there is good compliance with standards, and specify the actions needed to address any issues. Action plans need agreement from all or most of the stakeholders involved.

11. The clinical audit cycle demonstrates that improvement has been achieved and sustained. Re-auditing is required to complete the cycle unless all the standards were met in the initial audit.

EXERCISE 12.5

Consider our example of the clinical audit topic of hand hygiene. Who would you identify as the stakeholders? Who are the clinical stakeholders? Who are the non-clinical stakeholders? Would you include patients? If so, why? If not, why not?

The process of the audit involves measuring day-to-day practice and requires collection of valid and reliable data following ethical and confidentiality principles as set down by the organisation in which the audit is to be conducted.[10] In many cases, knowledge translation projects are classed as quality assurance and will not require ethical approval. The ethical conduct of the project, however, must always be considered. The aim here is to ensure that those involved are protected. Consent should be sought from the clinicians whose practice will be judged, and from patients if they are to provide any of their personal information. Anonymity should be maintained, and the methods used to maintain anonymity should be overt to the participants.[39] In addition to protecting the participants, they are more likely to provide accurate information if they know they cannot be identified. Permission to conduct this type of project should be sought first from senior clinicians of the unit involved, who should be able to advise what additional permissions should be sought. Contacting the organisation's safety and quality unit may be mandatory; but even if it is not, it is useful to let the unit know what you are planning. It may be aware of other units doing similar projects or be able to provide advice and assistance.

The 'valid and reliable data' that you collect for your audit or inquiry emerges from the 'tool(s)' that you use to collect it. Therefore, the tools of measurement should match with the question that you are asking. The question itself may be quantitative or qualitative in nature, and each type will require different approaches.

If there are 'best practice' indicators for the clinical situation to be audited, then the data collection tool should be reflective of these. This will then enable the easy recognition of whether or not best practice has been achieved. Once an audit topic has been agreed, the next step is to determine if there are any evidence-based standards that relate to it. These should be based on the best available evidence and should be definable and measurable. It is essential to provide specific details about the standard by which practice is to be evaluated. For example, for our topic of hand hygiene, the WHO (2009) evidence-based guidelines on hand hygiene provide standards of practice with sufficient detail to guide the measurement.[24] Similar standards need to be sourced for every audit topic. These standards then need to be developed into specific criteria against which practice will be compared.[40] Depending on the audit topic, it may also be necessary to succinctly describe exactly what should be happening in practice, as this description is what will be used to determine if practice meets the expected standard. Table 12.1 may be of use when translating evidence-based standards to specific measurable criteria to evaluate existing practice (p 288).[12] The example provided uses the standard related to pressure ulcer risk assessment to illustrate how the tool is used.

Standard statements are often quite broad and do not provide the level of detail required to measure practice. Standards criteria are more specific statements about how healthcare should be provided. For any given standard there may be multiple standard criteria. These criteria then need to be developed into appropriate audit criteria and then phrased as questions that can be answered without ambiguity.[12] The example in Table 12.1 looks at the assessment of pressure ulcer risk. Using the tool, a broad standard statement in the left column lacks specificity. The standard criteria provide more detail. The NPUAP/EPUAP guidelines indicate that a structured approach to risk assessment is required. They indicate that using a risk assessment scale would achieve this.[21] They do not, however, support any one risk assessment scale over another. Therefore, in the example, in the audit criteria the Braden scale is identified as the tool

TABLE 12.1

Example of translating a standard to an audit tool

Standard of care	Standard criteria	Audit criteria	Audit question	Data sources
Patients must be assessed for risk of pressure ulcer	A pressure ulcer risk assessment tool should be used to assess risk	The Braden scale should be used to assess risk of pressure ulcer	Has a Braden scale risk assessment been completed?	Patients' case notes
	Risk assessment should occur on admission and at regular intervals	Pressure ulcer risk assessment should be conducted on all patients within 8 hours of admission	Was the risk assessment completed within 8 hours of admission?	Patients' case notes
		Pressure ulcer risk assessment should be conducted on all patients weekly	Has there been a weekly risk assessment completed?	Patients' case notes

Source: *Adapted from R Wiechula, A Kitson, D Marcoionni, T Page, K Zeitz, H Silverston. Improving the fundamentals of care for older people in the acute hospital setting: facilitating practice improvement using a Knowledge Translation Toolkit.* International Journal of Evidence-based Healthcare *2009;7(4):288.*

sanctioned by the organisation where the audit is being conducted. This gives the audit the necessary detail required for an objective assessment of practice.

Once the standards and audit criteria are identified, the next critical stage of the audit process is the collection of the data that will be used to evaluate practice. There are many different ways by which data can be collected and the nature of the audit will determine which method is chosen. In general, the four ways of collecting information are by:

- observation
- questionnaire or survey
- interview
- documentation review.[36]

Observation

The benefit of observation is that it allows the observer to record events as they occur, rather than relying on someone's recollection.[41] Ideally, when conducting an observation the auditor should place themselves in a way that has the least impact on those being observed. The notion here is that a clinician is more likely to be compliant with the required care element when they know they are being observed (the so-called Hawthorn effect).[42]

Questionnaire/Survey

Questionnaires allow the gathering of large amounts of information from a large number of people, quickly, easily and with minimal expense. This type of data collection is useful when you want to investigate the knowledge and understanding of clinicians about an area of practice.[43] Questionnaires can also be used to measure outcomes. For example, patients can be surveyed to determine if they had been provided with appropriate discharge advice.[44] It is essential to pilot a questionnaire with a small percentage of the population or a group that has similar characteristics to the intended group. Most often the tools devised in this category contain either closed or open-ended questions. Closed questions require a 'yes' or 'no' answer, while open-ended questions require an opinion from the respondent.

Interviews

Interviewing allows a free interaction between the interviewer and the interviewee, and so allows a relationship to be established. This type of relationship may be important to establish, especially if sensitive issues are to be explored. Interviews can be structured, unstructured, or a combination of both methods. Ethical approval may be required to conduct and record interviews.[41]

Reviewing Documentation

There are many documents and records used in the delivery of nursing care that can contribute valuable information to a clinical audit. It is usual, however, to make use of the information from documentation alongside other methods of data collection. There are two types of documentation that can be used in a clinical audit: that which is already generated, and that which can be generated as a result of the audit.[45]

The first type may include:

- clinical records
- policies and procedure documents
- personal details of a patient
- annual reports
- committee and board meeting agenda and minutes
- statistical records.

The second type of documentation could include:

- journal or diary entries related to the focus of the audit
- accounts written by the participants in the audit (e.g. a focus group).

An enduring issue with many types of document sources is that the documentation may not be complete. It is possible to combine different data collection tools (i.e. observation with questionnaire, interview with a tick-box questionnaire to be completed by the auditor).

When we consider our hand hygiene example, the primary data collection method used for these audits is observation.

EXERCISE 12.6

Access the WHO Observation Form for Hand Hygiene, which can be found in the *Hand Hygiene Technical Reference Manual*.[46] Examine what data needs to be collected. The instructions about conducting the observation are also in the appendices of the document. Tour your unit and consider where you would place yourself to conduct the observation. This location needs to be at a distance where you would not be interfering with those providing care but you still have a good line of vision to be able to record activity accurately.

Once the data have been collected, analysis should be able to determine if clinicians are complying with the expected standard of practice and this is usually expressed as a percentage of compliance. Tables, graphs or diagrams are useful to display patterns and relationships between numerical data. Content analysis identifies the presence or absence of patterns or recurring themes from a text. It is important that results are presented in a clear and concise manner so that all involved can understand what is currently happening with the target area of practice.

If the results of the audit indicate that the current practices comply with 'best practice', then there is usually no further action required other than to provide this feedback to all stakeholders and those who participated in your audit. Typically, there will be some discrepancies between what is best practice and what is happening in reality. Recommendations for change should state some collaborative action for the future. This is examined in more detail in the following section.

IMPLEMENTING THE NECESSARY CHANGES

Do not underestimate the planning and preparation when beginning the implementation phase of a knowledge translation project. To ensure smooth implementation of practice change in any required area, it is essential to assess the environment in which the change is proposed and to develop the implementation plan based on these findings. The Promoting Action on Research Implementation in Health Services (PARiHS) framework considers three interacting elements that impact on successful implementation of best practice. These consist of evidence, context and facilitation. Each of these elements has sub-elements. The sub-elements of evidence include the research upon which the practice change is based, the clinical experiences of the practitioners, patient experience and local sources of information. Context sub-elements comprise the receptiveness of the context to change, organisational culture and leadership, and methods of evaluation utilised. The sub-elements of facilitation encompass the role, as well as the skills and attributes, of the facilitator.[14] A self-assessment tool has been developed, and this can be used to plan strategies for implementation of practice change. The premise for the PARiHS framework is strong evidence, and a receptive context provides the ideal situation for implementation of evidence into practice.[47]

EXERCISE 12.7

Using the references identified at the end of this chapter, access a copy of the PARiHS framework criteria. Review the descriptions and questions for each of the elements and sub-elements. Can you answer these questions for your organisation?[48–50]

There are many other knowledge translation methodologies, and a good overview of these can be found in the book by Strauss, Tetroe and Graham (2009),[51] listed in the references for this chapter. This reference contains examples of how knowledge translation models work.

As mentioned previously, all initial stakeholders will need to be involved in preparing an implementation plan. This list of stakeholders may also need to be revised to enable the identification of, and subsequent consultation with, all the people affected by the proposed change in practice.[10] Not all stakeholders will need to be involved in every aspect of the implementation process. Usually a smaller working party will coordinate the project. Others may be brought in for various aspects of the implementation. Still others may simply receive progress reports about what is happening. In keeping with the principles behind the PARiHS framework, it is important to consider who may be able to help facilitate the project.[48] A facilitator is someone who can advise and guide the project without necessarily leading it. This might be a clinician with previous experience in knowledge translation projects, or a member of the organisation's safety and quality unit, or an academic from a partner university with knowledge translation expertise.[31] Knowledge translation projects need to be planned and detailed, and able to work within an agreed structure. When the group meets for the first time they should agree on ways of working. Regular meetings should be scheduled; goals and timelines should be agreed to. The meetings should be documented, particularly in regard to what actions need to be taken and who is responsible for them. It is important at this stage to consider the scope of the implementation plan. This is a balance between what changes are required, based on the results of the initial audit, and what is feasible to achieve, given the time and resources available.[12]

In planning the strategies and interventions to be implemented, the elements of the PARiHS framework can provide a structure for the planning. There are many strategies that may be required to achieve the necessary change. Further information gathering may be necessary to determine which strategies are appropriate. For example, if we consider the element of evidence, the sub-elements here include the research upon which the practice change is based (external evidence), the clinical experiences of the practitioners, patient experience and local sources of information.[14,49] In planning the clinical audit, the external evidence to inform practice should have been accessed. It is important to review the guidance provided to staff to determine if it is evidence-based and matches the external evidence. When there are multiple types of guidance, they must be consistent. At a unit level, this may be a reasonably quick and simple process; however, if the area of practice is informed by an organisation-wide instruction the review and amendment of this material can take much longer. The clinical experience and knowledge of the clinicians needs to be taken into account. This may indicate a knowledge deficit, and an education program may need to be instigated. Patient experience should also be considered. This is particularly important in terms of prioritising which aspects of practice should be targeted for improvement first.

The sub-elements for context also provide us with information to plan the implementation strategies.[50] The receptiveness of the organisation to change must be gauged. Ways in which the existing structures will support or hinder change must be understood. For example, if new equipment must be purchased, are there resources available for this? Does the organisation have a culture that is conducive to change? Within any culture there are those who embrace change and those who resist change. It is important to know which individuals will be supportive and those that may be obstructive. Leadership is critical when attempting to change practice. Senior management must be kept informed of progress and will be required to approve the use of necessary resources. Informal leadership must also be considered. Non-designated leaders may wield considerable influence and they are not always easy to identify.[49,50]

Once the plan has been agreed on and the various elements have been put in place, there should be ongoing monitoring and evaluation of the project. Healthcare organisations are complex systems and unforeseen circumstances must be dealt with to ensure success. After a sufficient period of time, a formal evaluation must occur to measure the change in practice. The outcome of the follow-up audit will determine if there has been success or whether further action needs to be taken.[12,40]

SUSTAINING PRACTICE IMPROVEMENTS

At this point it is important to consider what needs to be done to ensure sustainability of the change. Many knowledge translation projects have initial success, but once the project finishes the enthusiasm wanes and practice returns to what was occurring previously. A number of strategies can be used to assist with sustainability. If there were resources required to purchase equipment or consumables, then there needs to be negotiation for ongoing funding. If the project was well documented with measurable improvements in practice, this will bolster the case for budget changes. If an education strategy was employed, it should be considered whether this should continue as mandatory professional development. There should be a plan for ongoing auditing either at a unit level or, ideally, within the organisation's audit program.

CONCLUSION

New graduates may feel that these activities are beyond their scope of influence; however, it is important to know that improving practice is part of the clinical role and, as such, should be conducted with the same degree of rigour as any other clinical practice. Healthcare organisations are frequently committed to capacity building of their staff – that is, the development of sustainable skills, structures, resources and commitment to health improvement.[52] Within every organisation there exist methods to improve practice, and these are the avenues to explore when practice improvement is required. Entities such as safety and quality committees, and utilising individuals as change champions such as link or liaison nurses, are common ways to improve practice standards and embed new practices. Participating in practice improvement also provides support for the nurse's professional portfolio and can be used as evidence of maintaining currency and utilisation of evidence to improve patient outcomes. Demonstrating a commitment to knowledge translation may also lead to recognition and assignment to link or liaison roles. Networking with academic staff from allied universities is also a way to ensure that practice change is facilitated and the methods of success are captured for replication with other topics.[12,31,53,54]

CASE STUDY 12.1

Caitlin's first placement as a new graduate is a busy surgical ward where there are many patients with wounds. On the evening shift she is instructed by the senior registered nurse to use a particular dressing for a patient's wound. The following morning, working with another registered nurse, Caitlin is given advice to use a different dressing for the same wound. It concerns her that the advice being given is not consistent. In her undergraduate program she remembers being told that variability in practice is usually not effective. She is uncomfortable about questioning either of these very experienced registered nurses.

REFLECTIVE QUESTIONS

1. How does Caitlin determine which advice to follow?
2. What objective sources of information might be available to her on the ward?
3. Consider how she might approach the two registered nurses to resolve this issue without causing offence.

CASE STUDY 12.2

Sam is a final-year nursing student working on a medical ward where many patients are nursed in 'isolation' due to norovirus gastroenteritis. He has noticed that many of the staff are not adhering precisely to care plan instructions about personal protective equipment.

REFLECTIVE QUESTIONS

1. What are Sam's responsibilities in dealing with this situation?
2. Who should Sam be talking with to improve the practice around personal protective equipment?

CASE STUDY 12.3

Maddy is a new graduate working on a ward that has been chosen for a knowledge translation project to improve hydration status in elderly patients. Maddy indicates that she thinks this is an important issue and wants to help with the project.

REFLECTIVE QUESTION

What part do you think Maddy would be able to play in this project?

RECOMMENDED READING

Harvey G, Loftus-Hills A, Rycroft-Malone J, Titchen A, Kitson A, McCormack B, et al. Getting evidence into practice: the role and function of facilitation. *Journal of Advanced Nursing* 2002;**37**(6):577–88.

Kitson A, Harvey G, McCormack B. Enabling the implementation of evidence based practice: a conceptual framework. *Quality in Health Care* 1998;**7**(3):149–58.

Kitson A, Rycroft-Malone J, Harvey G, McCormack B, Seers K, Titchen A. Evaluating the successful implementation of evidence into practice using the PARiHS framework: theoretical and practical challenges. *Implementation Science* 2008;**3**:1.

McCormack B, Kitson A, Harvey G, Rycroft-Malone J, Titchen A, Seers K. Getting evidence into practice: the meaning of 'context'. *Journal of Advanced Nursing* 2002;**38**(1):94–104.

Rycroft-Malone J, Seers K, Titchen A, Harvey G, Kitson A, McCormack B. What counts as evidence in evidence-based practice? *Journal of Advanced Nursing* 2004;**47**(1):81–90.

REFERENCES

1. Gerrish K, Ashworth P, Lacey A, Bailey J. Developing evidence-based practice: experiences of senior and junior clinical nurses. *Journal of Advanced Nursing* 2008;**62**(1):62–73.
2. Bonner A, Sando J. Examining the knowledge, attitude and use of research by nurses. *Journal of Nursing Management* 2008;**16**(3):334–43.
3. Dawes M, Summerskill W, Glasziou P, Cartabellotta A, Martin J, Hopayian K, et al. Sicily statement on evidence-based practice. *BMC Medical Education* 2005;**5**(1):1.
4. Straus SE, Tetroe J, Graham I. Defining knowledge translation. *Canadian Medical Association Journal* 2009;**181**(3–4):165–8.

5. Pearson A, Wiechula R, Court A, Lockwood C. The JBI model of evidence-based healthcare. *International Journal of Evidence-based Healthcare* 2005;**3**(8):207–15.

6. Straus SE, Tetroe J, Graham ID. Introduction: Knowledge translation: What it is and what it isn't. In: *Knowledge translation in health care.* John Wiley & Sons, Ltd; 2013. pp 1–13.

7. Estabrooks CA, Rutakumwa W, O'Leary KA, Profetto-McGrath J, Milner M, Levers MJ, et al. Sources of practice knowledge among nurses. *Qualitative Health Research* 2005;**15**(4):460–76.

8. Department of Health Western Australia. *Clinical Incident Management Policy.* Perth: Patient Safety Surveillance Unit, Performance Activity and Quality Division; 2014.

9. The Joint Commission. Sentinel Event Policy and Procedures. 2014 Available: <www. jointcommission.org/Sentinel_Event_Policy_and_Procedures/>.

10. Patel S. Achieving quality assurance through clinical audit. *Nursing Management (Harrow).* 2010;**17**(3):28–35.

11. Coombes ID, Reid C, McDougall D, Stowasser D, Duiguid M, Mitchell C. Pilot of a National Inpatient Medication Chart in Australia: improving prescribing safety and enabling prescribing training. *British Journal of Clinical Pharmacology* 2011;**72**(2):338–49.

12. Wiechula R, Kitson A, Marcoionni D, Page T, Zeitz K, Silverston H. Improving the fundamentals of care for older people in the acute hospital setting: facilitating practice improvement using a Knowledge Translation Toolkit. *International Journal of Evidence-based Healthcare* 2009;**7**(4):283–95.

13. Mokhtar IA, Majid S, Foo S, Zhang X, Theng YL, Chang YK, et al. Evidence-based practice and related information literacy skills of nurses in Singapore: an exploratory case study. *Health Informatics Journal* 2012;**18**(1):12–25.

14. Rycroft-Malone J, Seers K, Titchen A, Harvey G, Kitson A, McCormack B. What counts as evidence in evidence-based practice? *Journal of Advanced Nursing* 2004;**47**(1):81–90.

15. Martyn J, Terwijn R, Kek MY, Huijser H. Exploring the relationships between teaching, approaches to learning and critical thinking in a problem-based learning foundation nursing course. *Nurse Education Today* 2014;**34**(5):829–35.

16. Hastings C, Fisher CA. Searching for proof: creating and using an actionable PICO question. *Nursing Management* 2014;**45**(8):9–12.

17. Nadelson SG. Online resources: fostering students' evidence-based practice learning through group critical appraisals. Worldviews on Evidence-based Nursing/Sigma Theta Tau International. *Honor Society of Nursing* 2014;**11**(2):143–4.

18. Booth A. In search of the evidence: informing effective practice. *Journal of Clinical Effectiveness* 1996;**1**(1):25–9.

19. Khan KS, Kunz R, Kleijnen J, Antes G. Five steps to conducting a systematic review. *Journal of the Royal Society of Medicine* 2003;**96**(3):118–21.

20. Pearson A, Wiechula R, Court A, Lockwood C. A re-consideration of what constitutes 'evidence' in the healthcare professions. *Nursing Science Quarterly* 2007;**20**(1):85–8.

21. European Pressure Ulcer Advisory Panel and National Pressure Ulcer Advisory Panel. *Prevention and treatment of pressure ulcers: clinical practice guideline.* Washington, DC: National Pressure Ulcer Advisory Panel; 2009.

22. European Pressure Ulcer Advisory Panel and National Pressure Ulcer Advisory Panel. *Prevention and treatment of pressure ulcers: quick reference guide.* Washington, DC: National Pressure Ulcer Advisory Panel; 2009.

23. Graham ID, Harrison MB. Evaluation and adaptation of clinical practice guidelines. *Evidence-Based Nursing* 2005;**8**(3):68–72.

24. World Health Organization. *WHO guidelines on hand hygiene in health care.* Geneva: World Health Organization; 2009.

25. Gerrish K, Clayton J. Promoting evidence-based practice: an organizational approach. *Journal of Nursing Management* 2004;**12**(2):114–23.

26. Pravikoff DS, Tanner AB, Pierce ST. Readiness of U.S. nurses for evidence-based practice. *The American Journal of Nursing* 2005;**105**(9):40–51.

27. Thiel L, Ghosh Y. Determining registered nurses' readiness for evidence-based practice. Worldviews on Evidence-based Nursing/Sigma Theta Tau International. *Honor Society of Nursing* 2008;**5**(4):182–92.

28. Brady N, Lewin L. Evidence-based practice in nursing: bridging the gap between research and practice. *Journal of Pediatric Health Care* 2007;**21**(1):53–6.

29. Purcell GP. What makes a good clinical decision support system. *BMJ (Clinical Research Ed.)* 2005;**330**(7494):740–1.

30. AGREE Collaboration. Development and validation of an international appraisal instrument for assessing the quality of clinical practice guidelines: the AGREE project. *Quality & Safety in Health Care* 2003;**12**(1):18–23.

31. McLiesh P, Mungall D, Wiechula R. Are we providing the best possible pain management for our elderly patients in the acute-care setting? *International Journal of Evidence-based Healthcare* 2009;**7**(3):173–80.

32. National Guideline Clearinghouse. Pain management in older adults. In: *Evidence-based geriatric nursing protocols for best practice*. Rockville, MD: Agency for Healthcare Research and Quality (AHRQ); 8/23/2014. Available: <www.guideline.gov/content.aspx?id=43932>.

33. Royal College of Physicians, British Geriatrics Society and British Pain Society. *The assessment of pain in older people: national guidelines. Concise guidance to good practice series, No. 8*. London: RCP; 2007.

34. Healthcare Quality Improvement Partnership. *Patient and public engagment in clinical audit*. London: 2009a.

35. National Institute for Clinical Effectiveness. *Principles for best practice in clinical audit*. Radcliffe Medical; 2002.

36. NHS Blood and Transplant. *How to collect clinical audit data effectively*. Hertfordshire, UK: NHS Blood and Transplant; 2012.

37. Travaglia J, Debono D. *Clinical audit: a comprehensive review of the literature*. Sydney: Centre for Clinical Governance Research in Health, Faculty of Medicine, University of New South Wales; 2009.

38. Healthcare Quality Improvement Partnership. *Criteria and indicators of best practice in clinical audit*. London: 2009b.

39. Hughes R. Understanding audit: methods and application. *Nursing & Residential Care* 2009;**11**(2):88–91.

40. Cooper J, Benjamin M. Clinical audit in practice. *Nursing Standard* 2004;**18**(28):47–53.

41. Morrell C, Harvey G. *The clinical audit handbook: improving the quality of health care*. London: Balliere Tindall; 1999.

42. Yin J, Reisinger HS, Vander Weg M, Schweizer ML, Jesson A, Morgan DJ, et al. Establishing evidence-based criteria for directly observed hand hygiene compliance monitoring programs: a prospective, multicenter cohort study. *Infection Control and Hospital Epidemiology* 2014;**35**(9):1163–8.

43. Crawford NW, Yeo V, Hunt RW, Barfield C, Gelbart B, Buttery JP. Immunisation practices in infants born prematurely: neonatologists' survey and clinical audit. *Journal of Paediatrics and Child Health* 2009;**45**(10):602–9.

44. Thorne L, Ellamushi H, Mtandari S, McEvoy AW, Powell M, Kitchen ND. Auditing patient experience and satisfaction with neurosurgical care: results of a questionnaire survey. *British Journal of Neurosurgery* 2002;**16**(3):243–55.

45. Dixon N, Pearce M. *Guide to ensuring data quality in clinical audits*. Healthcare Quality Improvement Partnership; 2010.

46. World Health Organization. *Hand hygiene technical reference manual*. Geneva: World Health Organization; 2009.

47. Kitson A, Rycroft-Malone J, Harvey G, McCormack B, Seers K, Titchen A. Evaluating the successful implementation of evidence into practice using the PARiHS framework: theoretical and practical challenges. *Implementation Science* 2008;**3**:1.
48. Harvey G, Loftus-Hills A, Rycroft-Malone J, Titchen A, Kitson A, McCormack B, et al. Getting evidence into practice: the role and function of facilitation. *Journal of Advanced Nursing* 2002;**37**(6):577–88.
49. Kitson A, Harvey G, McCormack B. Enabling the implementation of evidence based practice: a conceptual framework. *Quality in Health Care* 1998;**7**(3):149–58.
50. McCormack B, Kitson A, Harvey G, Rycroft-Malone J, Titchen A, Seers K. Getting evidence into practice: the meaning of 'context'. *Journal of Advanced Nursing* 2002;**38**(1):94–104.
51. Straus SE, Tetroe J, Graham I. *Knowledge translation in health care: moving from evidence to practice.* 2nd ed. Oxford, UK: John Wiley & Sons, Ltd; 2013.
52. Hawe P, King L, Noort M, Jordens C, Lloyd B. *Indicators to help with capacity building in health promotion.* North Sydney: NSW Health Department; 2000.
53. Gordge L, De Young J, Wiechula R. Reducing functional decline of older people in an acute-care setting: are we providing adequate care to maintain/optimise the functional status of our elder patients? *International Journal of Evidence-based Healthcare* 2009;**7**(3):181–6.
54. Kitson A, Silverston H, Wiechula R, Zeitz K, Marcoionni D, Page T. Clinical nursing leaders', team members' and service managers' experiences of implementing evidence at a local level. *Journal of Nursing Management* 2011;**19**(4):542–55.

CHAPTER 13

Perspectives on quality in nursing

Cathy Jones

LEARNING OBJECTIVES

When you have completed this chapter you will be able to:

- describe the key components of a quality improvement program
- identify approaches to measuring quality in health from an individual and system-wide perspective
- describe the activities implemented by nurses to measure and enhance quality
- discuss the importance of consumer perspectives in the measurement and improvement of the quality of nursing care
- reflect on practice and be ready to implement the practice tips provided

KEYWORDS: clinical indicator, consumer, patient safety, quality, clinical risk management

INTRODUCTION

In every successful business, attention needs to be directed to ensuring that products and services are of high quality and appropriate for the market. Organisations have adopted increasingly stringent standards to ensure that quality is achieved and maintained through models such as Continuous Quality Improvement and Total Quality Management. The impetus for quality in business began in earnest in the 1940s and 1950s, with Juran, Crosby and Deming being the founding experts. While the early focus was on cost,[1] the definition has now broadened to include compliance with defined specifications or standards, with quality being measured as compliance with these standards.[2] However, these definitions were not always appropriate for service organisations, including healthcare, and quality was expanded to include a focus on meeting or exceeding customer expectations.[3]

Health services are committed to providing quality care, and the concepts defined in other industries have been adapted to measure the performance and outcomes in healthcare, both at a patient and organisational level. Different but legitimate perceptions of the critical aspects of quality vary according to various stakeholders such as patients, healthcare workers, healthcare managers, policy makers and governments.[4,5,6] Nevertheless, attempts have been made to elicit the key dimensions of quality in healthcare and these are seen to include (but are not limited to) safety, effectiveness, appropriateness, consumer participation, access and efficiency.[3] These dimensions are often included in the frameworks and criteria organisations that governments use to measure quality in healthcare.[7]

Despite the wealth of knowledge and research about quality of healthcare, it cannot be taken for granted in any organisation. Two key obstacles to quality and safety remain:

- Best practice – research evidence is not always implemented.[5,8]
- Patients continue to suffer harm from healthcare interventions.[4,9]

Ensuring patient safety has become a major concern of governments, healthcare providers and the public in developed countries. Patient safety has emerged as a compelling healthcare issue and an international priority research field.[10] New ways of addressing patient safety problems and seeking their solutions have emerged, with the most powerful aspect of the reforms being to shift blame from individuals to systems, and an emphasis on investigating 'how people do things', rather than 'what people do'.[9]

The Australian Commission for Safety and Quality in Healthcare (ACSQHC) is the Australian government agency that sets the healthcare quality agenda for Australia. The Commission leads and coordinates national improvements in safety and quality in healthcare, while supporting healthcare workers and organisations. The Commission focuses on specific priority areas such as patient identification, medication safety, clinical handover, healthcare-associated infection, open disclosure, accreditation, falls prevention, credentialling and antimicrobial stewardship, and a number of other areas. Its website is the first place to visit for the latest evidence on these specific quality and safety issues.

Newly qualified nurses are often put off the concept of quality and safety by the plethora of acronyms and jargon that are used. These include Total Quality Management (TQM), Quality Assurance (QA), Continuous Quality Improvement (CQI), Quality Control (QC), Statistical Process Control (SPC), Quality Cycle, Quality Circle and Six Sigma. Although these may sound daunting, all mean approximately the same thing. Throughout this chapter, the simple terms *quality* and *safety* will be used.

The aim of this chapter is to discuss what quality means in the context of nursing care. Clinical, organisational and consumer perspectives of quality relating to healthcare in general, and nursing care specifically, will be discussed. Newly qualified nurses are encouraged to integrate quality and safety into their practice by implementing the practice tips given throughout this chapter.

CLINICAL GOVERNANCE

One of the most popular quality-related terms in healthcare today is clinical governance. Healthcare organisations have always been responsible for corporate governance, which includes providing strategic direction and ensuring that operational, financial and risk management systems are in place to meet required corporate standards.[11] Clinical governance 'is an umbrella term for everything that helps to maintain and improve high standards of patient care'.[12] It draws together a range of quality and safety activities (such as incident monitoring, risk management, auditing, morbidity and mortality meetings) in a way that ensures an organisational focus on the development of a culture, systems and processes that promote quality of care as the main focus of the organisation.[3]

The landmark study *To Err is Human: Building a Safer Health System* quantified the extent of errors and adverse events in hospitals and identified a plan of action to enhance patient safety.[10] As well, inquiries into reported poor care both in the United Kingdom and Australia have resulted in governments realising the need for healthcare organisations to focus on clinical as well as corporate governance.[13]

Clinical governance within an organisation is an all-encompassing concept and incorporates all of the concepts discussed within this chapter.

HOW DO WE MEASURE QUALITY?

The measurement of quality is facilitated by the use of standards, performance indicators and outcome measures. The first documented example of quality in nursing is credited to Florence Nightingale. She identified principles of care, which she developed into the standards she used to measure the structures and processes by which care was provided in military hospitals. Methods of evaluating care have increased in sophistication and precision since that time, and nurses have realised the diversity of ways in which quality of care can be measured and predicted.[14] Each member of the healthcare team has an important role to perform in maintaining the momentum by identifying problems and contributing to solutions to establish effective systems and processes.

The measurement of quality in healthcare varies depending on whether you are looking at an entire population, a healthcare provider level or an individual level:

- *Population:* This level includes entire nations, or broad groups and communities such as newborn babies or indigenous communities.
- *Organisation:* This level includes any organisation that provides healthcare, such as a hospital, community health service or diagnostic imaging practice, to groups of consumers.
- *Individual:* This level includes nurses, allied health professionals, medical practitioners and anyone who provides healthcare interventions in partnership with individual consumers, patients and carers.

Population Measures

In Australia, performance in the health system is measured and reported against three broad domains described by the national health performance framework.[4] Each domain has multiple dimensions that direct development of specific standards that can be implemented at national, state and local levels. The first of the three domains, health status, addresses policy on the general health of Australians – for example, Indigenous mortality rates. Reporting against the outcomes provides data to identify the relative health status of groups or regions, and identifies opportunities for improvement. The second domain, determinants of health, takes into account factors that influence the health status of Australians – for example, smoking rates and obesity. The third domain, health system performance, measures variables such as access to and equity of service provision, safety and sustainability – for example, screening rates for breast cancer.

Organisational Measures

There are many ways of measuring quality and safety in healthcare organisations. Most quality and safety systems in an organisation will include some or all of the following:[3]

- external accreditation/inspection against a set of recognised standards – for example, hospitals in Australia use the National Safety and Quality Health Service Standards (NSQHSS)
- internal audit against standards and policies
- patient/consumer feedback – for example, surveys
- clinical and other performance indicators
- incident and adverse event monitoring
- patient health outcome measures – for example, the Functional Independence Measure for rehabilitation patients.

Criteria and procedures for the accreditation of programs,[15] standards of practice, competencies for practitioners and indicators of outcome have been developed to provide a measure against which the quality of clinical performance by all care providers and outcomes of organisations can be judged. A brief description of the quality measures used is provided below.

The new graduate has a responsibility to identify the accreditation programs, standards of practice, competencies and indicators of outcome that are used in their practice setting. If these tools are not being used, the nurse may have a facilitative role in the establishment of these quality measures in a particular practice setting.

Practice Tip: Find out how your organisation measures quality and safety. If one of the elements listed above is not evident, ask why not.

Individual Measures of Nursing Quality

Nationally established professional nursing standards are a useful starting point and can provide the benchmark for healthcare organisations with regard to standards of care, competency-based education and quality. It is important to note that, while clinical practice may differ across settings, the standards continue to serve as a unifying link for nursing practice, regardless of the setting.

In addition, nurses are increasingly being urged to demonstrate the quality of their practice in terms of its effect on consumers,[14,16] and they have responded by taking a proactive role in the development of mechanisms to assure quality, such as nursing indicators and patient experience scores.[17]

Once the performance standard has been established, the level of competence (knowledge, skills and abilities) necessary to achieve the standard can be described. In healthcare, the development of competency standards provides a measure of quality against which practitioners and organisational policy are measured with regard to three key elements: attributes (knowledge, skills, attitudes and abilities), performance and standards.[18] The Australian Nursing and Midwifery Council has developed standards of competence for registered nurses,[19] enrolled nurses,[20] midwives[21] and nurse practitioners.[22] These documents, which are customised for each group, present the core competency standard against which the performance of practitioners is assessed to obtain and retain a licence to practise. A measure of performance and accountability is articulated which can be used to promote and demonstrate best practice, to guide occupational classification and restructuring, and as a basis for education and training.

Ensuring competence at the point of entry to the profession and on an ongoing basis benefits the nurse, the profession, the community and employers. Over the past two decades, most regulated professions in Australia have developed statements of competence, including the majority of disciplines associated with health. All accredited nursing courses preparing registered and enrolled nurses in Australia are required by the nurse-registering authority, the Nursing and Midwifery Board of Australia,[23] to reflect the Australian Nursing and Midwifery Council competency standards.

Competency standards can be used to differentiate between levels of competence and, in doing so, provide an objective measure against which nurses can be judged for recognition of advanced and/or specialist practices, skills or knowledge.

Credentialling is the process by which an individual's performance is measured against relevant practice standards. It is a peer review process which requires an individual nurse to present evidence that he or she has achieved the prescribed level of competence (attitudes, skills and standards) for recognition as a specialist practitioner. The main objective of credentialling practitioners is to ensure high-quality care and to provide a process by which:

- the profession can extend expectations of clinical practice
- clinical standards can be scrutinised
- the nursing role in healthcare can be promoted
- nurses can demonstrate their accountability
- nurses can work within the boundaries of their skills and expertise
- professional education can be planned.[24]

Specialty nursing groups around the world have developed standards, competencies and credentialling procedures, driven by the desire of advanced practitioners to be recognised for the contribution they make to nursing and healthcare.

Credentialling provides a process by which specialisation and advanced practice can be recognised and the image of nursing enhanced. National registration for health professionals facilitates specialist organisations to form associations with a central registering body to control and monitor practice.

Practice Tip: Are there are any nurses within your workplace who are credentialled to practise beyond the basic level of nursing care? How did they get this qualification/credentialling?

QUALITY STANDARDS

Standards are developed for two primary reasons: (1) to protect the public from harm; and (2) to improve the quality of services.[13,25] A standard is defined by Standards Australia as:

> ... a document, established by consensus and approved by a recognized body, that provides, for common and repeated use, rules, guidelines or characteristics for activities or their results, aimed at the achievement of an optimum degree of order in a given context.[18]

Standards reflect values because they are statements derived from a consensus of professional thinking, and are based on research, expert opinion and observation.[26] Standards determine what and how performance will be measured.[18]

Standards provide a framework that identifies the boundaries and essential elements for practice, and in doing so links three key professional practice accountabilities: care, quality and competence.[19,26] Standards are key to the success of nursing as healthcare evolves, monitoring the roles and settings of nursing practice and thus providing the link between institutional standards of care, competency-based education programs and quality assurance activities.[14]

Accreditation

Accreditation is a mechanism whereby an external body assesses an organisation to determine its performance and compliance with agreed standards. Accreditation procedures measuring the quality of hospital and community-based healthcare are well established in Australia. The aim of accreditation is to ensure and improve quality.

Generic accreditation programs with application to health facilities include the International Standards Organisation (ISO 9001).[27] The ISO 9001 provides independent accreditation to certify organisations against international standards to ensure they remain competent to perform their functions.

There are several sets of standards and accreditation programs that have been specifically designed for healthcare and are mandatory in Australia for certain sectors, including hospitals, pathology and diagnostic imaging. The National Safety and Quality Health Service (NSQHS) standards were developed by the Australian Commission on Safety and Quality in Healthcare and were introduced in 2013.[13,18] These standards are applicable for hospitals, day procedure centres and dental practices.

The ten NSQHS standards provide a nationally consistent guide to the best practice care consumers can expect from healthcare organisations. Typically, organisations go through a three- or four-year cycle of self-assessment, organisation-wide survey and periodic review to meet the standards.[28]

Practice Tip: Find out when your workplace was last accredited, by whom, and what recommendations were made by the accrediting body.

Evidence-based Practice

Evidence-based practice is the deliberate use of current best research evidence in making decisions about the care of individual patients. Clinical practice guidelines are designed to translate findings from medical research into clinical practice. When properly implemented, guidelines have been shown to improve health outcomes.[29]

However, it is well known that there is a gap between the evidence available and clinical practice in many areas of healthcare. Various studies claim that only 50% of clinical care is based on treatments that have been shown to be effective.[30,31] Reducing this evidence–practice gap has been associated with a reduction in morbidity and mortality.[32]

While ensuring that nurses are appropriately credentialled for the roles and functions they undertake is one way to ensure quality care, outcomes will also be enhanced by attention to clinical procedures and processes. Evidence-based practice is a philosophy that ensures all practice, clinical policy and guidelines are based on scientific evidence where available.[6] The emergence, and current prominence, of evidence-based practice has compelled clinicians to reflect on the origins of their practice techniques and procedures. The ready availability of the Cochrane Collaboration and online nursing evidence databases such as EBSCO and the Joanna Briggs Institute has provided a unique opportunity to pursue this ideal with some vigour.

Clinical practice guidelines and pathways are a form of evidence-based practice that have been developed to improve the care received by patients by promoting the use of interventions with proven benefits and discouraging ineffective interventions.[33] Clinical guidelines function as education resources for clinicians and consumers by providing evidence for clinical decision making and information about treatment options, services and standards of care.[34,35]

Guidelines are developed from research, expert opinion and clinical experience, often in combination.[36] Research has demonstrated that the development and use of clinical guidelines can change the process of health and improve health outcomes; however, the potential for health gain is dependent on the quality of the evidence and acceptance by clinicians. Development of evidence-based guidelines requires extensive financial and human resources to complete the research process that is required.

While there is evidence about effective ways to encourage clinicians to change practice when appropriate,[37] there continues to be a gap between the evidence and actual clinical care, and researchers, managers and clinicians are turning their attention to identifying the barriers and incentives to change practice.[38] The development, implementation and evaluation of clinical guidelines have application across a wide range of health services, and are fundamental to narrowing the theory–practice gap and promoting best practice.

Practice Tip: Find out when the clinical guidelines in use within your workplace were last updated, and whether they are based on the latest evidence and research.

INDICATORS OF QUALITY

Clinical Indicators

A clinical indicator is simply a measure of the clinical management and/or outcome of care. It is a quantitative measurement that can be compared over time or with other services that use the same definition. Indicators provide a useful method of assessing the quality and safety of care at a system level. When applied to healthcare, indicators can measure outcome (e.g. the number of deaths due to falls in hospitals), process (e.g. the number of completed falls risks assessments) or structure variables (e.g. the establishment of a falls coordinator position) to monitor the performance of healthcare facilities and the clinical practice of health professionals.[18]

A well-designed indicator should screen, flag or draw attention to a specific clinical issue. Indicators usually identify the rate of occurrence of an event, and are expressed as the percentage of events in a population. For example, one indicator of quality in surgery is the percentage of patients who require an unplanned return to theatre in the population of all patients undergoing surgery.

Indicators are designed to indicate potential problems that might need addressing. They demonstrate statistical outliers or variations within data results, rather than provide qualitative information about the actual issue identified. Nevertheless, indicators are useful as a tool to assist in assessing whether or not a standard in patient care is being met and also in monitoring changes over time.[25,39]

Increasingly, clinical indicators are being published online for consumers, funders, governments and the general public to access. The MyHospitals website lists all public and many private hospitals in Australia and published the first data in 2011. The MyHospitals indicators include measures such as emergency department waiting times, unplanned hospital readmission, hand hygiene and infection rates.[40] Private hospital providers in Australia also publish performance data online, with Healthscope the leader in the publication of consumer-focused quality data, showing trends over time and comparison to established benchmarks.[41]

Practice Tip: Find out which clinical indicators your workplace collects. Does your nursing practice have any impact on these indicators? Can your nursing practice help to improve the rate?

Outcome Measures

Clinicians and managers realise that it is important to assess not only how healthcare is delivered, but also to assess changes in clients' condition as a result of these interventions.[26] The potential for those data to inform clinical decision making underpins the increasing interest in valid outcome indicators of care.[42]

The need for healthcare providers to demonstrate the quality of services is paramount in the quest for good practice, professional standing, accreditation and, ultimately, funding. The shift in focus to include outcomes as well as process means that nurses must develop measures and reporting mechanisms that will enable them to demonstrate the benefits of nursing interventions to patients.[37]

Global outcome measures such as Health of the Nation Outcome Scales (HONOS) and Functional Independence Measure (FIM) provide a measure of outcome from the patient perspective. It is often difficult to separate this from the outcome of nursing interventions.

Monitoring clinical indicators is considered to have the potential to stimulate a variety of quality activities within healthcare organisations, including changes to procedures and policy.[42]

The development and use of clinical indicators can positively influence clinical practice. The Australian Council on Healthcare Standards (ACHS) liaises with medical colleges, associations and societies to develop clinical indicators. Both hospital-wide and discipline-specific sets of clinical indicators have been developed.[39] It is important to use valid and reliable tools and processes for documentation and retrieval of data.[43] Nurses are often involved in manual data collection in the workplace for various clinical indicators and patient administration systems, and coding data are also used for organisation-wide data.

Practice Tip: Talk to one of your patients to find out what they would define as a good indicator of a positive outcome of their healthcare.

Benchmarking

Quality can be measured against the performance of similar organisations through benchmarking activities against standards established by external accrediting bodies.

Benchmarking is defined as:

> ... an improvement tool whereby a company measures its performance or process against other companies' best practices, determines how those companies achieved their performance levels, and uses the information to improve its own performance.[7]

Benchmarking is one of the foundations of a comprehensive quality program. There are many different models for a successful benchmarking exercise,[44] but the following four stages are typically followed:
1. Choose a range of indicators or topic areas to look at and measure.
2. Compare your workplace to other similar workplaces, using these measures.
3. Identify your weaknesses and their strengths.
4. Learn from others how they achieve their results and how you can improve.
Benchmarking should be restricted to comparable agencies. Issues such as size and location of the agency, as well as the target population and the types of services delivered, must all be considered. If benchmarking indicators, the same definitions must be used.

For nursing, benchmarking can sometimes be a starting point for producing or improving clinical guidelines for high-quality nursing care.[45] This involves determination of the clinical guidelines to be measured, the measuring of these guidelines, the production of data, and the implementation of the clinical change required to bring a service into step with best-practice guidelines.

Clinicians and managers recognise the importance of ensuring consistently high-quality care but need also to be acutely aware of competing priorities in health. In order for a service to remain sustainable, hard decisions must sometimes be made around issues such as levels and mix of staff, case mix and priority services.

Benchmarking criteria that have an impact on quality and govern cost-effectiveness include staffing levels, average length of stay, infection rates, mortality rates, readmission rates and staff absenteeism. Although the majority of nurses are removed from decisions regarding the distribution of a health services budget, they can be directly involved in providing the clinical measures necessary to inform managerial decisions about budgetary and quality of clinical care issues.[44]

CLINICAL RISK MANAGEMENT

Clinical risk management is the systematic approach to developing strategies that enable healthcare organisations and clinicians to learn from past events in order to minimise future risk.[46] While clinical risk management encompasses some of the topics already discussed in this chapter, such as credentialling, evidence-based practice and clinical guidelines, it primarily focuses on monitoring adverse events and incorporation of risk management methodology into clinical care.[47]

Incident Reporting

There will always be errors (usually called incidents) in health, and some will become adverse events. Incidents are any failure of a planned or expected action to be completed as intended.[9] Adverse events are defined as a consequential bad outcome, an injury to the patient, in response to an error that occurs during care.[9] An incident does not lead to an adverse event in all cases.

In most healthcare organisations, formal incident-reporting systems have been implemented. Incident-reporting systems ensure that individual incidents are reviewed by senior staff and action is taken both for the individual event and to prevent similar incidents from recurring. Nurses need to be vigilant in identifying potential errors or near misses, and in recognising errors when they occur.[48] It is the responsibility of all healthcare professionals to be part of a culture that strives to provide quality care; however, some staff are reluctant to report incidents when they occur[49] and, as a result, the occurrence of incidents is underreported.[16]

The roles and responsibilities of nurses place them in a perfect position to recognise and intercept incidents and errors.[50] In most healthcare organisations, nurses report the vast majority of clinical incidents and are well placed to identify and implement strategies for prevention. The more incidents that are identified and analysed, the more likely an organisation will be able to improve patient safety and prevent future adverse events by putting preventive strategies in place.

The most serious incidents will need to be analysed using root cause analysis methodology, where the aim is to find out what happened, why it happened and how it can be prevented from happening again.[51,52] Nurses participating in root cause analysis need to have the knowledge, skills and training to identify causes and contributing factors of errors. Ensuring a safe environment for clinicians and people who use the health system is paramount in the design and planning of health services. Nurses have direct and continuous contact with patients, and therefore they can play a vital role in the development of an organisation that promotes safety. Within that environment nurses must be, and indeed will be, empowered to speak out, prepared to report errors and near misses when they occur, and able to analyse situations and events to discover why errors occur and to change systems when necessary.

Practice Tip: Next time you report an incident or near miss, ask your manager to explain to you the outcome and any preventive action taken.

Risk Management

Incident analysis can lead to identification of specific systemic risks across an organisation – for example, patient falls. Multiple incidents can indicate a systemic risk that can be stratified using a risk assessment matrix to quantify the consequences and likelihood of such incidents recurring. This enables a numerical risk rating, typically consequences multiplied by likelihood. The Australian risk management standard[53] is a generic guide that provides a framework and practical steps for identifying, analysing, evaluating and treating risks.[2,27] The framework, with its emphasis on ongoing monitoring and review, is well suited for use in healthcare.

CONSUMER PERSPECTIVES

Consumers play a pivotal role in measuring the quality of care.[54] Traditionally, the term *patient* has implied a passive recipient of healthcare. The word *consumer* is more frequently used today, as it implies agency, choice and voice in choosing and using healthcare services.

The views of consumers provide crucial information for service development and quality review. This feedback has traditionally been gained from complaints and satisfaction surveys, but increasing emphasis is being placed on various forms of consumer participation as a more effective means of including the consumer perspective in healthcare.[54] This participation applies at an individual patient level, with involvement in their own care; but also, importantly, it promotes participation in organisational services, education, quality improvement, planning and strategy.

Complaints

A quality improvement approach promotes the integration of complaints management into a comprehensive quality program. Similar to the approach taken with adverse events, the systemic analysis of complaints is an important component of clinical risk management.[55] Nurses must be aware of the need for open communication with patients and carers when things go wrong, and of the need to promote a culture that ensures complaints and consumer feedback generate opportunities for learning at both an individual and organisational level.[56,57]

A number of early, but still influential, studies heightened concerns about unacceptable levels and rates of adverse events in hospitals.[58,59] These studies, coupled with the response to the increased awareness of complaints and complaints handling in healthcare, led to the establishment of a healthcare complaints commission in each Australian state and territory.[13,58]

Practice Tip: If a patient makes a complaint, first always say, 'Sorry.' Then address the issue as soon as possible, or pass it on to the person who is best able to help.

Consumer Surveys

Consumer satisfaction and experience surveys have frequently been used by clinicians, facilities and government to provide a quality measure. Results are used to monitor performance, identify trends, inform policy and service development, assess the effectiveness of policies and programs, benchmark with similar health services and identify opportunities for improvement.[59,60] However, satisfaction survey results can be limited to numeric or quantitative scores, and do not always uncover the reasons for consumer dissatisfaction.[61]

Consumer surveys are a valuable means for measuring, over time, if areas targeted for improvement, such as discharge planning or preadmission clinic, have in fact improved.

Practice Tip: Find out what area had the lowest satisfaction score in your workplace's most recent survey. Get involved in improving this issue.

Consumer Participation

Consumer participation is driven by a patient-centred care philosophy. Patient-centred care is healthcare that is responsive to and respectful of the needs, values and rights of consumers and carers.[60,61] Involvement of consumers in their own care has also been frequently shown to improve safety.[62]

Consumers need to be heard, and mechanisms beyond surveys must be in place to ensure that their suggestions are considered for action. The NSQHS Standards have an entire standard (standard 2) devoted to consumer participation and involvement in decisions about healthcare and organisational planning.[18]

There are various levels at which consumers can participate in healthcare, ranging from inclusion in decision making about their personal healthcare to being members of peer support groups, acting as consumer representatives on boards and committees, and taking on the role of consultants and advocates (using their own experience and knowledge) in service development.[63]

Practice Tip: Once a week, ask one of your patients to tell you what would improve their experience at your healthcare organisation. Incorporate their views into your practice.

CONCLUSION

Quality and safety is not an add-on to basic nursing care; it is an integral part of day-to-day practice. Incorporating the practice tips within this chapter will assist newly qualified nurses to integrate quality and safety principles into their everyday patient care. And for those nurses who see quality as the most important aspect of their practice, there is always an opportunity to become involved more formally with quality programs within the workplace. This could be done through conducting a quality improvement activity, attending a medication safety working group, reviewing the national falls prevention standard, or helping to redesign a clinical pathway based on evidence. In this way, your contribution to quality and safety does not just benefit the patients receiving your direct care, but also all of the patients in your workplace and into the future.

The future challenge for nurses is to continue to be vigilant in their pursuit of quality and diligent in their efforts to develop and implement reliable and valid measures. It is a challenge that clinicians, educators and researchers in nursing must embrace to promote the professionalism of nurses and the clinical value of nursing care. The additional challenge for new graduates is to develop an awareness of quality issues within the clinical setting, and to become actively involved in the process of measuring and evaluating quality activities.

CASE STUDY 13.1

Ruby is completing the final rotation of her graduate year in a medical ward at a tertiary referral hospital when she is invited to join the Quality Improvement Committee established by the director of nursing. Ruby has been asked to talk to other registered nurses on her ward, and to compile a list of the quality indicators used in that area to monitor the quality of nursing care.

REFLECTIVE QUESTIONS

Answer these questions based on your recent experiences in clinical areas.

1. What nursing indicators are typically collected, monitored and measured at ward level?
2. How could these indicators be used to improve quality?

CASE STUDY 13.2

At a recent meeting of the Quality Improvement Committee, the group was addressed by a representative from the hospital's consumer participation network, who spoke about the ways consumer feedback can be obtained and information used to improve the quality of care.

REFLECTIVE QUESTIONS

Answer these questions based on your recent experiences in clinical areas.

1. How can consumer feedback be obtained in clinical settings?
2. How could a consumer be involved in evaluating quality at a clinical level?

CASE STUDY 13.3

Ruby has been asked to review the ward clinical guidelines for removal of sutures, removal of indwelling catheters and administration of intravenous antibiotics.

REFLECTIVE QUESTIONS

Answer these questions based on your recent experiences in clinical areas.

1. What are the sources of evidence used to develop or locate existing evidence-based clinical guidelines?
2. Who should Ruby consult in the review of the guidelines?

RECOMMENDED READING

Agency for Healthcare Research and Quality. Available: <www.ahrq.gov>.

Australian Commission on Safety and Quality in Healthcare. Available: <www.safetyandquality. gov.au>.

Australian Council on Healthcare Standards. *Risk management and quality improvement handbook.* Sydney: Australian Council on Healthcare Standards; 2013.

Balding, C. *Create a great quality system in six months.* Melbourne: Qualityworks; 2013.

Institute for Healthcare Improvement. Available: <www.ihi.org>.

REFERENCES

1. Kelemen M. *Managing quality: managerial and critical perspectives.* London: Sage Publications; 2003.
2. Standards Australia and Standards New Zealand. *AS/NZS ISO 9001: 2006 Quality management systems – fundamentals and vocabulary.* Sydney: Standards Australia and Standards New Zealand; 2006.
3. Australian Commission on Safety and Quality in Healthcare. *Australian safety and quality framework for health care.* Sydney: Australian Commission on Safety and Quality in Healthcare; 2010.
4. Australian Commission on Safety and Quality in Healthcare. *Windows into safety and quality in health care 2010.* Sydney: Australian Commission on Safety and Quality in Healthcare; 2010.
5. Institute of Medicine. *Crossing the quality chasm: a new health system for the 21st century.* Washington, DC: National Academy Press; 2001.
6. Schouten L, Hulscher M, van Everdingen J, et al. Evidence for the impact of quality improvement collaboratives: systematic review. *BMJ Online First [serial on the Internet]* 2009. Online. Available: <www.bmj.com/content/336/ 7659/1491.full.pdf>.
7. Australian Council on Healthcare Standards. *Risk management and quality improvement handbook.* Sydney: Australian Council on Healthcare Standards; 2013.
8. Titler MG. The evidence for evidence-based practice implementation. In: Hughes RG, editor. *Patient safety and quality: an evidence-based handbook for nurses.* Rockville, MD: Agency for Healthcare Research and Quality; 2008.

9. Kohn L, Corrigan J, Donaldson M. *To err is human: building a safer health system.* Washington, DC: Institute of Medicine; 2000.

10. Drosler E, Klazinga N, Romano P, et al. Application of patient safety indicators internationally: a pilot study among seven countries. *International Journal of Quality in Health Care* 2009;**21**:272–8.

11. Callaly T, Arya D, Minas H. Quality, risk management and governance in mental health: an overview. *Australasian Psychiatry* 2005;**13**:16–20.

12. Royal College of Nursing. *Clinical governance: how nurses get involved.* London: RCA Publications; 2000.

13. Australian Commission on Safety and Quality in Healthcare. *Developing a safety and quality framework for Australia.* Sydney: Australian Commission on Safety and Quality in Healthcare; 2008.

14. Farquhar M, Kurtzman E, Thomas A. What do nurses need to know about the quality enterprise? *Journal of Continuing Education in Nursing* 2010;**41**:246–56.

15. Australian Nursing and Midwifery Council. *Standards and criteria for the accreditation of nursing and midwifery courses leading to registration, enrolment, endorsement and authorisation in Australia – with evidence guide.* Canberra: Australian Nursing and Midwifery Council; 2009.

16. Johnstone MJ, Kanitsaki O. Patient safety and the integration of graduate nurses into effective organizational clinical risk management systems and processes: an Australian study. *Quality Management in Health Care* 2008;**17**:162–73.

17. Montalvo I. The National Database of Nursing Quality Indicators™ (NDNQI®). *Online Journal of Issues in Nursing* 2007;**12**: Manuscript 2.

18. Australian Commission on Safety and Quality. *National Safety and Quality Health Service Standards.* Sydney: Australian Commission on Safety and Quality; 2011.

19. Australian Nursing and Midwifery Council. *National competency standards for registered nurses.* Canberra: Australian Nursing and Midwifery Council; 2006.

20. Australian Nursing and Midwifery Council. *National competency standards for the enrolled nurse.* Canberra: Australian Nursing and Midwifery Council; 2006.

21. Australian Nursing and Midwifery Council. *National competency standards for the midwife.* Canberra: Australian Nursing and Midwifery Council; 2006.

22. Australian Nursing and Midwifery Council. *National competency standards for the nurse practitioner.* Canberra: Australian Nursing and Midwifery Council; 2006.

23. Nursing and Midwifery Board of Australia. About the Board. 2014. Online. Available: <www.nursingmidwiferyboard.gov.au/> [Viewed 28 August 2014].

24. Queensland Department of Health. *Credentialing and defining the scope of clinical practice.* Brisbane: Queensland Department of Health; 2013.

25. Quality Improvement Council. *Health and community services standards.* 6th ed. Melbourne: Quality Improvement Council; 2010.

26. National Health Information Standards and Statistics Committee (NHISSC). *The National Health Performance Framework.* 2nd ed. Sydney: NHISSC; 2009.

27. Standards Australia and Standards New Zealand. *Quality Management Systems AS/NZS ISO 9001: 2008 Self assessment checklist.* Sydney: Standards Australia and Standards New Zealand; 2008.

28. Australian Council on Healthcare Standards. *EQuIP5.* Sydney: The Australian Council on Healthcare Standards; 2010.

29. Grimshaw JM, Russell IT. Effect of clinical guidelines on medical practice: a systematic review of rigorous evaluations. *Lancet* 1993;**342**(13):17–22.

30. Bryant J, Boyes A, Jones K, Sanson-Fisher R, Carey M, Fry R. Examining and addressing evidence-practice gaps in cancer care: a systematic review. *Implementation Science* 2014;**9**:37.

31. Cochrane LJ, Olson CA, Murray S, Dupuis M, Tooman T, Hayes S. Gaps between knowing and doing: understanding and assessing the barriers to optimal health care. *Journal of Continuing Education for Health Professionals* 2007;**27**(2):94–102.

32. McCullough ML, Patel AV, Kushi LH, Patel R, Willett WC, Doyle C, et al. Following cancer prevention guidelines reduces risk of cancer, cardiovascular disease, and all-cause mortality. *Cancer Epidemiology, Biomarkers and Prevention: A Publication of the American Association for Cancer Research, Cosponsored by the American Society of Preventive Oncology* 2011;**20**(6):1089–97.

33. National Health and Medical Research Council. *Procedures and requirements for meeting the 2011 NHMRC standard for clinical practice guidelines.* Canberra: Commonwealth of Australia; 2011.

34. The Guidelines International Network. The Guidelines International Network. 2010. Online. Available: <www.gin2010.org/?page_id=33>.

35. National Institute of Clinical Studies (NICS). Clinical practice guidelines portal. Australian Government; 2010. Online. Available: <www.clinicalguidelines.gov.au/>.

36. Pearson A, Field J, Jordan Z. *Evidence-based clinical practice in nursing and health care. Assimilating research, experience and expertise.* Melbourne: Blackwell; 2007.

37. Doran D, Harrison M, Laschinger H, et al. Nurse-sensitive outcomes data collection in acute care and long-term-care settings. *Nursing Research* 2006;**55**:S75–81.

38. Fong J, Marsh GM, Stokan LA, et al. Hospital quality performance report: an application of composite scoring. *American Journal of Medical Quality* 2008;**23**:287–95.

39. Australian Council on Health Care Standards. *Clinical indicator program information.* Sydney: Australian Council on Health Care Standards; 2014.

40. National Health Performance Authority. Myhospitals: About the data. 2014. Available: <www.myhospitals.gov.au/about-the-data#a10> [Viewed 25 August 2014].

41. Healthscope. MyHealthscope. 2014. Available: <www.MyHealthscope.com.au> [Viewed 25 August 2014].

42. Fung C, Lim Y-W, Mattke S, et al. Systematic review: the evidence that publishing patient care performance data improves quality of care. *Annals of Internal Medicine* 2008;**248**:111–23.

43. Albanese MP, Evans DA, Schantz CA, et al. Engaging clinical nurses in quality and performance improvement activities. *Nursing Administration Quarterly* 2010;**34**:226–45.

44. Guven-Uslu P. Benchmarking in health services. *Benchmarking: An International Journal* 2005;**12**:293–309.

45. Wait S, Nolte E. Benchmarking health systems: trends, conceptual issues and future perspectives. *Benchmarking: An International Journal* 2005;**12**:436–48.

46. Hovenga E, Kidd M, Garde S, et al. Resource, quality and safety management. *Studies in Health Technologies & Informatics* 2010;**151**:360–84.

47. NSW Health. *Performance management framework.* North Sydney: NSW Department of Health; 2009.

48. Johnstone M-J, Kanitsaki O. Processes influencing the development of graduate nurse capabilities in clinical risk management: an Australian study. *Quality Management in Health Care* 2006;**15**:268–78.

49. Wakefield JG, Jorm CM. Patient safety – a balanced measurement framework. *Australian Health Review* 2009;**33**:382–9.

50. Hughes R, Clancy C. Nurse's role in patient safety. *Journal of Nursing Care Quality* 2009;**24**:1–4.

51. Middleton S, Chapman B, Griffiths R, et al. Reviewing recommendations of root cause analyses. *Australian Health Review* 2007;**31**:288–95.

52. Woloshynowych M, Rogers S, Taylor-Adams S, et al. *The investigation and analysis of critical incidents and adverse events in health care.* Contract No. 19. London: National Health Service; 2005.

53. Standards Australia and Standards New Zealand. *AS/NZS ISO 31000: 2009 Risk management principles and guidelines.* Sydney: Standards Australia and Standards New Zealand; 2009.

54. Greco M. Raising the bar on consumer feedback – improving health services. *Australian Health Consumer* 2006;**3**:11–12.
55. Romios P, Newby L, Wohlers M, et al. *Turning wrongs into rights: learning from consumer reported incidents, summary annotated literature review.* Canberra: Department of Health and Ageing, Commonwealth of Australia; 2003.
56. Australian Commission on Safety and Quality in Health Care (ACSQHC). *Australian Open Disclosure Framework.* Sydney: ACSQHC; 2013.
57. Iedema R, Jorm C, Wakefield J, et al. Practising open disclosure: clinical incident communication and systems improvement. *Sociology of Health & Illness* 2009;**31**:262–77.
58. Health Care Complaints Commission. *Understanding and managing patient complaints.* Sydney: NSW Government; 2008.
59. Burford B, Bedi A, Morrow G, et al. Collecting patient feedback in different clinical settings: problems and solutions. *The Clinical Teacher* 2009;**6**:259–64.
60. Luxford K, Safran DG, Delbanco T. Promoting patient-centred care: a qualitative study of facilitators and barriers in healthcare organisations with a reputation for improving the patient experience. *International Journal of Quality in Healthcare* 2011;**23**(5):510–15.
61. Australian Commission on Safety and Quality in Health Care (ACSQHC). *Patient centred care: improving quality and safety through partnerships with patients and consumers.* Sydney: ACSQHC; 2011.
62. Mohsin-Shaikh S, Garfield S, Franklin B. Patient involvement in medication safety in hospital: an exploratory study. *International Journal of Clinical Pharmacy* 2014;**36**(3):657–66.
63. Gregory J. *Conceptualising consumer engagement: a review of the literature.* Melbourne: Australian Institute of Health Policy Studies; 2007.

CHAPTER 14

Managing emotional reactions in patients, families and colleagues

Paul Morrison and Christine Ashley

LEARNING OBJECTIVES

When you have completed this chapter you will be able to:

- identify causes of emotional stress in nursing
- examine your responses to emotional conflict
- develop a greater level of self-awareness
- explore ways of managing emotional reactions in yourself and others
- take a positive and constructive approach to dealing with conflict.

KEYWORDS: conflict, coping, interpersonal skills, self-awareness, strategies for managing conflict

INTRODUCTION

The care context is a microcosm of society. It exposes us to the whole gamut of stresses and strains that unfold during a person's lifetime. But it does so in an intense way and sometimes over a very short and compressed period of time. Whether you work primarily in a hospital or community setting, you will be exposed to a wide range of stressful events that elicit attendant emotional reactions and upset in you and others. You will also have to learn to cope with the routine tensions that affect us all outside work. How you deal with these will have an impact on how you deal with work-related issues. Learning to cope with and respond positively to the emotional side of things will not only help you to function more effectively at work; it will also help you to stay healthy.

STRESS AND YOU

One useful way of considering how much stress you are under is to use the life events scale developed by Holmes and Rahe some years ago.[1] Take a few minutes to rate yourself on the life events scale and calculate your overall score.

EXERCISE 14.1

Mark each item on the list that has occurred in your life during the past 12 months. Then add the points together.

Life Events Scale

Life event	Lifechange unit	Life event	Lifechange unit
Death of spouse	100	Trouble with in-laws	29
Divorce	73	Outstanding personal achievement	28
Marital separation	65	Spouse begins or stops work	26
Imprisonment	63	Begin or end school	26
Death of close family member	63	Change in living conditions	25
Personal injury or illness	53	Revision of personal habits	24
Marriage	50	Trouble with boss	23
Dismissal from work	47	Change in work hours or conditions	20
Marital reconciliation	45	Change in residence	20
Retirement	45	Change in schools	20
Change in health of family member	44	Change in recreation	19
Pregnancy	40	Change in church activities	19
Sexual difficulties	39	Change in social activities	18
Gain of new family member	39	Minor mortgage or loan	17
Business readjustment	39	Change in sleeping habits	16
Change in financial state	38	Change in number of family reunions	15
Change in number of arguments with spouse	35	Change in eating habits	15
Major mortgage	32	Vacation	13
Foreclosure of mortgage on loan	30	Christmas	12
Change in responsibilities at work	29	Minor violation of the law	11
Son or daughter leaving home	29		

Source: *Reproduced from TH Holmes, RH Rahe, The social readjustment rating scale.* Journal of Psychosomatic Research *1967;11:213–18, with the permission of Elsevier Science.*

The life events scale lists 41 positive and negative common occurrences that require adjustment and affect your risk of illness. A score of over 300 in 1 year greatly increases your chance of illness. A score of 150–299 reduces the risk by 30%, and less than 150 indicates a small risk of illness. However, even if you are at great risk due to major changes in your life, you can reduce that risk through the use of effective stress management techniques.

We respond to these sorts of pressures in individual ways as we evaluate the impact they will have on our lives and our capacity to cope effectively with them over time. Not all stress is bad. The normal stress in our lives – called eustress – helps us to perform and achieve things on a daily basis. The process of appraising the tasks facing us, and our capacity to deal with these effectively, helps us to identify support networks and personal resources that may be helpful. These networks, coupled with an optimistic attitude, tend to promote good coping in student nurses.[2]

Some coping strategies may create more problems; for example, excessive use of alcohol, food, recreational drugs and tobacco can lead to additional problems in your work life, and at home with your partner and children. They will also have a negative impact on your identity and general wellbeing. Consider how you tend to cope with these general stresses. It is important to develop an awareness of the sorts of things that you find especially stressful, and learn positive ways of coping with them. Self-awareness is perhaps one of the first steps in this direction. Being aware of the difficult issues and having someone to talk to will help. It is surprising how taking the time to complete a simple scale like the one you have just done can provide helpful feedback that raises awareness and generates personal insight. This is an important step in promoting change and positive coping.

EMOTIONAL REACTIONS IN NURSING PRACTICE

There are many potential sources that elicit emotional reactions at work. We have divided some of these into three major categories, but in reality they blend into each other depending on the complexity of the situation. In addition, you will probably be able to generate your own list of emotionally trying situations from your clinical experiences and those of your close colleagues. The examples outlined below should provide a realistic flavour of some of the common issues that provoke strong emotions.

Patients and Clients

We use the terms *patient* and *client* here to reflect the different work environments in which you may find yourself. In the acute hospital sector the word *patient* will prevail; while in other areas of health, such as the community or mental health, the term *client* may be preferred. Patients or clients can be a major source of emotional reactions in you. One of the main reasons for this is the changing nature of healthcare, with a greater emphasis on the professional relationship and more active patient participation within a patient-centred model of care.[3] Consider a few scenarios. A mother and child with a relatively minor complaint have to wait in the accident department for 2 hours because the staff is busy following a major road accident. As you walk by, the mother complains in a rude and hostile manner that her child has not yet been examined and may be seriously ill. She describes the nurses as 'arrogant bitches'. On other occasions you may come across people who are drunk or on drugs and demand immediate attention. Some patients may have unrealistic expectations about what you can do and the level of resources at your disposal. They simply assume that you can give them what they want promptly.

In emergency situations such as resuscitation or dealing with major traumas, people's emotions will be working overtime. Verbal assault, and occasionally physical assault, are almost inevitable in some areas of healthcare, especially in the emergency department. It is wise to prepare for these.[4] It is also vital that, if this happens to you or to a colleague, the incident is reported and dealt with appropriately. This includes you, or the colleague who has been exposed to verbal or physical assault, being provided with support and care.

CASE STUDY 14.1

Jane was a new graduate in her first week on a medical ward. During an evening shift, an elderly man was admitted to the ward from the emergency department suffering from severe head and facial injuries and fractured ribs. The patient had been the victim of a brutal attack during a robbery in his home.

During the attack, the man's wife was killed. The man was accompanied by a police guard and by members of his family. During the first two shifts that Jane cared for this patient, she was kept very busy dealing with the victim's physical injuries. The family members were cared for by the senior nurses, who organised support and counselling. The man gradually regained consciousness, and it was then that the full horror of the incident became apparent to Jane. She listened to a description of the events leading up to the assault, and she stayed with the patient as he begged to be allowed to die. He did not want to live without his wife, he said. Jane also found the constant presence of the police officers an intrusion on the nurse–patient relationship.

By the fourth day, Jane realised that she was becoming emotionally drained by nursing the patient, dealing with his distress and trying to comfort the family. She broke down on the ward and found it hard to come back to work the next day, thinking that she was not cut out for nursing. A senior nurse on the ward recognised that several other nurses were also experiencing similar distress. She organised for a counsellor from a support group for victims of crime to hold a debriefing session for staff. Everyone attended, including several of the police officers.

Jane found great comfort in being able to recognise that the trauma associated with such violence was a normal reaction, and that her response did not indicate weakness on her part. She felt much stronger as a result of the counselling session and returned to caring for the victim with increased empathy and understanding.

REFLECTIVE QUESTIONS

1. What struck you personally about Jane's story?
2. What does the story illustrate about the difficulties of dealing with the victims of crime?

There are times when you will come across people from different cultures whose language, value system and beliefs are all different from yours. This can create enormous difficulties in communication and arriving at a mutual understanding of events, needs and expectations. It can be a major source of frustration in you and others. From time to time, you may come across the victims of serious crimes such as rape, domestic violence and torture, or people who have attempted suicide or the relatives of those who have committed suicide. All of these people will elicit strong emotional responses in you as a nurse and as a person.

Families

Dealing with the families of patients can be an additional pressure. One of the most difficult aspects of working with families is having to give them bad news about the results of tests, or telling them that a family member has just died. You may be torn between the need to inform them and your desire to shield them from the pain that will inevitably follow your disclosure. It is an unsolvable dilemma.

However, we all have to face the inevitability of death in our families. Most family members respond to bad news with great courage; however, sometimes they react by blaming you and the hospital, and this can cause great distress. As you spend time with family members of dying patients you will inevitably get to know them and share some of their grief and the sense of loss they are experiencing.

The parents of very sick and dying children will need psychological support and help. Watching parents spend time with a dying child (or any member of the family, old or young) can be especially traumatic. If you happen to be a parent, too, then it is an even more difficult experience. The sense of crushing vulnerability[5] you will experience as a parent and nurse may help you to empathise more fully with the family. Personal pain and vulnerability are undeniable aspects of your role.

CASE STUDY 14.2

'We have to be real as nurses. We've moved a long way from the days when it was unacceptable for nurses to express emotions when caring for people. The day I don't feel will be the day I won't do this work anymore. But I always remember the children are not mine. There is a professional intensity and closeness; we get to know the child and their family incredibly well. Families remember everything about the care of their child, but I don't. I move on and bring that level of intensity to the next family ... Getting that balance right comes from experience, but developing really good knowledge and skills about how to care for yourself from the beginning is very important,' says Karyn Bycroft, a New Zealand nurse practitioner who cares for dying children.[6]

REFLECTIVE QUESTIONS

1. Think of a client or patient you felt close to during your clinical work. What was it about the context and the person involved that enabled that closeness to be established?
2. How did the closeness influence the care you provided?
3. How did you manage to move on from that momentary closeness?

Colleagues

This category may seem slightly strange and out of place here for someone working in a 'caring' profession such as nursing. However, as you become more experienced you will find, if you have not done so already, that colleagues and other members of the healthcare team can be a major source of conflict in your working life.[7] Sometimes managers, supervisors or colleagues make unfair demands on you: asking you to work unreasonable rosters or ignoring your requests for special shifts; or you may feel unreasonable pressure to come to work when you are unwell. In the workplace, you may feel that your contributions to discussions relating to patients' issues or ward management are being deliberately ignored. In other words, you feel undervalued or 'picked on' in your workplace. *Horizontal violence* is the term used to describe intergroup conflict of this nature.[7,8]

There may also be times when you come into conflict with colleagues from other disciplines. For example, you may feel that an elderly patient with terminal cancer should be allowed to die in peace, while the surgeon insists on performing another traumatic and expensive operation in the hope that it might prolong the patient's life for another 6 months.

It can be very difficult to challenge another colleague in a situation like this because of the power differences that exist. Nurses often just accept the situation without question, and this may be part of the hidden curriculum they have been exposed to as students or new graduates – that is, not to question the doctor or other senior colleagues. However, a clash of values, especially if they occur in a particular workplace setting, needs to be dealt with constructively or people will feel very stressed and disempowered and their effectiveness will deteriorate.

There may be times when a situation at work raises ethical dilemmas for you. You may suspect that a colleague (and friend) may be taking medications from the ward and using or selling them. Yet, you have no proof. Do you confront your friend and run the risk of ruining the friendship? Or do you report your suspicions to the supervisor? Both options carry the risk that your friend's career may be in jeopardy. Yet, you also have a responsibility to the patients whose medication your friend may be stealing by falsifying their medication records. As a registered nurse you must report any incident of this nature. Reporting another health professional who is acting inappropriately or unethically is now a legal requirement for registered nurses.[9]

CASE STUDY 14.3

Sue started work in a busy mental health ward in a regional hospital. She had gained a year's experience in a large city centre after completing her postgraduate studies in mental health nursing. There were several nursing practices in the new workplace that Sue knew were outdated and not evidence-based. She spoke to the nurse manager about these and asked if she could revise them. The manager told her that the current practices worked very well and she saw no reason to revise them.

From then on, the manager often ridiculed Sue in front of her fellow workers and gave her tasks to do with unrealistic timeframes. Sue began to feel intimidated and lost confidence in her abilities. When she confided in her fellow workers, she was told, 'If you want a quiet life, keep your head down and do as you're told.' Senior nurses on the ward also constantly made sly comments about her psychiatric training, saying that she thought she 'knew it all' because she had attended university.

Sue became so depressed about her work situation that she contemplated leaving nursing, until a colleague from her student days advised her of some strategies to use, and told her about the role of anti-harassment officers in the workplace. As a result, Sue was able to learn some skills for dealing with conflict in the workplace, and also gained comfort from learning about her legal rights and the steps she could take if the situation became untenable.

Gradually, over a period of time, the other staff members accepted Sue. Later, another new staff member experienced the same difficulties, and Sue was able to assist her by sharing her own experiences.

REFLECTIVE QUESTIONS

1. Think of a time when you felt in some way undermined or diminished as a person in a clinical setting. How did you manage to get through this difficult period?
2. What skills and resources did you evoke to help you at the time?
3. What would you like to share with other less experienced students about how to overcome these difficult moments at work?

Personal Dilemmas

There may be times when you have to make important decisions that affect your ability to balance a career and personal life successfully. Getting married, deciding to start a family or to return to full-time study, taking on a mortgage or working overseas for a few years can all interrupt your career, sometimes with negative consequences. There are no right answers here. Lots of people, in an effort to be supportive, will tell you what to do. This type of advice is rarely helpful. What is very important is for you to explore different perspectives in order to clarify your values and long-term goals. When you are clear about these you will be able to make informed choices that suit you and those closest to you. Important decisions are never easy. Whatever circumstances might emerge, it is important to remember that humans have a great capacity to adapt and find happiness and contentment in life.[10]

STRATEGIES FOR MANAGING CONFLICT CONSTRUCTIVELY

Acknowledge the Conflict

The situations described above may all be considered sources of conflict that elicit strong emotional reactions – such as feelings of anxiety, tension, guilt, depression, or anger and hostility – for those involved. These occurrences can range from minor discomforts, incidents and misunderstandings to serious crisis situations that can have an impact on a whole ward team and across disciplines. Most importantly, these forms of emotional reactions will often lead to stress, sour relationships and poor work performance.[11] Acknowledging a conflict or situation is important because it will help you to make sensible plans to address the issue and to arrive at a point where you feel a stronger sense of self-control.

Deal with Emotional Reactions

Emotions play an important role in how you manage work and the people you encounter. Becoming more self-aware and learning about your emotional self will enable you to manage your emotions at work more effectively and at the same time help you to be more aware of other people's reactions. This enhanced awareness will help to build more productive relationships and manage conflict at work in a calm and constructive fashion and is referred to as 'emotional intelligence'.[12]

EXERCISE 14.2

Take a few moments to think about a situation that elicited strong emotions in you, then complete the following activities.

1. Describe a situation and identify the people involved.
2. Describe your emotional reaction and label the feelings you experienced during and after the situation. What changes did you notice in your breathing, heart rate and stomach during the event?
3. Describe how you responded to the situation. How did you behave? What did you say and do?
4. Describe how the situation was resolved or managed. Did you react negatively or constructively?

Notice how completing a short exercise like this may evoke some of the feelings, thoughts and bodily experiences that you felt at the time of the incident. If it has, then it suggests that this incident is a form of 'unfinished business' and you may need to continue to work through this, perhaps by talking with a supportive friend, if you are to move forward at work.

Take Care of Yourself

Unfortunately, many nurses downplay the effects of emotional abuse or violence in the workplace. Exposure to this sort of working environment, in the long term, will have a very negative effect on your performance both at work and at home.[13] If you are a victim of violence or abuse of any sort, the literature is clear in advocating that you will benefit from debriefing and post-trauma counselling.[14] In many cases, the support of peers and workplace colleagues can facilitate a positive outcome in the short term. However, 'spot debriefing' is often not enough, and more formal follow-up should be sought. Unfortunately, in rural or remote areas there is often inadequate support available. It is important, though, if your employer is unable to provide you with follow-up, that you seek professional help from your doctor, counsellor or another health professional.

You can also take care of yourself by ensuring that you have a balanced lifestyle. Avoid overworking, overeating and overdrinking, and take regular exercise. Make sure that you take all the vacation time that you are entitled to, and that you get enough sleep and relaxation. Plan to review your work situation and lifestyle at three or four points in the year. Too many people fail to take time out to reflect on how things are and where they are headed. If you find that some people or situations are continually causing you to feel overwhelmed and exhausted, do something about it. Learn how to say 'no' (and mean it) to taking on more than you can reasonably deal with. Where possible, avoid interacting with those people who add to your stress at work. Focus on a small number of priorities – do not try to do everything at once. Work on being happy and take steps that will help with this goal.[15,16]

Know Your Rights

Employers in Australia are required under workplace health and safety legislation in each state and territory to provide a safe place of work and to provide and maintain a safe system of work. Equal employment and anti-discrimination legislation also protects you from unfair discrimination and certain objectionable conduct. So, if you work in a situation that, in your opinion, leaves you exposed to physical risks or sexual or emotional abuse, you have a right to take this up with your supervisor or employer.

Perhaps you are working in a rural or remote setting on your own at weekends. You are caring for several potentially aggressive patients, and you have limited access to back-up in an emergency. You consider you are potentially at risk, but you do not want to appear to your colleagues as if you cannot cope. Do not assume that, because no one else has done anything about the situation, you should avoid doing anything, too. Remember: you have a right to feel safe at work. You also have a responsibility to your patients, to your profession, and to yourself and your family. It is vital that you discuss the situation with your supervisor, and try to be constructive in your discussions. Remember that knowing that the law is on your side is, in itself, empowering.

Use Interpersonal Skills and Build Rapport with Others

How you cope with a given situation will depend very much on how you interact with others in the workplace. In a complex social environment such as a hospital or healthcare centre, working cooperatively and being able to get along with others is vital. Understanding how you interact is important if you are to develop skills to deal with conflict. Learning to enhance your awareness of your interpersonal approach and skills is an ongoing process. Try Exercise 14.3 below for yourself. The items are adapted from the Opener Scale.[17]

Now that you have considered your own strengths and weaknesses more carefully, you can use this information to improve your skills in dealing with conflict. Having the ability to listen and be empathic is important in all aspects of nursing, not least when we are expected to resolve conflict or defuse emotionally charged situations. When attempting to manage a conflict, it is really important to develop a clear understanding

EXERCISE 14.3

- People often tell me about themselves
- I like listening to people's stories
- People trust me with their secrets
- I am very accepting of others
- People feel comfortable around me

Consider each of these statements in turn along a continuum from 'very much like me' to 'not at all like me' and ask yourself the following questions:

1. To what extent is this statement a good description of me at work?
2. Are there things I would like to change? If so, why? If not, why not?
3. How does this description of me shape how I relate to others at work?
4. How does this description of me shape how others relate to me at work?
5. Do you see this description of you as a strength or a weakness in your approach to others? If so, why? If not, why not?

of the other people involved and their particular wants and needs. This takes time and patience and very good communication skills. The ability to empathise with the other parties is fundamental. Remember, too, that people may have very good reasons to be angry, so it is important to explore the situation from different perspectives. Being able to take on board the perspectives of others will help you to acknowledge and accept that some stresses cannot be avoided, mishaps and mistakes are inevitable, and learning to forgive is an important skill in successful coping and promotes health and wellbeing.[18]

Realise Your Potential as a Professional and a Person

Part of dealing effectively with challenging situations as a nurse comes about through life's experiences over time and developing personal maturity. Most new graduates are concerned by their lack of experience; however, remember, while you may lack extensive clinical expertise, your ability to deal with delicate situations comes about not only through knowledge gained at university and on clinical placements but also through the experiences you have gained throughout your life. Travel, working in other environments and dealing with family crises are important in developing coping skills and shaping you as a person. So, when opportunities present themselves, always consider the potential benefits that may result from, for example, an overseas trip or the invitation to be part of a childcare centre management committee. These opportunities will increase your self-esteem and self-awareness, and provide you with unexpected extra knowledge and skills.

As you prepare to embark on your career as a nurse, you will be experiencing the relief of having come to the end of several hard years of study. However, do not make the mistake of thinking that your studying days are over! Sociologists tell us that we will be likely to undergo several career changes during our working lives, so it is vital to recognise the importance of continuing professional development as part of your working life. Learning is a lifetime commitment, so seize opportunities as they arise and keep yourself informed and up to date. Look upon the acquisition of knowledge and skills as the key to your long-term success in the future.

Learn to Live with Pressure

Living with pressure and coping with rapid change is now a routine requirement in most professional careers. Many of us view 'pressure' as a stress that can lead to conflict in our daily lives. Part of learning to cope with pressure at home, at university and at work is to recognise that pressure can also be a stimulus for enhancing our performance – some anxiety helps us to perform better. However, too much pressure for lengthy periods of time becomes exhausting and leads to deterioration in performance.

Similarly with change: we all need to accept change as a positive experience rather than something that should be avoided or that can have only negative consequences. Consider the following example: as a cost-cutting exercise, the staffing on your ward has been cut by one registered nurse on the evening shift. At first, you feel overwhelmed at the thought of how you will get through the resulting extra work, and you worry through your days off about returning to the workplace. This is responding negatively to change and pressure. However, when you start to consider what you normally do each shift, you begin to realise that much of the evening work is done simply because that's the way it has always been done, rather than being based on evidence for best practice. By using your professional judgment and some creative skill you realise that, in fact, you can work more efficiently and effectively than before, and with fewer staff. Change, in this case, has had a good outcome, and you have responded to the pressure positively.

Some of us thrive on pressure – we all know the old saying that if you want something done, you go to the busiest person. Yet others are not able to cope so well. It is important that you know your own capabilities, and do not expose yourself to unnecessary pressure. Do not fall into the 'Messiah trap'[19] and get caught up in the belief that you are 'indispensable' and everyone else's needs must come before your own. Being a Messiah can make you feel indispensable, but it can also leave you feeling worthless, unimportant and isolated because your personal needs are being ignored.

Berry[19] describes the 'Messiah trap' as a two-sided lie into which many caring people fall:

Side 1	If I don't do it, it won't get done. (You take responsibility for everything and feel indispensable.)
Side 2	Everyone else's needs take priority over mine. (You believe you are expected to put everyone else first at the expense of caring for yourself.)

Nursing will always involve a certain amount of pressure in any specialty, but some clinical settings are recognised as high-stress areas, such as emergency departments and intensive care units. If you know you do not cope well with these highly stressful clinical areas, use this knowledge to guide you as you choose your career path. If you are starting to feel 'burnt out' by your work, then recognise this as a sign that you are not coping well with pressure. Depending on its severity, dealing with burnout may involve debriefing with colleagues, seeking counselling from a professional, having a well-earned holiday or even reviewing your place of work.

Find Your Niche

Sometimes we find roles and areas for which we are really well suited, and sometimes we do not. For example, it was found that those who were more effective helpers in professions like the clergy and teaching were more likely to view the world from a basically person-centred perspective. It may come as no surprise to hear that many people in professions like nursing and social work change their career and enter counselling. Their system of beliefs may be in conflict with the daily practices of their former profession.[20] However, the search may be a long and arduous one and many blind alleys may have to be explored first. Not everyone finds the niche they hope for.

CONCLUSION

In this chapter we have examined a number of areas that have the potential to elicit strong emotional reactions in clients, patients and relatives, and in us as professional carers. Emotional stress is a byproduct of nursing work and cannot be avoided. However, it can be managed effectively through the development of self-awareness and good interpersonal skills. These skills are prerequisites for establishing sensible boundaries to protect yourself against the inevitable stresses that will emerge in clinical work. They can help to 'inoculate' you against the negative consequences of emotional stress and to be an assertive professional. Changes in organisational culture and an increasing awareness of employment safety issues will also help to alleviate stress and conflict in the workplace. Work should be challenging, but it should also be rewarding and fulfilling.[21] Developing positive strategies to deal with emotional reactions in yourself and others will help to ensure that this is the case for you.

~~~~~~

CASE STUDY 14.4

During her first week on placement on a busy ward environment, Jacinta found that some of her new colleagues continued to refer to her as a student. On the third day she asked a senior registered nurse for advice on whether or not to give a patient PRN Seroquel when the patient reported feeling very agitated. The senior registered nurse said: 'I'm busy. You should know what to do anyway.'

REFLECTIVE QUESTION

How would you support Jacinta in this instance?

~~~~~~

CASE STUDY 14.5

Six months after graduating and completing mental health and surgical placements, Oisin found that the key skills that helped him to cope with the challenges in that time were reflection and journalling of his experiences, feelings and thoughts on a regular basis. Moreover, he found himself rereading old notes and revisiting things that he had not fully understood as a student. Oisin found this very odd; during his undergraduate years he had failed to see the point of reflection!

REFLECTIVE QUESTION

What questions would you like to ask Oisin?

CASE STUDY 14.6

As part of her graduate program, Jill has just completed a 6-month allocation in a small country hospital, working in various settings, including the emergency department, operating rooms and the general ward. She has been collating various incidents for her professional portfolio and recalls that there have been two episodes where she has witnessed nursing staff bullying other members of the team. Although she has not experienced this directly herself, she feels on reflection that she needs to record these events in her portfolio and examine what affirmative action she could have taken.

REFLECTIVE QUESTIONS

1. What steps could Jill take in terms of developing her skills to handle bullying at work?
2. How could these events best be recorded in a professional portfolio in order to provide evidence of reflective learning?

RECOMMENDED READING

Albom M. *Tuesdays with Morrie.* London: Time Warner Books; 2003.

Blumenthal E. *Believing in yourself: a practical guide to building self-confidence.* Oxford, UK: Oneword; 1997.

Burns GW, editor. *Healing with stories: your casebook collection for using therapeutic metaphors.* Hoboken, NJ: John Wiley; 2007.

McEwan K. *Building resilience at work.* Bowen Hills, Qld: Australian Academic Press; 2011.

Potter-Efron RT, Potter-Efron PS. *Letting go of anger.* 2nd ed. Oakland, CA: New Harbinger Publications; 2006.

Sarma K. *Mental resilience: the power of clarity.* Novato, CA: New World Library; 2008.

Seligman MEP. *Flourish: a visionary new understanding of happiness and well-being.* Sydney: Heinemann; 2011.

REFERENCES

1. Holmes TH, Rahe RH. The social readjustment rating scale. *Journal of Psychosomatic Research* 1967;**11**:213–18.
2. Gibbons C, Dempster M, Moutray M. Stress and eustress in nursing students. *Journal of Advanced Nursing* 2007;**61**:282–90.

3. Kitson A, Marshall A, Bassett K, Zeitz K. What are the core elements of patient-centred care? A narrative review and synthesis of the literature from health policy, medicine and nursing. *Journal of Advanced Nursing* 2013;**69**(1):4–15.

4. Flores N. Dealing with an angry patient. *Nursing* 2008;**May**:30–1.

5. Morrison P. *Understanding patients.* London: Bailliere Tindall; 1994.

6. O'Connor T. Caring for children who are dying: a nurse practitioner has found her nursing niche caring for dying children. *Kai Tiaki Nursing New Zealand* 2014;**20**(4):22–3.

7. Hubbard B. What can be done about horizontal violence? *Alberta RN* 2014;**69**(4):16–18.

8. Longo J. Horizontal violence among nursing students. *Archives of Psychiatric Nursing* 2007;**21**:177–8.

9. AHPRA. 2010. Online. Available: <www.ahpra.gov.au/Legislation-and-Publications/AHPRA-FAQ-and-Fact-Sheets.aspx> [Viewed 20 September 2014].

10. Peterson C. *A primer in positive psychology.* Oxford, UK: Oxford University Press; 2006.

11. Cornelius H, Faire S, Cornelius E. *Everyone can win. Responding to conflict constructively.* 2nd ed. Sydney: Simon & Schuster; 2006.

12. Goleman D. *Emotional intelligence: why it can matter more than IQ.* New York: Bantam Books; 1995.

13. Hegney D, Tucket A, Parker D, Eley R. Workplace violence: differences in perceptions of nursing work between those exposed and those not exposed: a cross-sector analysis. *International Journal of Nursing Practice* 2010;**16**:188–202.

14. Weinand M. Horizontal violence in nursing: history, impact, and solution. *The Journal of Chi Eta Phi Sorority* 2010;**54**(1):23–6.

15. Myers D. *Psychology.* 10th ed. New York: Worth Publishers; 2013. Chapter 12.

16. Fredrickson BL. *Positivity.* New York: Three Rivers Press; 2009.

17. Weiten W, Dunn DS, Hammer EY. *Psychology applied to modern life: adjustment in the 21st century.* 10th ed. Melbourne: Cengage Learning; 2012.

18. Lawler KA, Younger JW, Piferi RL, Billington E, Jobe R, Edmondson K, et al. A change of heart: cardiovascular correlates of forgiveness in response to interpersonal conflict. *Journal of Behavioral Medicine* 2003;**26**(5):373–93.

19. Berry CR. *When helping you is hurting me: escaping the Messiah trap.* New York: Cross Roads; 2003.

20. Combs AW. What makes a good helper? *Person-Centred Review* 1986;**1**:51–61.

21. Csikszentmihalyi M. *Finding flow: the psychology of engagement with everyday life.* New York: Basic Books; 1997.

CHAPTER 15

Clinical leadership

Debra Thoms and Christine Duffield

LEARNING OBJECTIVES

When you have finished this chapter you will be able to:

- understand the responsibility everyone has for leadership
- identify how transformational leadership behaviours can be implemented and the need to be able to adapt these to address difficult issues
- identify opportunities to display leadership behaviours relevant to responsibility and accountability
- start building your own leadership capability
- recognise the role that emotional intelligence has in leadership.

KEYWORDS: leadership behaviours, transformational leadership, emotional intelligence, new registered nurse, capability

INTRODUCTION

Health systems today still have hierarchical structures, and the nursing profession is no exception. While senior managers may be the most visible leaders in the nursing work environment, it is important to note that they are not the only people who can and do display leadership. In this chapter, we show that everyone, including newly registered nurses, has an important part to play in nursing leadership. We also consider some simple strategies you can use to increase your leadership knowledge and skills in the nursing work environment. Good leadership encompasses a range of capabilities, including communication and social awareness. You will have read about a number of these capabilities in other chapters. A continuing challenge for health systems and the staff within them is the need to respond and adapt to change. Understanding the links between various leadership capabilities and the ability to adapt will assist in identifying how to build your own leadership skills. In your first few weeks of practice you may not be called on to take on roles such as team leader, or to be in charge of a shift. However, you should consider taking the opportunity when asked to take on these roles, as this will build your leadership capabilities from an early stage. As a consequence, you will find yourself in a better position to adapt to the challenge that you will find such a role presents initially.

THE LEADERSHIP RELATIONSHIP

Health systems are complex organisations and working within them brings many challenges. At times the management and leadership of an organisation can appear to be rigid and somewhat mechanistic (also described as 'bureaucratic'). While this may be how a unit or service may appear, organisations are also capable of adapting and shifting to meet new challenges. There may be opportunities for local solutions to be developed and implemented. Often these may appear to be the informal structures sitting alongside the more formal structures. Within these settings, leaders have an important role to play. Leaders create and support the environment that allows the team to find the solutions and put them into action.[1] Within your workplace, you may find opportunities to contribute to the development and implementation of solutions while enhancing your growth as a leader.

Leaders do not exist without followers, and at various times and depending on the circumstances we can be either the leader or the follower. However, as Kouzes and Posner show in their research, in order for leaders to be followed, they have to create a relationship with other people who are willing to follow them to progress to a desired goal.[2] While at this stage of your career you may find yourself predominantly in the role of follower, there will be opportunities to lead in various activities and functions within your unit. By creating good relationships with team members and your unit manager from the beginning, you may be able or may be asked to take on leadership activities, which will assist you in building your leadership capability. At other times, you may find yourself taking on an informal leadership role with a small group of staff on a particular activity. By increasing your understanding of leadership, you will be better able to take advantage of these opportunities if and when they arise. This will also assist when you are placed in roles such as being in charge of a team or shift at what you may feel to be an early point in your career. Having well-developed positive relationships can enhance the team's support for you in challenging times. As you develop these leadership capabilities, we would encourage you to review your understanding of transformational leadership and the role of emotional intelligence, both of which are covered here. We would also suggest you consider how you are able to work with and support people to address some of the difficult problems and issues in your workplace.

TRANSFORMATIONAL LEADERSHIP AND ADAPTIVE LEADERSHIP

In 1978, James McGregor Burns wrote about the need to bring together conceptually the role of the leader and that of the follower.[3] He defined leadership as 'leaders inducing followers to act for certain goals that represent the values and the motivations – the wants and needs, the aspirations and expectations – of both leaders and followers'.[3] Adaptive leadership is defined as 'the practice of mobilising people to tackle tough challenges'.[4] Working to clarify your own values and understand those of the team with which you work will assist in reaching solutions to these challenges and is part of providing adaptive leadership.[5] It is about trying, and if it does not quite work the way you thought then adapting and trying again.

As a newly registered nurse, there will be opportunities for you to facilitate a small group of staff (possibly as part of a team) to achieve common goals, and in this way you will be building your leadership capability. At times, the team may include various levels of staff, such as enrolled nurses and assistants in nursing, who will have different competencies and skills. Your interaction and work with these staff members will be enhanced if you can successfully engage them in achieving your common goal of good patient care. One way in which this may be done is by recognition of shared values and a common purpose – namely, to make patient care the best that it can be within the given constraints of practice.

You may have heard the term *transformational leadership* during your studies, and read about it elsewhere in this book. Once again, it was Burns who first distinguished between transformational and transactional leadership. He defines 'transactional leadership' as 'when one person takes the initiative in making contact with others for the purpose of an exchange of valued things' and that this exchange can be 'economic or political or psychological in nature'.[3] Transactional leadership is found in all organisations and has an important place in many interactions, such as those requiring adherence to standards or procedures. However, the transactional model tends to be associated with lower levels of staff satisfaction and innovation than the transformational model, and, for this reason, transformational leadership is often emphasised.

Transformational leadership occurs when 'one or more persons engage with others in such a way that leaders and followers raise one another to higher levels of motivation and morality'.[3] In this situation the purpose of both the leader and the follower is shared, and the leader acts to inspire the follower to greater creativity and originality. As mentioned above, researchers have found that nurses who work with transformational leaders tend to report higher levels of satisfaction and lower rates of turnover.[6–8] For these reasons, it is especially important that newly registered nurses aiming to develop their leadership skills pay particular attention to transformational leadership characteristics. While you may find that you work with some nurse leaders who display more transactional leadership behaviours than transformational, this does not necessarily prevent you from endeavouring to work in a more transformational way with other members of staff.

EXERCISE 15.1

1. Think about leaders and managers you have encountered and the type of leadership they demonstrate. Which did you prefer, and why?
2. Think about your own values, and then those of the team with whom you work. Do you know what values other team members hold?
3. How well do your values and those of the team fit with each other? Does this enable and support you all to work together to achieve change and manage the challenges of your day-to-day work?

BUILDING TRANSFORMATIONAL LEADERSHIP CAPABILITY

A number of writers have identified capabilities for transformational leadership, and it is possible to consider how these can be developed and applied as a newly registered nurse.[6,9–11] This may at times be challenging, particularly early in your first year, when you will be coming to terms with a wide range of issues and may occasionally find that some staff are less supportive than you would desire. Nevertheless, even in such difficult situations, it is still possible to consider the various strategies that transformational leaders use, and to think about these as you grow and develop your overall practice. In addition, by giving consideration to the values that various staff and teams hold, you will be able to better understand and perhaps find strategies to address issues more effectively. In the next sections, we list some important strategies that transformational leaders employ. We will describe how effective leaders apply these strategies, and put forward some ideas about how you might use these in your practice.

Get to Know Your People

A key strategy for leaders is to get to know their staff. This involves simple approaches, such as greeting people each day; taking an interest in their lives outside the workplace; listening to ideas and seeking input; and letting them know they make a contribution.[12] These conversations will also assist you in understanding the values that people hold and in identifying how you may be able to work together to solve shared problems. By greeting people each day and taking an interest in them and their lives, you will not only build this capability as a leader for the future, but will also be creating positive relationships with other staff. Additionally, by listening to and asking questions of more experienced staff members, you can build your clinical knowledge and skills. At times, you may not be met with a positive response from some staff members. However, this should not discourage you. If your inquiries are met with negative feedback from some staff, this may simply alter those from whom you seek advice and information. By actively asking and questioning, you will grow in knowledge and skill, knowing that you are building your leadership capabilities at the same time.

Help People to Learn and Develop

People generally like to learn, and as a transformational leader an environment that supports and encourages learning should be developed. Additionally, as a leader it is important to model a desire and willingness to learn and discover. By setting such an example, you will help encourage other staff members to learn.[12]

Naturally, there will be much to learn within your work environment as a newly registered nurse. However, as you become more comfortable and confident, it is important to look for further opportunities to develop professionally. This may be achieved through attending in-house learning programs or tutorials and seminars. There may also be external conferences and short courses that you may find of benefit. Consider and demonstrate your commitment to your own ongoing professional development by being prepared to contribute your own time and resources to participate. Good leaders seek not only to further their own professional development, but also to motivate and inspire other staff to seek such opportunities. Therefore, when working with other staff members take opportunities at appropriate times to encourage them to participate as well. Nonetheless, it is important to have created a good working relationship with your co-workers (see 'Get to know your people', above) before sharing your knowledge or suggesting future opportunities for them.

Give Plenty of Feedback

People in leadership roles need to provide appropriate feedback to team members in a timely way. It is as important to give positive feedback (e.g. praising a staff member for high-quality work) as it is to give negative feedback (such as advising a staff member to take additional care with tasks). When providing negative feedback, this should be done in private, whereas positive feedback can often be shared more publicly. When giving feedback, it is important to use active listening. Active listening incorporates both verbal skills (such as asking open-ended questions, and providing summaries and clarification) and non-verbal skills (such as using open body language) and helps to show that you are paying attention to the other person.[13,14] It is a particularly helpful skill if giving negative feedback.

In the early stages of your career as a newly registered nurse, it is likely that you will not have to give feedback regularly. It is much more probable that you will be receiving feedback, rather than providing it. Nonetheless, in some circumstances, newly registered nurses may find themselves in a position where they are expected to provide feedback to team members. The strategies outlined above provide some guidance on how to give feedback effectively; however, importantly, they can also be used when receiving feedback. For instance, it is relevant for both those giving and receiving feedback to listen actively. The giver of the feedback should ask questions to ensure that the receiver understands the message being given, while the receiver should seek clarification to make sure that he or she has accurately grasped the speaker's meaning.

Give Responsibility and Status

This is achieved by delegation, which helps to support the growth and development of individuals. In delegating, it is important to understand the individual's knowledge of the job, and provide the person with the opportunity to ask questions so that he or she feels comfortable with undertaking these new responsibilities.

Delegation can be one of many challenging areas that you will come across as a newly registered nurse.[15] Initially, you may not find yourself in a position to be delegating to others, but that will change rapidly. Make use of tools such as the decision-making framework available on the Nursing and Midwifery Board of Australia website (www.nursingmidwiferyboard.gov.au),[16] as this will assist you in understanding how to make a decision to delegate, and what your responsibilities are when delegating to another team member.

It is important that you have a good understanding of the skills and capabilities of those you are working with before you delegate. This may mean that you need to familiarise yourself with the education programs undertaken by enrolled nurses and assistants in nursing, so that you have a sound knowledge of their abilities.[17] Additionally, you should ensure you are familiar with any policies that guide the roles of staff members within your particular organisation. When you have delegated an activity and the staff member has performed well, remember to thank the person and offer positive feedback if possible (see 'Give plenty of feedback', above).

Give Your People Rewards

Identify strategies such as giving credit for good work and providing development opportunities as ways of rewarding people.[12]

Again, as a newly registered nurse or new member of a team, you may find you have limited opportunity to reward people in comparison to more senior staff. Remember, though, that a positive word or sincerely felt thank you to someone who assists you is a form of reward. Simple expressions of gratitude will encourage people to continue their good work, and improve staff morale. Giving thanks also allows you to practise providing positive feedback in a natural and genuine manner. This is an important skill to have, especially as you develop and move into more formal leadership positions. Providing genuine support and encouragement to staff members will be seen as a positive behaviour, which will contribute to your capacity to motivate staff.

Strategies for Communicating Information

There are two important strategies here. The first is developing trust through creating a positive communication atmosphere. The second is inclusive communicating, which involves sharing information with all relevant staff, not just a few. Communicating information as soon as possible through a range of methods such as meetings, newsletters, bulletins and email lists is an important aspect of transformational leadership. Good communicators are skilled not only in delivering information, but also in receiving information, so once again, being a good listener is vital.[12]

Communication is a key capability no matter what role you find yourself undertaking. It is important to develop your skills in this area from the beginning of your career. Be prepared to admit if you do not know something and to actively seek assistance from others. Although some staff may respond to your inquiries negatively, do not see this as a reason not to seek advice in the future (see 'Get to know your people', above). Instead, you may wish to think about different ways of communicating with those whom you find challenging, or perhaps seek advice from other staff members. Succeeding in finding good strategies at this stage will contribute to your career as it develops. Also, be willing to share information that you may have learnt about a patient or the activities of the unit.

EXERCISE 15.2

Think about how you might be able to apply these strategies in your workplace. Consider the barriers and enablers to you applying them, and how you might manage the barriers and use the enablers to develop your leadership capabilities further.

EMOTIONAL INTELLIGENCE

Being emotionally intelligent is useful for everyone in day-to-day work and enhances the skills and capabilities of leaders. Emotional intelligence is about managing our feelings in an effective way so that we can work well with people and enhance the ability of people to work together.[18] Emotional intelligence is something that can be learnt and, while it will continue to develop throughout our life, we can assist that growth in understanding and capability.[16] Daniel Goleman outlines the main domains of emotional intelligence, which follow.[19,20]

Knowing One's Emotions (Self-awareness)

The ability to monitor your feelings with insight and understanding is a crucial element of emotional intelligence. Self-aware people have an in-depth understanding of their emotions, strengths and limitations, as well as their values and motives. This self-knowledge assists them in making decisions. Goleman suggests that people who have greater certainty about their feelings are better able to steer their lives in the direction they wish.[19]

Self-management (Being Able to Handle Feelings Appropriately)

Unless we have a good understanding of our feelings, we will not be in a good position to be able to manage them well and in a positive manner. 'Self-management' refers to being in control of your feelings, rather than letting your feelings control you. If we do not manage how we feel, this can have a major impact on others (such as colleagues or patients), and so it is important to be able to recognise and respond to our own positive or negative emotions.[20]

Social Awareness (Empathy)

Empathic people are able to recognise when others need or want something – they are able to 'put themselves in the other's shoes', and to respond accordingly.[19] In terms of leadership, this means taking into account how others feel, and making intelligent decisions that recognise those feelings.[20] Being empathic will help you to respond better to patient needs, but also to manage some of the more challenging behaviours you may experience from other staff.

Relationship Management

Relationship management is the final domain of emotional intelligence. In managing relationships, there is a need to manage people's emotions. However, this must be done with authenticity and genuineness. By being aware of their own values, leaders skilled in relationship management are able to articulate a vision, and to share that with others. Additionally, such leaders are skilled at managing conflict and change, and are able to use their capacities to build teams, encourage collaboration and help team members develop their skills.

As a newly registered nurse it is useful to understand these domains, because, as Goleman indicates, the skills and capabilities that contribute to emotional intelligence can be learnt.[19,20] Even when not in a leadership role, emotional intelligence is critically important. You can begin building your emotional intelligence by identifying your capacity in each of the domains and endeavouring to increase your skills. For example, if you are experiencing negative emotions about your work or an incident in your life, using your emotional intelligence can help you to deal with these feelings in an appropriate way. This is important, as your actions and emotions affect not only you, but also have an impact on your co-workers and the patients for whom you may be caring. We believe that, while emotional intelligence is particularly important for leadership, it is also important for all staff, and can enhance how the whole team works.

EXERCISE 15.3

Consider each of the domains and think about how well you meet them. Reflect on this and consider how you might develop your capabilities further.

CONCLUSION

It is hoped that, through reading this chapter and undertaking the exercises, you will have identified opportunities to develop your leadership capability at this early stage of your career. You should also recognise that, although you may not be in a formal leadership position, you still have an opportunity to display leadership capacity, and this will stand you in good stead as you progress in your nursing career.

CASE STUDY 15.1

Mary has just started work at a small country hospital in the mixed medical and surgical ward. John is the nursing unit manager and has not worked with newly registered nurses before; this is the first time the hospital has employed a new registered nurse. John has a quick chat with Mary after about 4 weeks and does not seem entirely happy with her, but Mary is unsure what the issues are.

REFLECTIVE QUESTIONS

1. How often should Mary expect to receive feedback from John? What are the important aspects for Mary to develop in her practice as a registered nurse?
2. What should Mary do about the 'quick chat' that John has had with her?
3. Mary feels that perhaps staff have a limited understanding of her education and clinical experience. What could she do to address their knowledge deficit?

CASE STUDY 15.2

Mark is a newly registered nurse of 4 weeks. He is working with two other staff – Susan, an eighth-year registered nurse in charge on night duty, and Diane, a very experienced enrolled nurse.

REFLECTIVE QUESTIONS

1. How will Mark respond if Susan delegates tasks to him that he does not feel able to do?
2. Diane offers to assist Mark with some activities, but he is not sure of the scope of practice of the enrolled nurse. What should he do?
3. Mark notices that some care is not being carried out according to the required standard. What should he do?

CASE STUDY 15.3

Jill is a very experienced clinical nurse educator on a rehabilitation ward. She has been working with Libby, a newly registered nurse, for a few weeks now. Jill believes that Libby is performing at a very high level for a new nurse; in fact, she thinks that Libby is more productive than many of the more experienced registered nurses on the ward.

REFLECTIVE QUESTIONS

1. Jill asks the nursing unit manager to let Libby lead a team on morning shift to develop her capabilities further. How will Libby respond to the other registered nurses in her team who may be more experienced?
2. What could Libby have done to place her in the best position to perform most effectively when placed in charge of the shift and to lead those she is working with to solve the challenges that arise throughout the shift?
3. Libby sometimes finds herself in conflict with one very experienced registered nurse who does not seem to recognise Libby's skills. What should she do?

RECOMMENDED READING

Anonson J, Walker ME, Arries E, Maposa S, Telford P, Berry L. Qualities of exemplary nurse leaders: perspectives of frontline nurses. *The Journal of Nursing Management* 2014;**22**(1):127–36.

Clark CC. *Creative nursing leadership and management.* Sudbury, MA: Jones & Bartlett Learning; 2009.

Garber PR. *Giving and receiving performance feedback.* Amherst, MA: HRD Press; 2004.

Heifetz R, Grashow A, Linsky M. *The practice of adaptive leadership.* Boston: Harvard Business Press; 2009.

Moss MT. *The emotionally intelligent nurse leader.* San Francisco: John Wiley; 2009.

Shaw S. *International Council of Nurses: nursing leadership.* Oxford, UK: Wiley Blackwell; 2007.

REFERENCES

1. Wheatley M. *Finding our way: leadership for an uncertain time.* San Francisco: Berrett-Koehler; 2005.
2. Kouzes J, Posner B. *The leadership challenge.* 3rd ed. San Francisco: Jossey-Bass; 2003.
3. Burns J. *Leadership.* New York: Harper; 1978. pp 3–19, 20.

4. Heifetz R, Grashow A, Linsky M. *The practice of adaptive leadership*. Boston: Harvard Business Press; 2009. p 14.

5. Heifetz RA. *Leadership without easy answers*. Cambridge, MA: Harvard University Press; 1994. p 23.

6. Weberg D. Transformational leadership and staff retention: an evidence review with implications for healthcare systems. *Nursing Administration Quarterly* 2010;**34**:246–58.

7. Gardner BD. Improve RN retention through transformational leadership styles. *Nursing Management* 2010;**41**:8–12.

8. Tomey AM. Nursing leadership and management effects work environments. *Journal of Nursing Management* 2009;**17**:15–25.

9. Failla KR, Stichler JF. Manager and staff perceptions of the manager's leadership style. *Journal of Nursing Administration* 2008;**38**:480–7.

10. Govier I, Nash S. Examining transformational approaches to effective leadership in healthcare settings. *Nursing Times* 2009;**105**:24–7.

11. Aarons GA. Transformational and transactional leadership: association with attitudes toward evidence-based practice. *Psychiatric Services* 2006;**57**:1162–9.

12. Cottingham C. Transformational leadership: a strategy for nursing. In: Hein E, Nicholson M, editors. *Contemporary leadership behavior*. Selected readings. 4th ed. Philadelphia: J.B. Lippincott; 1982.

13. Fassaert T, van Dulmen S, Schellevis F, et al. Active listening in medical consultations: development of the Active Listening Observation Scale (ALOS-global). *Patient Education and Counseling* 2007;**68**:258–64.

14. Derkx H, Rethans J, Maiburg B, et al. Quality of communication during telephone triage at Dutch out-of-hours centres. *Patient Education and Counseling* 2009;**74**:174–8.

15. Bittner NP, Gravlin G. Critical thinking, delegation, and missed care in nursing practice. *The Journal of Nursing Administration* 2009;**39**:142–6.

16. Nursing and Midwifery Board of Australia. A national framework for the development of decision-making tools for nursing and midwifery practice. Available: <www.nursingmidwiferyboard.gov.au/Codes-and-Guidelines.aspx>; 2013.

17. Keeney S, Hasson F, McKenna H, et al. Nurses', midwives' and patients' perceptions of trained health care assistants. *Journal of Advanced Nursing* 2005;**50**:345–55.

18. Goleman D. *Working with emotional intelligence*. New York: Bantam; 1998.

19. Goleman D. *Emotional intelligence: why it can matter more than IQ*. London: Bloomsbury; 1995.

20. Goleman D, Boyatzis R, McKee A. *Primal leadership: learning to lead with emotional intelligence*. Boston: Harvard Business School Press; 2002.

SECTION 3
ORGANISATIONAL ENVIRONMENTS

CHAPTER 16

Excellence in practice: technology and the registered nurse

Alan Barnard

LEARNING OBJECTIVES

When you have completed this chapter you will be able to:

- ▲ discuss the meaning and implications of technology for nursing care
- ▲ outline concepts for appropriate use and integration of technology in clinical practice
- ▲ discuss strategies for developing technology skills and knowledge
- ▲ debate technology in relation to the organisation of nursing and healthcare
- ▲ reflect on the relation between technology and person-focused care.

KEYWORDS: technology, knowledge, skills, clinical practice, technique, technological competency

INTRODUCTION

Technology is everywhere. We nurses use it to care for people and manage our working day. Nurses talk about technology, develop skills and knowledge to apply technology, praise the qualities of the latest technology development and sometimes blame it for the demise of human contact. In addition, we write about technology, attend courses to learn about new equipment, work within highly organised healthcare systems, and live in a world that is organised increasingly in accordance with efficiency and logical order. Healthcare is becoming more and more technology-dependent, and understanding the influence and impact of technology is essential for effective clinical practice.

Technology has often been interpreted as machinery and equipment; however, it is much more than the things we use. Our meaning of technology also needs to include the knowledge and skills used to apply, develop, design and assess objects, and the development of a human, organisational and political system aimed at the maximisation of efficiency. Technology is in fact a complex interrelationship between a range of important elements, including machinery, equipment, tools, utensils, automata, apparatus, structures, people, organisations, science, culture, systems, gender, values and politics. Technology assists with many diagnostic, assessment and treatment responsibilities, but at the same time it can challenge our moral, cultural and social development. It remains an important component of nursing practice and is valued highly, since technology provides us with evidence for patient care, extends communication and treatment options, assists us to organise time-consuming responsibilities, and is used as part of a number of hospital and community activities in healthcare.

This chapter explores technology and the beginning registered nurse in acute and hospital-based care with specific reference to skills and knowledge development for patient care delivery. The primary goal is to unite examples of practical issues common to clinical nursing practice with theoretical concepts in order to assist beginning registered nurses to work better with technology. The chapter examines the meaning of technology and the various types of technologies typical of acute care. It also explores issues related to skill and knowledge development with specific emphasis on the personal implications of working with the influence of technology.

WHAT IS TECHNOLOGY?

The word *technology* refers to the practical arts, and the knowledge and/or activity of a group (i.e. technologist). Technology is more than the sum of all the equipment we use in healthcare, the latest piece of machinery or the internet. Technology has associated characteristics that include the development of skills, knowledge, and the incorporation of social and cultural values.[1-3] One way to portray this interpretation of technology is as three concentric circles (see Figure 16.1). Concentric circles highlight the characteristics of technology that together emphasise a characterology of the phenomenon. The concentric circles focus our attention not only on the 'things' of nursing at the centre, but also on their relations with other characteristics such as skills change, knowledge development, gender and cultural differences, competency development, and a growing emphasis on efficiency and rational order. (The term *rational order* means the organisation of behaviours, actions, and ways of thinking about nursing into preplanned and predictable processes.)

Artifacts and Resources

The smallest and central concentric circle depicted in Figure 16.1, entitled 'Artifacts and resources', is technology at its most obvious and refers to the integration, use and application of the 'things' of nursing. Rinard[4] noted that in modern nursing three key periods of change have been significantly influenced by technology. The first period was from 1950 to 1960, and was characterised by new medical techniques and a significant introduction of pharmaceuticals to care. The second period identified was from 1965 to 1980, and was associated with increasing machinery and specialisation. The third period was from 1980 to 1995, and was associated with increasing technical control, streamlining and prediction of care. Although not noted by Rinard, a fourth period of change has emerged that could be characterised as a period of information access, retrieval and computerisation of care. We each have greater knowledge availability and communicate with more immediacy, and there is a perceived link between quality care, sophisticated technology and knowledge access.

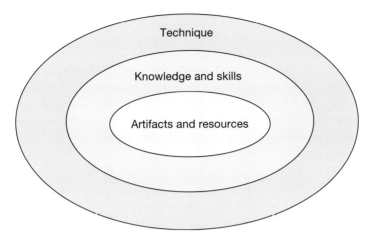

Figure 16.1
A characterology of technology

Knowledge and Skills

The second, or middle, concentric circle portrays technology as knowledge and skills. The care we provide is in many ways determined by the knowledge and skills we develop; as such, we have to include knowledge and skills as part of technology. Without the required knowledge and skills, we have limited ability to meet the needs of patients. For example, without the knowledge and skills to use an intravenous pump correctly, it is of no use as a piece of equipment for your care delivery and consequentially becomes a technology of potential danger for a patient. Nursing is a practical occupation and our knowledge is expressed most often through the way we perform our work. Failure to establish and develop knowledge and skills is inadequate for the quality of nursing practice, your patients, the colleagues with whom you work, the requirements of the healthcare sector and the equipment you hope to use. Technological knowledge takes many forms and relates not only to hands-on competency but also to knowledge of organisational policy, current research and changing evidence.

Technique

The influence of technology on nursing practice is illustrated and described in a broader sense by the third and most inclusive concentric circle, entitled 'Technique'. The third concentric circle extends our characterology of technology to include the way policy, politics, economics, ethics, culture, organisational management and human behaviour are organised for the benefit of technology. The way nursing practice is organised for, as well as by, artifacts and resources is as much technology as the first and second levels of meaning. 'Technique' does not refer to one specific thing. It describes a way of thinking about the way we do things and go about our daily care. It describes an attitude and tendency in clinical practice towards changing previously instinctive, reflexive, natural and particular practices for individuals and cultures into organised methods, behaviours and protocols. In automated and tightly regulated technological environments, differing cultural and social values have a tendency to be replaced by a dependency on predetermined actions and protocols, and this is increasingly the case with nursing practice.

Technique is complex and has three subtle, yet important, characteristics. First, technique adheres to a primacy of reason to govern practice. It is a way of thinking, acting and organising care by which there is an attempt to control the personal, passionate and emotional world of everyday nursing practice via protocols, rules, evidence and general observance of a predetermined logical order.

Second, it requires a desire for efficiency in order to assist its goal and to justify its activity. The desire for efficiency is akin to the inventor or factory owner who seeks to streamline methods and actions in order to obtain certain outcomes that simplify and make predictable previously uncontrolled or random activity. It must be stressed that there is nothing wrong per se with a desire for planned activity or efficiency. In fact, there is nothing new about efficiency as a reasonable and worthwhile goal. The desire for efficiency and systems to control actions and activity has guided invention throughout human history, and, after all, who wants to be exposed to ineffective care? However, the third characteristic of technique brings about new and different experience, because it stresses primacy of efficiency in every realm of human activity and thinking.

Technique has become so prevalent in nursing and society that many people are increasingly incapable of thinking outside its boundaries in their search for meaning. In this environment the importance of human experience and caring are marginalised by an emphasis on control, efficiency and logical order.[5-9] Technique reduces human-centred activities such as caring in nursing to measurable and predictable outcomes. That is, technique brings about qualitative transformation(s) in care that impact directly on you and your patients.

Together all the concentric circles shown in the figure highlight that technology is as much about, for example, pieces of equipment, as it is about our knowledge and skills and how we organise care. The concentric circles highlight that a full understanding of technology must include understanding that it can have a direct impact on, for example, cultural differences and how we each express our nursing practice. A common experience is that there is growing reliance on efficiency and logical order, sometimes at the cost of advancing human-centred care.

NURSING AND TECHNOLOGY

Nurses have always used tools, chemicals, potions, equipment and machines to provide care for people. Nursing technology includes any technology that we use and/or claim to be fundamental to our daily practice. Depending on context, there are at least 12 different types of nursing technologies (Table 16.1), even though a lot of nursing technology is not immediately evident to us. Interestingly, a lot of nursing technology is not recognised as such by nurses both in clinical practice and in nursing literature. For example, there is sometimes in the literature an overemphasis on sophisticated computer technology and an uncritical lack of emphasis on technology associated with the 'dirty work' of nurses (e.g. bed pans). The reasons for this lack of recognition are numerous but include: (1) an overemphasis on, and excitement about, new and

TABLE 16.1

Examples of types of technology associated with nursing practice

Types of technology	Examples
Clothes	Shroud Pyjamas
Utensils	Bedpan Kidney dish
Structures	Hospital ward Isolation room
Apparatus	Jordan frame Patient transport trolley
Utilities	Electrical power Gas services
Tools	Wheelchair Urinary catheter Sphygmomanometer
Resources	Pharmaceuticals Sterile dressing
Machines	Intravenous infusion pump Mechanical ventilator
Automata	Computer Call bell Refrigerator
Tools of doing used to enact clinical practice	Nurse's watch Stethoscope
Objects of art or religion	Nurse's uniform
Toys (e.g. diversional therapy)	Chessboard

sophisticated machinery and equipment; (2) our inclination to focus on new technology and to take for granted older and simpler technologies; and (3) the lack of research and scholarship examining technology within nursing.[6,10–14] In fact, it can be argued that inadequate appreciation of the breadth of technology used in nursing has restricted our capacity to interpret the influence of technology on our profession and healthcare more generally.

The 12 types of technology listed in Table 16.1 emphasise technologies that are simple, sophisticated, old, new, unique and commonplace. Given that nursing technologies have not been examined adequately,[6,15–17] the types of nursing technology proposed highlight both the strongly technological basis of nursing and the diverse range of technologies that come together to assist practice. Over time, many types of technology (e.g. tools) evolve from being external and hand-held to becoming machinery and/or automata that operate independently. Witness, for example, the evolution of blood pressure monitoring from the hand-held sphygmomanometer to electronic devices. Technology often evolves from being human-powered to being controlled by alternative power sources such as electric motors and computers. Much of the hands-on manipulation of technology has reduced, as evidenced by the hospital bed that can be adjusted automatically, computer-based nursing/medical records, and vital signs which are accessible at distance.

While an extended debate could be undertaken to examine what technologies are specific to nursing, it must be acknowledged that the breadth of nursing technology needs to be better acknowledged as significant to nursing practice, as this assists us to increase our clarity, understanding and participation in its use.[18,19] There remains a lack of reflection on the types and importance of technology in clinical practice, and this lack of recognition affects how we think about and understand nursing practice.

EXERCISE 16.1

What types of technologies are part of your clinical area? Next time you are engaged in clinical practice, make a mental note of the various technologies you use in your clinical practice.

EXERCISE 16.2

Reflecting on your experience, do you think technologies such as tools, machines and automata are more highly valued than technologies that are less sophisticated? Why do you get this impression? What does this tell you about nursing and healthcare? Make a list of how these values might influence nursing practice and professional goals.

READINESS FOR CLINICAL PRACTICE: SKILLS AND KNOWLEDGE

The seminal work of Patricia Benner[20] described different levels of clinical performance and expertise among nurses. Her work, together with that of Bondy[21] and Krichbaum,[22] provided an understanding that at different stages in our careers, nurses approach the delivery of care in different ways. For a beginning registered nurse in Australia, a systematic approach where goals and stages of care provision are explained is beneficial for safety as they assist to guide the completion of less familiar roles and responsibilities, whereas the more experienced nurse in the same context may require less direction to assess practice principles and priorities of practice. This is normal, but both instances emphasise that it is essential in practice to direct our nursing gaze to the principles that underpin a skill or procedure.

Advancement of competency needed for the use of technology in patient care is crucial to foster clinical excellence. Beginning nurses often find that they lack the experience, skills and knowledge required to practise with technology in specialist areas. In addition, beginning nurses are often required to be at ease with the use of technical equipment before they have developed higher-level critical thinking and decision-making skills. As we saw in our characterology of technology, the need to integrate technology in our care before developing skills and knowledge to employ it thoughtfully can compromise quality of care. For example, it is easy to turn on an oxygen saturation monitor, place the transducer on a person's finger and read the number displayed on the machine's gauge/display. Higher-level skills include interpreting the information, knowing whether the information being received is accurate, and responding to it in an appropriate manner. Ongoing education and a commitment to personal development are essential for effective clinical practice. It is not good enough to know how to use the machinery if the nurse cannot use the information obtained accurately, safely and with appropriate effect.

Technological advances in care provision such as microsurgery, eHealth and tele-health are exciting, but place unprecedented demands on each nurse to maintain and foster new knowledge and competence. Knowledge and skills alter regularly, and thus an active commitment to maintaining and advancing competence is a sign of a caring and responsible nurse. Attitudes that reflect an offhand and neglectful interest in updating knowledge and skills are inadequate and reflect a failure to value the profession. Competence reduces anxiety and fear, and increases the likelihood of successful care.

Competency standards associated with technology in general and advanced practice are part of, for example, the current Australian Nurses Federation competency standards for registered nurses.[23] Technology-related knowledge and skills are clearly a major focus, and the standards are a useful framework that describes appropriate nursing practice related to, for example, decision making, communication, assessment and ethical behaviour.[23] Achieving and maintaining Australian standards need to be the goals of each nurse and relate directly to technology integration in the care you provide.

The standards highlight the central importance of developing skills and knowledge. For example, standard 1.4 specifies that a registered nurse in general practice must recognise and respond to the need for ongoing education and training to maintain competence for nursing practice. For the advanced registered nurse, practice competency standard 6 highlights, for example, that each nurse must seek out and integrate evidence from a range of sources to improve healthcare outcomes based on experience, clinical judgment, and statutory and common-law requirements where a decision by an individual or group contravenes safe practice.[23] Numerous standards emphasise the central role and responsibility of nurses in appropriate skill development and knowledge acquisition, and a significant part of this development has a direct association with technology.

Even though specialist knowledge and skills are needed in a lot of nursing contexts, there are many technologies that are commonplace and integral to the complex practices of all nurses (e.g. stethoscope, thermometer). As a beginning nurse, it is worth remembering that there was a time when even these technologies were challenging. (Do you remember the first time you tried to measure a patient's blood pressure manually?) As a registered nurse, you have, and must acquire, knowledge and skills necessary to practise using all the commonplace machinery, equipment and resources of nursing in your context of practice. While a personal goal to develop the necessary ability to practise with advanced technology is appropriate, this goal should be balanced with suitable appreciation of your existing capabilities and competency. Technology provides new options in clinical practice and acts to extend skills. You must know how to apply knowledge and skills to all technology in a capable and appropriate manner in addition to fostering new clinical skills and knowledge.

'They do things differently from the way I was taught'

A beginning registered nurse will witness variations in how different nurses complete clinical activities and, on first experience, you might think that perhaps you were not taught correctly during your undergraduate degree. You may witness slight differences in the way a simple dressing technique is performed and ask yourself: Are these differences important? Is my practice adequate? Do these differences breach nursing standards?

In most cases, the differences you will come across will not be a problem. One reason for perceived differences can be an overemphasis on behavioural action, rather than on principles of practice. Fuszard[24] suggested that nurses have tended historically to perform clinical skills based on behavioural rules learnt from teachers and mentors during the formative phase of a career. During their formative years, nurses learnt rules through a process of modelling that was often based on the cultural traditions of an institution, teacher or mentor.[25] For example, there are practice principles such as asepsis that are central when performing a simple dressing. These principles have at times been overshadowed by the traditions of specific employers and institutions, spawning an emphasis on behavioural steps based on preference and context rather than research evidence.

Many generations of nurses have accepted institutional preference as the way to execute skills and complete procedures. An often-heard observation expressed by a registered nurse might be: 'That's not how we do it here.' Non-divergence from behavioural steps was interpreted as the right way to perform a nursing task, and clinical assessment of students based on rules tended to reinforce confusion between rules and practice principles. In addition, many nursing procedure manuals utilised expert opinion but lacked the advantage of nursing research. Tradition and personal experience tended to be the primary foundation for the establishment of procedural steps, in association with the preferences of employers, medicine, individuals and other professional groups. These influences need to be critically considered when establishing how practice principles should be applied in practice, especially since our professional environment now emphasises personal responsibility, evidence-based practice and awareness of litigation.

From Rules to Evidence

In reality, there may be no single correct behavioural rule for performing a range of skills and/or procedures, but there are principles of practice embedded in actions that need to be understood and enacted for safe care. In fact, behavioural rules as a basis for your action without equal clarity about the principles that inform action and technology practice are potentially unsafe and unhelpful. When principles are clearly explained and understood, it becomes easier to differentiate practice principles from procedural rules and to accept variations in the ways of doing a procedure. Preferences when performing (doing) a simple dressing can be adopted; however, it is important to ensure that, embedded in the preferred procedural steps, the principle of asepsis (for example) is maintained at all times. On this basis, performance of actions by different nurses associated with a procedure can vary with no real problem.[26]

Healthcare providers today often seek external accreditation from groups such as the Australian Council on Healthcare Standards (ACHS),[27] and this development is to your advantage because the process of accreditation helps to clarify and improve clinical practice. In Australia the ACHS Evaluation and Quality Improvement Program (EQuIP 4) standards provide a clear indication that procedures, and clinical practice more broadly, need to be evidence-based,[27] and highlight the need to move away from behavioural rules applied simply as procedural steps. In practice, you must think critically and make your best judgment based on evidence, reflection and the advice of experienced colleagues. A beginning point for achieving excellence in your practice is to think through the reasons for a specific clinical intervention being undertaken, contrast practice(s) with known evidence, and decide on the legitimacy of actions in line with the principles that should be employed.

EXERCISE 16.3

As a student nurse, you would have been taught principles of wound management. Can the principle of asepsis be applied absolutely in a practice environment? Think about managing a large sacral pressure area for a patient who is incontinent of faeces. Is asepsis likely to be possible when cleaning the wound? The context of your practice and the presentation of each person's health condition will dictate the best use of technology.

Experience teaches each nurse to adapt practice by critically engaging with principles to bring about the best possible outcome(s) in specific clinical situations.

Reflect for a moment on your practice. Can you think of instances where behaviours and practice principles were adapted for a particular situation? What were the reasons for the modification to clinical practice, and what has this type of experience taught you?

Troubleshooting: Problem-solving Technology

When technology functions inadequately and does not operate in the way it should, the experience of using technology can be one of frustration. If not resolved quickly and with competence, inadequate patient care can occur as a result of decreased efficiency and clinical effectiveness.[16,28–33] Technology can become a burden and is potentially unsafe if it is not maintained well, is inadequate for the job at hand, or is inappropriate for a practice environment. The following quotation from an experienced nurse highlights a typical clinical scenario when technology is not well maintained:

> ... you wonder sometimes – like, some machines need to have more time spent with them because they're just not the right design. Some machines are easier and more useful than others, obviously ... just even yesterday ... we had to use a pulse oximeter in a medical ward – a guy with COAD [chronic obstructive airways disease], asthma and a chest infection; they [doctors] wanted to know what his oxygen sats were going to be. You know they're not going to be fantastic but, anyway, they want to know what it is now, and the machine, well, I put it on and they [other nurses] said, 'Well, you've got to fiddle with the thing to make it go' and of course I'm fiddling with the thing – 10 minutes I think I fiddled with it. I couldn't get the signal properly, and they said, 'Well, you've got to do it like this' and then I got somebody else and they had a go and they couldn't do it, and then another girl came and finally she said, 'Yes, I got it.' That's great, but that took half an hour to get one reading, and I said, 'Can't you send it down to the workshop to get it fixed?' He said, 'It spends all its life down at the workshop getting fixed.' And then they said, 'Well, you can go and borrow the one from the ward next door,' and I thought oh, no. You know. In that way I think it would make life more difficult. I mean, I spent a lot of time trying to get the machine to work. I got two other people involved in it. I could have had another ward involved in it [as well].[19]

Technology needs appropriate resources (e.g. space, power supply) to function in an efficient and effective manner, and so when technology is defective or deficient the practice of nursing can become time-consuming, difficult and distracted.[6,34] Immediate reporting of faulty equipment and replacement of inadequate technology are essential, as is clear understanding of the ways that each specific technology operates. It is essential to develop the necessary skills to manipulate machinery and equipment and problem solve their operation. Problem solving the efficient operation of technology is a prerequisite skill for practice, and it is the case that many of these skills can only be learnt 'on the job'. The activity of fixing technology such as machinery and equipment while they are in use within a clinical area is commonly known as troubleshooting. The following nurse explained her role when troubleshooting technology:

> ... you end up being the trouble-shooter, Miss [Mr] Fix-it-type person, and you're supposed to have a competency to look after, say, somebody with an epidural or to change the PCA [patient-controlled analgesia] syringe. Sometimes you might be the only person on the ward who knows how to fix it, who is allowed to do it or who does really know how to work the machinery. You spend quite a lot of time with them.[19]

It is important to learn from experienced colleagues but not to develop an unhealthy reliance on the Miss/Mr Fix-it in your clinical environment. As explained by the nurse above, reliance creates a significant burden. Time spent managing technology leaves less time to be with people[34] and consumes the time and expertise of those nurses who have to assist you. An inability to troubleshoot technology leaves less time to manage

TABLE 16.2

Strategies to develop troubleshooting skills

Activity	Strategies
Education prior to using technology	Identify technologies common to clinical context. Read operating manuals/other relevant resources. Observe expert nurses. Attend in-service sessions. Ask a lot of questions.
Practise using technology	Operate first when it is not in clinical use. Identify clinical opportunities to employ it. Seek supervision and feedback in the initial phase.
Reflect on technologies employed	Keep a diary of things to remember. Reflect on the effectiveness of technologies. Identify benefits of correct usage.

other aspects of nursing practice and can compromise patient care. Merely hoping to solve problems without a clear understanding of the technology does not foster the behavioural patterns needed to face future challenges, and will not advance your professional reputation or trust. Table 16.2 outlines strategies you can employ to develop troubleshooting skills and knowledge.

Solving technical problems appropriately ensures that clinical treatment is delivered in a timely manner, the condition of patients is monitored properly, patients do not become anxious about their care because they trust you, safety standards are maintained because you know what you are doing, and excessive time is not taken away from you attending to your other roles and responsibilities. Technology will operate incorrectly due to factors such as inadequate resources, incorrect settings, inexperienced staff and malfunction. Failure to develop troubleshooting skills and knowledge will not foster autonomy in your practice. For this reason, although there will probably be a Miss or Mr Fix-it in your clinical area, it is best to view this person as a mentor who can foster the development of your own troubleshooting skills, rather than as a long-term solution to your technology problems.

EXERCISE 16.4

Make a note of any unfamiliar technology that you have come across in clinical areas. Increase your knowledge and skills by talking with an expert nurse about his or her use of the technology. Take time to practise the operation of any unfamiliar machinery, automata or equipment, read relevant literature and observe nurses troubleshooting. Remember to ask questions, watch every step, and make notes for you to review at a later time.

We work in changing and demanding environments, often with patients who have a high acuity (i.e. a high level of care requirement in terms of symptom management, care needs and healthcare condition). Increasing roles and responsibility require you continually to improve your skills, knowledge and clinical expertise. Knowledge takes many forms and relates to organisational policies, research evidence, scope of practice, ethical standards and hands-on knowledge such as troubleshooting technology. Growing your experience through ongoing education, personal reflection and assistance from colleagues is valued highly in healthcare.[28,31] In contrast, failure to establish and develop knowledge and skills is inadequate for your practice and unhelpful to patient care and the team with which you work.

EXERCISE 16.5

Nurses can sometimes be seen pressing buttons in the hope that a machine will eventually do what they want it to do. If the same problems arise again and the nurse employs the same behaviour, how should this form of troubleshooting be interpreted? Is it always easier to read the manual first? What management strategies could you implement in clinical settings to ensure that all nurses can learn to troubleshoot?

TECHNOLOGY AND CLINICAL ASSESSMENT

As demonstrated by our characterology (see Figure 16.1), technology is more than individual pieces of equipment, machinery and related resources, and has to be understood in a holistic way. As a registered nurse you must focus not only on the skills and knowledge of technology usage, but also on the patients within the healthcare organisation.[6,31,35] Numerous nurses have highlighted problems that arise as a result of the relationship between technology and nursing behaviour.[36–43] Technology will influence professional values, practices, skills, knowledge and the environment of care. For example, clinical environments such as intensive care and medical units are noteworthy for their use of technology and constant demands on your skills and knowledge.

Nurse clinicians and researchers continue to stress the importance of achieving an appropriate balance between nursing the patient and integrating technology into daily care.[38,39,44] It is the case that nurses sometimes can be distracted by the demands of machinery and equipment and by the ways that organisational departments are organised.[45] On busy days, basic patient needs such as daily living requirements can become secondary to a focus on maintaining and using technology and, in extreme cases, the experience of a patient can seem less important than information obtained from technology. Subjective experience and clinical presentation of the patient can become secondary to evidence obtained from technology.[2,5,7,31,34,35,46–48] It is easy to be caught up in attending to technology rather than with the experience and presentation of a person. One nurse explained a typical clinical situation she had experienced as follows:

> ... you have a baby in the nursery on monitors and some people, when the alarm goes off, go and check the monitor to see what it is doing, but with the pulse oximeter and a baby, if they move, shake, rattle or roll, they will set it off [pulse oximeter alarm], so it's more important to go and check what the baby is doing. Is it breathing or shallow breathing? ... it is more important to go and look at the baby than look at the machine. Yes, the monitor can say, come and see what is happening, but you should see what is happening with the baby, not what is happening with the machine ... we forget that they are here to alert us to the patient.[19]

Machinery and equipment do not always provide the irrefutable evidence necessary for diagnostic accuracy and best nursing intervention. It is you – not technology – that is responsible for clinical assessment and decision making, even though at times technology assists you in the process. In fact, confounding processes in the body can mask the information provided by technology to you as evidence. It is not appropriate for any healthcare professional to replace, justify or bolster assessment skills through reliance on information from machinery and equipment. The following nurse explained her experience:

> I have seen younger, newer nurses who have gone, oh, that patient is in atrial fibrillation, and you say, well, are they? And they say, the machine [said it], you know (rather than because they had completed a full patient assessment). And particularly, I think, in the ward area, if a patient has chest pain and people do not feel really comfortable with the technology, or with what's happening to the patient because they're unstable, they may tend to rely on the technology a little bit.[19]

Clinical evidence obtained from technology that informs your assessment, practice choice(s) and clinical judgment is important to care. Assessment based on a patient's symptoms, signs and clinical history needs to be balanced with information from technology and consultation with colleagues. There can sometimes be a tendency to respond to information from technology alone, rather than to integrate it into a comprehensive assessment structure. Interpreting information provided by technology involves ensuring it is accurate and responding to it in an appropriate manner. For example, a pulse oximeter may indicate that the oxygen saturation for a person is only 78% when physical assessment demonstrates no shortness of breath or evidence of cyanosis. In this case, it is not appropriate to record the oxygen saturation unthinkingly as 78%. Making a clinical assessment in isolation from other assessment findings will lead to inappropriate conclusions and care. Indeed, physical assessment of the person should cause you to consider why the information from the equipment did not fit (align) with the clinical presentation of the patient.

Information from technology is of benefit and is effective when evaluated in relation to the experience, needs, physical condition, cultural background and desires of the patient. Technology used appropriately can help to reduce suffering and assist to bring about humane care and excellence in clinical practice. Locsin[46] states that technological competence, as a form of caring, is expressed as an authentic desire and intention to use technology expertly for the betterment of each individual. What determines whether a technology depersonalises care or marginalises the person being treated is not the technology per se, but rather how individual technology is used in specific contexts, the meanings attributed to information gained from the technology, and the skills and knowledge of the healthcare worker(s).[49] Your nursing intervention and treatment must be guided by compassion, skill, knowledge, appropriate assessment, and an understanding of each person's experience and physical condition.

EXERCISE 16.6

Registered nurses who are new to a clinical area can sometimes place their clinical trust in technology, rather than in other forms of patient assessment. In addition, a great deal of time may be spent examining and responding to the operation of technology. Over time, as familiarity with technology improves, there is a (re)focus on human (patient) experience. However, when new technologies are introduced, we once more focus on their use.

With your colleagues, discuss and make a list of strategies that could be implemented to assist student and registered nurses to familiarise themselves better with technology and encourage holistic patient assessment skills.

NURSING PRACTICE WITH TECHNOLOGY

Nurses are often the only healthcare workers who possess the skills required to use technology in clinical environments. Your expertise can lead to increasing involvement in decision making, autonomous practice, professional recognition and collegiality. Technology is of value to the healthcare sector and society, and this quality of value transfers to those individuals who use it.[6,11,14,50] However, true expertise and quality of value are achieved when all aspects of our care are enhanced and balanced as part of our clinical role. For example, if you use technology efficiently but fail to ensure adequate care (e.g. mouth care) for your patient, you have missed the point of nursing. Nurse authors have argued consistently for the centrality of the person in nursing practice.[6,11,34,44,45,51] Failure to focus on the person is not necessarily caused by technology, and may more accurately reflect the way nursing is organised and the priorities that are rated most highly at any one time. Authentic respect and autonomy come from a consistent excellence in nursing practice, appropriate use of technology, and a willingness to resolve challenges that lead to unacceptable standards of care.

For example, while education, experience and commitment will focus your attention on professional responsibility, the push for new or increased skills and knowledge will not always make clinical practice less busy or demanding. It is a fact that, on some days, an outcome of increasing technology will mean that your clinical environment can be so demanding that the human focus of nursing is subsumed in a haze of activity. Under these conditions, it is difficult to focus on human experience and nurses develop various strategies to compensate for the challenge, as described by the following registered nurse:

> Other days you work your butt off, get through the day and you know. Sometimes I'll stay back after work, in my own time, just to talk to someone because I felt like I cheated them a bit, I wasn't there for all their needs.[19]

While it is noteworthy that this specific nurse gave her own time back to her patients because she could not give it during her working hours, there are other ways of meeting the needs of patients without having to stay late at work. A less desired strategy that nurses often employ is to complete their day's work when technology places high demands on their energies; a task-based instrumentalist approach to care. This strategy focuses primarily on those patients who are most in need of physical assistance, and on simply getting jobs done. More often than not, the strategy successfully relieves a demanding work situation, but it does not lead to excellence in care. Alternative strategies for addressing the issue are listed in Table 16.3 and may help in managing and improving your practice.

Increasing technology in the workplace actually acts to organise our labour. It is important to be involved in decision-making processes that influence the purchase, assessment, research, education and future use of technology since it directly influences your practice.[38] Technology purchase, use and integration are influenced by political and economic agendas and decisions. Therefore, an important activity for nurses is to become actively involved in assessing the safety, skills and knowledge implications of new technology.[31,32,41–43,52] For example, one way of engaging in this activity is through

TABLE 16.3

Strategies to manage technology during your working day

Activity	Strategies
Maintain the knowledge base	Actively seek education on technology. Develop skills in utilising technology. Establish troubleshooting capacity.
Choose wisely	Assess the usefulness of technology. Consider the practice environment. Only employ technologies if they definitely: ■ help to provide care ■ save time.
Maintain the environment	Lobby[6,31] for a clinically relevant resource base which considers: ■ appropriately trained staff ■ patient acuity ■ agreed standards of care. Replace inefficient technology. Remove non-essential technology.

involvement in economic and organisational decisions related to the ongoing use and purchase of technology. A starting point is to make known your interest in helping to integrate useful technology better into the clinical practice environment.

EXERCISE 16.7

Reflect on your nursing experience. Do you have any recommendations for integrating technology with nursing practice that would improve care? Think of an example from your own experience, and discuss what changes are needed to nursing policy.

CONCLUSION

Technology has a direct influence on the knowledge, skills, practice, values, ethics and politics of nursing. As such, the meaning and implications of technology for your nursing practice must be considered in relation to all aspects of nursing and healthcare. As the contexts of nursing practice alter with the needs of a changing society, your roles and responsibilities will change. New graduates and more experienced nurses need to foster insight into the ongoing challenges that technology brings to nursing practice, skills development, knowledge and standards of patient care. Nursing practice has altered as much, and as quickly, as the types of technology that are now integrated into care. You must be diligent to use all your skills and knowledge in order to advance clinical excellence and the best care outcomes for each person.

CASE STUDY 16.1

John is a 3-year-old boy with severe cerebral palsy. He has been in hospital for an extended period of time but is now being discharged home, with his family providing his primary care. He is in a permanent wheelchair and has partial ventilator support.

Sarah is new to her registered nurse position in her ward and wants to ensure that John and his family are supported to provide best care.

REFLECTIVE QUESTION

To ensure that both John and his family are supported, what pre-discharge considerations and discharge plans should Sarah put into place so that the family can best provide care at home for this ventilator-dependent child?

CASE STUDY 16.2

During Greg's second rotation in his transition year he is assigned to an acute 32-bed respiratory medical ward in a large metropolitan hospital. On arrival for duty, he is unsure about the correct use of a lot of the equipment used for care on the ward. Greg decides it is an opportunity to set about familiarising himself with all the available technology. He learns that most of the registered nurses employed on the ward also have limited experience.

REFLECTIVE QUESTION

What strategies and resources could assist Greg to prepare for this clinical role and his responsibilities?

CASE STUDY 16.3

After completing her new graduate program, Amal secures a permanent position in the intensive care unit. Many of the patients admitted to the unit require management of acute and chronic medical conditions. After witnessing a number of events that occurred in the unit, Amal believes that a lot of the healthcare team tend to rely too much on information from technology when undertaking patient assessment, rather than also seeking evidence directly from their patients. Amal is eager to encourage a more holistic approach to the management of patients and to improve the level of patient-focused care and assessment.

REFLECTIVE QUESTIONS

1. Who should Amal speak to about her perception of patient care in the unit?
2. How could Amal begin to express her views in a supportive and constructive manner?
3. In a small group, discuss your experiences of technology. List strategies to improve understanding and appropriate use of technology in clinical practice, and discuss them with others.
4. In small groups, list three potential technology- and nursing-related research studies. In a larger group, report on your proposed studies. Rank the cumulative list of research studies for their relative priority. Why have certain studies been ranked above others?

RECOMMENDED READING

Australian Nurses Federation. *Competency standards for nurses in general practice.* Available: http://anmf.org.au/pages/competency-standards [Viewed 22 August 2014].

Barnard A, Locsin RC, editors. *Technology and nursing practice.* London: Palgrave-Macmillan; 2007.

Barnard A, Sandelowski M. Technology and humane nursing care: a(n) (ir)reconcilable or invented difference? *Journal of Advanced Nursing* 2001;**34**:367–75.

Bridges J, Nicholson C, Maben J, Pope C, Flatley M, Wilkinson C, et al. Capacity for care: meta-ethnography of care nurses' experiences of the nurse–patient relationship. *Journal of Advanced Nursing* 2013;**69**(4):760–72.

Marck PB. Recovering ethics after 'technics': developing critical text on technology. *Nursing Ethics* 2000;**7**:5–14.

REFERENCES

1. Feenberg A. *Questioning technology.* New York: Routledge; 1999.
2. Pacey A. *Meaning in technology.* Cambridge, MA: MIT Press; 1999.
3. Winner L. *Autonomous technology.* Cambridge, MA: MIT Press; 1977.

4. Rinard R. Technology, deskilling, and nurses: the impact of the technologically changing environment. *Advances in Nursing Science* 1996;**18**:60–70.

5. Barnard A. On the relationship between technique and dehumanization. In: Locsin R, editor. *Technology, caring and nursing.* Westport, CT: Greenwood; 2001. pp 96–105.

6. Barnard A, Locsin RC, editors. *Technology and nursing practice.* London: Palgrave-Macmillan; 2007.

7. Clifford C. Patients, relatives and nurses in a technological environment. *Intensive Care Nursing* 1986;**2**:67–72.

8. Fairman J, D'Antonio P. Virtual power: gendering the nurse–technology relationship. *Nursing Inquiry* 1999;**6**:178–86.

9. Purcell C. *White heat: people and technology.* London: BBC Publications; 1994.

10. Barnard A, Cushing A. Technology and historical inquiry in nursing. In: Locsin R, editor. *Technology, caring and nursing.* Westport, CT: Greenwood; 2001. pp 12–21.

11. Fairman J. Watchful vigilance: nursing care, technology, and the development of intensive care units. *Nursing Research* 1992;**41**:56–60.

12. Pelletier D. Health care technology: sharpening the definition and establishing aspects of the social context. *Australian Health Review* 1989;**12**:56–64.

13. Reverby S. *Ordered to care: the dilemma of American nursing, 1850–1945.* Cambridge, UK: Cambridge University Press; 1987.

14. Sandelowski M. *Devices and desires: gender, technology and American nursing.* Chapel Hill, NC: University of North Carolina; 2000.

15. Fairman J. Response to tools of the trade: analysing technology as object in nursing. *Scholarly Inquiry for Nursing Practice* 1996;**10**:17–21.

16. McConnell EA. The impact of machines on the work of critical care nurses. *Critical Care Nursing Quarterly* 1990;**12**:45–52.

17. Sandelowski M. Tools of the trade: analysing technology as object in nursing. *Scholarly Inquiry for Nursing Practice* 1996;**10**:5–16.

18. Barnard A. Technology and nursing: an anatomy of definition. *International Journal of Nursing Studies* 1996;**3**:433–41.

19. Barnard A. *Understanding technology in contemporary surgical nursing: a phenomenographic examination.* Nursing Inquiry, Volume 6, Issue 3, pages 157–166, September 1999.

20. Benner P. *From novice to expert: excellence and power in clinical nursing practice.* Menlo Park, CA: Addison-Wesley; 1984.

21. Bondy KN. Criterion-referenced definitions for rating scales in clinical evaluation. *Journal of Nursing Education* 1983;**22**:376–82.

22. Krichbaum K. Clinical teaching effectiveness described in relation to learning outcomes of baccalaureate nursing students. *Journal of Nursing Education* 1994;**33**:306–16.

23. Australian Nurses Federation. *Competency standards for nurses in general practice.* 2014. Online. Available: http://anmf.org.au/pages/competency-standards [Viewed 22 August 2014].

24. Fuszard B. *Innovative teaching strategies in nursing.* Gaithersburg, MD: Aspen; 1995.

25. Aviram M, Ophir R, Raviv D, et al. Research briefs. Experiential learning of clinical skill by beginning nursing students. 'Coaching' project by fourth-year student interns. *Journal of Nursing Education* 1998;**37**:228–31.

26. Potter PA, Perry AG. *Fundamentals of nursing: concepts, process, and practice.* St Louis, MO: Mosby; 1997.

27. Australian Council on Healthcare Standards (ACHS). *EQuIP 4: Standards and guidelines for the ACHS.* Sydney: ACHS; 2007.

28. Barnard A, Gerber R. Understanding technology in contemporary surgical nursing: a phenomenographic examination. *Nursing Inquiry* 1999;**6**:157–70.

29. Carnevali DL. Nursing perspectives in health care technology. *Nursing Administration Quarterly* 1985;**9**:10–18.

30. Pelletier D. Technology. In: Romanini J, Daly J, editors. *Critical care nursing.* Sydney: Harcourt Brace; 1994. pp 1039–63.
31. Pelletier D, Duffield C, Mitten-Lewis S, et al. Australian nurses and device use: the ideal and the real in clinical practice. *Australian Critical Care* 1998;**11**:10–14.
32. Pillar B, Jacox AD, Redman BK. Technology, its assessment, and nursing. *Nursing Outlook* 1992;**38**:16–19.
33. Almerud S, Alapack RJ, Fridlund B, Ekebergh M. Caught in an artificial split: a phenomenological study of being a caregiver in the technologically intense environment. *Intensive and Critical Care Nursing* 2008;**24**:130–6.
34. Barnard A. Alteration to will as an experience of technology and nursing. *Journal of Advanced Nursing* 2000;**31**:1136–44.
35. Pelletier D. Diploma-prepared nurses' use of technological equipment in clinical practice. *Journal of Advanced Nursing* 1995;**21**:6–14.
36. Brown J. Nurses or technicians? The impact of technology on oncology nursing. *Canadian Oncology Nursing Journal* 1992;**2**:12–17.
37. Cooper MC. Care: antidote for nurses' love–hate relationship with technology. *American Journal of Critical Care* 1994;**3**:402–3.
38. Kiekkas P, Karga M, Poulopoulou M, Karpouhtsi I, Papadoulas V, Koutsojannis C. Use of technological equipment in critical care units: nurses' perceptions in Greece. *Journal of Clinical Nursing* 2006;**15**:178–87.
39. Kongsuwan W, Locsin R. Thai nurses' experience of caring for persons with life-sustaining technologies in intensive care settings: a phenomenological study. *Intensive and Critical Care Nursing* 2011;**27**:102–10.
40. Merideth C, Edworthy J. Are there too many alarms in the intensive care unit? An overview of the problems. *Journal of Advanced Nursing* 1995;**21**:15–20.
41. McConnell E. How and what staff nurses learn about the medical devices they use in direct patient care. *Research in Nursing and Health* 1995;**18**:165–72.
42. Darbyshire P. Rage against the machine? Nurses and midwives' experiences of using computerized patient information systems for clinical information. *Journal of Clinical Nursing* 2003;**13**:17–25.
43. Keefe-McCarthy SO. Technologically-mediated nursing care: the impact on moral agency. *Nursing Ethics* 2009;**16**:786–96.
44. McGrath M. The challenges of caring in a technological environment: critical care nurses' experiences. *Journal of Clinical Nursing* 2008;**17**(8):1096–104.
45. Bridges J, Nicholson C, Maben J, Pope C, Flatley M, Wilkinson C, et al. Capacity for care: meta-ethnography of care nurses' experiences of the nurse–patient relationship. *Journal of Advanced Nursing* 2013;**69**(4):760–72.
46. Locsin R. Machine technologies and caring in nursing. *Image: Journal of Nursing Scholarship* 1995;**27**:201–3.
47. Locsin R. Technologic competence as caring in critical care. *Holistic Nursing Practice* 1998;**12**:50–6.
48. Green A. How nurses can ensure the sounds patients hear have a positive rather than negative effect upon recovery and quality of care. *Intensive and Critical Care* 1992;**8**: 245–8.
49. Sandelowski M. A case of conflicting paradigms: nursing and reproductive technology. *Advances in Nursing Science* 1988;**10**:35–45.
50. Barnard A, Sandelowski M. Technology and humane nursing care: (ir)reconcilable or invented difference? *Journal of Advanced Nursing* 2001;**34**:367–75.
51. Barnard A. Towards an understanding of technology and nursing practice. In: Greenwood J, editor. *Nursing theory in Australia: development and application.* 2nd ed. Sydney: Prentice Hall; 2000. pp 377–95.
52. Henderson A. The evolving relationship of technology and nursing practice: negotiating the provision of care in a high tech environment. *Contemporary Nurse* 2006;**22**:59–65.

CHAPTER 17

Establishing and maintaining a professional identity: portfolios and career progression

Susan Alexander and Lyn Stewart

LEARNING OBJECTIVES

When you have completed this chapter you will be able to:

- discuss the importance of maintaining a professional identity
- develop and maintain a professional portfolio
- clearly explain the preparation required for an interview for a professional appointment
- demonstrate an understanding of the importance of ongoing professional development
- articulate the significance of lifelong learning in career planning and development.

KEYWORDS: professional portfolio, curriculum vitae (CV), interview, career planning, lifelong learning

INTRODUCTION

Although an achievement of which you can be justifiably proud, the completion of a bachelor's degree is only the foundation in your development as a professional nurse or midwife. As you embark on this journey from beginning practitioner to becoming an expert in your chosen field, it is vital that you establish and develop your identity as a professional.

There are a number of attributes associated with being a professional. Two attributes that are particularly relevant to the topic of this chapter are lifelong learning and autonomy. As the name suggests, lifelong learning represents the continual process of learning throughout life. However, as students near the end of preregistration education, the short-term goal of obtaining employment as a registered nurse or midwife tends to be the paramount focus. Often, little thought is given at this stage to the long-term career plan or commitment to professional development. This development can occur either passively through gaining experience in the workplace or actively through undertaking workplace professional development opportunities as well as postgraduate education. The professional attribute of autonomy is applicable to the development of your professional identity because you are the person primarily responsible for its development. As a result, you need to develop your own career plan that enables you to maximise all formal and informal learning opportunities.

It is also important that you keep a record of your developing professional identity. Documentary evidence of your knowledge, experience, skills and competence will assist you when applying for employment or promotion as your career develops. It will also assist you in demonstrating compliance with Nursing and Midwifery Board of Australia (NMBA) requirements, particularly those associated with continuing professional development (CPD). In addition, it is important to demonstrate ability to apply the graduate attributes associated with your tertiary education provider. These attributes typically include characteristics such as professional communication, teamwork, accountability, ethical practice and appreciation of diversity.

To assist you in developing and tracking your professional identity, this chapter will provide information about applying for nursing or midwifery positions, as well as the establishment and maintenance of a professional portfolio. There will be some discussion on the topics of lifelong learning and CPD; however, as these topics are discussed in other chapters, they will not be addressed in depth in this chapter.

PLANNING THE DEVELOPMENT OF YOUR PROFESSIONAL IDENTITY

In much the same way that your career will only develop with a plan, goals and strategies, the development of your professional identity will also require a strategic approach. Laker and Laker[1] illustrated this need for planning when they stated, 'For most [university] students, lack of career planning wastes time and resources and may result in years of "career drift"' (p 128). They also emphasise that what you are doing today was influenced by what you did five years ago and, in turn, will influence what you are doing in five years' time. So, you need to start planning your career and your professional identity *now*. The portfolio will help you to do this, but some other strategies that you might access include role models or mentors, researching areas of interest, clinical experience (paid or voluntary), and seeking the advice of career advisors.

DEVELOPING AND MAINTAINING A PROFESSIONAL PORTFOLIO

Portfolios are becoming an increasingly valuable asset for professionals. Although, in Australia, it is only mandatory at this point in time for nurse practitioners to maintain a portfolio, the possibility of extending this requirement to all nurses is already being considered.[2] Outside of regulatory requirements, Capan and colleagues[3] found that nursing portfolios were a valuable tool for showcasing achievements, encouraging continued professional growth and supporting annual performance reviews. Development of a portfolio is not a discrete undertaking, but rather an ongoing process that requires regular updating.[4] The basic interpretation of the term *portfolio* is 'a receptacle for information'.[5] However, a professional portfolio is much more than a collection of certificates and other relevant documents.[2] It is a comprehensive collation of biographical and other evidence that maps your career trajectory as it summarises and reflects upon who you are, what you have learnt, your career development to date and what you have planned for the future.[5,6] The portfolio enables you to showcase your abilities and achievements. It can be a critical tool in obtaining employment or supporting your application for a grant or scholarship. It is also a means of keeping track of your learning and career development to date.[4] Maintaining your CPD records in one location will also assist you to ensure you comply with governance requirements. For example, the NMBA requires that registered nurses and midwives and enrolled nurses undertake at least 20 hours of CPD per annum and keep written documentation of that CPD. A portfolio is the ideal vehicle for keeping track of CPD. The NMBA will audit nurses periodically to ensure that CPD requirements are being met. See Table 17.1 for a full list of the benefits of establishing and maintaining a professional portfolio.

TABLE 17.1

Benefits of portfolios

Efficiency	Learning opportunities
Information all in one repository	Personal empowerment
Easier to maintain and update	Flag a learning event/reflect later/focus thinking
Accessible anytime, anywhere (e-portfolio)	Process of learning can be seen, as well as outcomes
Identification of education requirements	More rapid feedback
Allows for input from multiple sources	Creativity in selection of evidence
Structure enhances organisation and readiness	Assists the planning and organisation of learning
Provides a timeline for learning	Easier to link evidence
Allows the reader to navigate between sections	Easier to reflect on value of evidence
Maintains technological currency (e-portfolio)	Assists in development of self-awareness and self-assessment
Individualised and dynamic presentation	Enhanced technological skills
Interactive through the use of a variety of multimedia resources (e-portfolio)	Enhanced presentation skills
	Autonomy and accountability reflected in ownership of learning
	Fosters lifelong learning

Sources: *Adapted from F Timmins, A Duffy,* Writing your nursing portfolio: a step-by-step guide. *Maidenhead, UK: Open University Press; 2011; S Reed,* Successful professional portfolios for nursing students. *Exeter, UK: Learning Matters; 2011.*

EXERCISE 17.1

Access a copy of the relevant competency standards for registered nurses or midwives and list how you think you can provide evidence of beginning competency in each of the areas. Consider how you could plan to comply with the competencies once you have completed your graduate year as a registered nurse. In addition, reflect on how you are continuing to develop the graduate attributes that you acquired during your tertiary education.

Electronic Professional Portfolios

The term *portfolio* derives from the Latin *portate* which means 'to carry', and *foglio,* which means 'a sheet'[5] (p 2). As the technological imperative gains speed, however, there is less paper and less to 'carry', as portfolios are increasingly being established and maintained online. Benefits of an e-portfolio include the possibility for requisite sections to be easily compiled into a smaller portfolio that can be customised to support specific employment, promotion or grant applications. E-portfolios have the added benefit of being easily accessible at any time from any place across the globe, making them easy to update and share.[3] Even in instances where technology is not available, the e-portfolio can be adapted to hard copy if required. Within contemporary professional practice in an era of rapidly changing technology, the majority of recruitment processes now require online submission. Because the e-portfolio aligns with this process, the ensuing discussion will focus on e-portfolio development.

There are a wide range of platforms that can assist with e-portfolio establishment. These include: educational, institution and alumni sites such as Pebble Pad and Mahara. There are also professional sites available to subscribing members of professional nursing organisations such as the Australian College of Nursing (ACN). In addition, there are a variety of web-based resources such as GoogleSites, Weebly, Wordpress and Wix that do not require payment and are easy to use. The choice of platform will depend on individual requirements and preference.

Preparing the Components of Your Portfolio

Whichever platform is selected, the portfolio will need a framework for structuring the content and presenting it in a cohesive and professional style.[5] Furthermore, as preparing a portfolio can be a time-consuming task, it is a good idea to break it down into manageable steps.[5] The use of the FOLIO acronym as a guideline can assist in this process:

- **F**ind what others have advised about format and content.
- **O**nline or paper-based?
- **L**ist what sections to include.
- **I**nsert information into each section.
- **O**ptimise your opportunities by reviewing regularly.

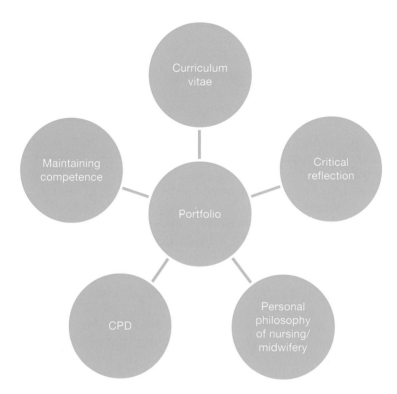

Figure 17.1

Portfolio development mindmap

Sources: *Adapted from F Timmins, A Duffy,* Writing your nursing portfolio: a step-by-step guide. *Maidenhead, UK: Open University Press; 2011; S Reed,* Successful professional portfolios for nursing students. *Exeter, UK: Learning Matters; 2011.*

Getting Started

Even with a structure, it may be difficult to know where to start. Try mindmapping or brainstorming (see Figure 17.1 for an example). You may prefer to use the traditional pen-and-paper model; however, there are many software programs available, such as Popplet lite, that can assist in this process. Following the brainstorm, transform each idea into a section or subsection where you can commence inserting information. Recommended contents can include:

- table of contents
- timeline of your achievements
- personal profile
- educational background
- educational transcripts and qualifications
- employment history
- career goals
- continuing professional development
- conference/workshop/seminar presentations or attendance

- strategies to achieve identified learning requirements
- awards and certificates
- letters of appreciation and commendation
- participation in professional organisations
- peer and performance appraisals
- evidence of achieving graduate attributes and nursing or midwifery competency standards
- professional organisation and journal subscriptions
- relevant details of appropriate referees
- evidence of reflection on learning and practice
- participation in health-related research projects
- publications and reports
- other documents that demonstrate professional growth.

(Timmins & Duffy;[5] Reed;[6] Andre & Heartfield;[7] Dempsey;[8] Johnson;[9] Mannix & Stewart;[10] Howatson-Jones[11])

In this chapter, the focus will be on the development of the professional profile, curriculum vitae (CV), CPD and evidence of reflection.

Professional Profile

Traditionally, when applying for a position, an applicant submitted a CV and cover letter. However, contemporary employers are increasingly trending towards a brief profile supported by a detailed account addressing position criteria. The profile provides a short, sharp outline of you as a professional. It spotlights your personal attributes, academic and employment achievements, career goals, and strategies for complying with professional codes and guidelines. The profile is often the first part of an e-portfolio that is read by a prospective employer. Therefore, it needs to be professional and sufficiently enticing to encourage the reader to learn more about your credentials and your ability to fulfil the position or grant application criteria. If you choose to include a photograph, this image must reflect the expected professional standard. See Box 17.1 for a sample profile.

BOX 17.1 Example of a professional profile

I am a recently graduated registered nurse (or midwife) who is passionate about the profession of nursing and eager to develop competence in a clinical environment. My personal philosophy incorporates a commitment to engage collaboratively and professionally with patients and other members of the multidisciplinary healthcare team to ensure optimal health outcomes for the patient. Strategies to uphold this philosophy include: compliance with Nursing and Midwifery Board of Australia codes and guidelines; practice based on the best available evidence; critical reflection on my practice; and continued development of my knowledge and competencies. As part of my journey towards becoming an experienced practitioner, I will also be working towards my goal of clinical nurse consultant in neonatal nursing. I have three years' experience as an assistant in nursing at a residential aged care facility and intend to enrol in postgraduate education in the next 1–2 years.

Curriculum Vitae

A key aspect of your career development involves maintaining a current record of your education, qualifications and employment history. This information is kept in your CV. Although the CV is sometimes referred to as a 'résumé', it should be noted that these terms are not interchangeable. Contemporary understanding is that the CV includes detailed information about your education, employment, research, publications and professional development. In contrast, a résumé is a summary of your professional history, often limited to one or two pages in length and tailored for a specific purpose, such as a promotion. A résumé can be developed from information contained in the CV.

As a registered nurse beginning your professional career, your CV may be brief in relation to clinical nursing or midwifery experiences. However, it is important to note that some preregistration experiences can be included in your CV. A good example would be employment in a service-based environment requiring collaborative interpersonal skills. This information will alert prospective employers to knowledge and skills also applicable to professional nursing and midwifery practice. Your CV represents a pivotal opportunity to impress potential employers, and, as such, needs to showcase your capabilities in relation to the position for which you are applying. Highlighting your strengths and key qualifications will enhance your chances of success. Regardless of the format, your CV should be succinct, factual, clear, and free of grammatical and spelling errors.[7] Providing personal information such as your age, marital status and country of birth is unnecessary in your CV. In fact, providing such information may detract from the professional impression you are hoping to provide to potential employers.[10]

When developing your CV, it is suggested that you present your information in the following order, ensuring that the most recent information is listed first in each section:

- name and contact details (including phone and email addresses)
- details of professional registration
- education qualifications. Include the name of the qualification, the institution conferring it and the year it was conferred
- any professional prizes or awards you have received
- professional employment history, beginning with your current position. If you have experience outside nursing, it can also be included. In this section include position title, organisation, dates of employment, and a brief description of the role and associated responsibilities and achievements
- professional development, including professional memberships, professional presentations, publications and research projects. You may also include in this section any continuing education that you have completed that did not lead to a formal educational qualification
- committee memberships
- specific skills and attributes that will assist you in a professional setting – for example, fluency in a second language, advanced computing skills
- overseas placement experience; work with non-government organisations (NGOs)
- voluntary work
- interests, particularly those that indicate good teamwork or leadership

■   a list of referees. Be sure to select suitable referees. For example, a nurse manager
or supervisor will be a more appropriate referee than a colleague at a similar level
of employment. Most employers contact referees directly, either by phone or email.
Therefore, it is imperative that you provide accurate referee contact details.
Remember to seek the permission of potential referees prior to including their
contact details in your CV.

Continuing Professional Development

It is a requirement of all professional disciplines that members commit to a minimum
level of CPD. Ongoing development enables professionals to maintain and improve
their knowledge, skills and competence for contemporary practice. For nurses and
midwives practising in Australia, the mandatory requirement is at least 20 hours per
year.[12] For practitioners holding dual registration, the requirement is 40 hours per
year.[12] Nurses in New Zealand are required to undertake 60 hours of CPD every
three years to demonstrate competence across the scope of midwifery practice.[13]

Approved CPD may include formal and informal activities such as accredited
courses, attendance at conferences and seminars, participation in professional groups
where a certificate of compliance/completion is awarded, mandatory workplace
learning, service to the profession, reviewing scholarly literature, other self-directed
learning or any other structured learning activities.[11] As a professional, it is important
to maintain up-to-date records of all CPD activities and to scan valid documents into
the portfolio. Stages in the CPD cycle include reviewing practice, identifying learning
needs, planning and participating in relevant learning activities across the domains of
practice, and reflecting on the value of those activities.[11]

Reflection

The commitment to continually reflect on practice is another attribute of professionals.
For nurses in Australia, the *Code of Professional Conduct for Nurses in Australia*[14] and
the *National Competency Standards for the Registered Nurse*[15] outline the expectation
that nurses will practise reflectively and ethically. By examining experiences, reflection
assists practitioners to gain insight into themselves and to illuminate blind spots, thus
advancing their personal and professional development.[7,11] It is a natural human
activity, but is typically unstructured. In the case of professionals, however, reflection is
deliberate and structured, often following a predetermined model.[5,11]

Reflection is a critical component of your professional portfolio because it identifies
and examines your learning and areas that require further development, thus
strengthening the link between theory and practice.[11,16] It also demonstrates your ability
to reflect on your practice.[5] As a record of learning and career development, it is
imperative that your portfolio includes reflection on personal learning;[7,11] its use as a
development tool is otherwise limited and it runs the risk of being just a description of
what you have done.[6,8]

When reflecting, select a specific event upon which to reflect; otherwise, your
reflection may be vague and lacking in meaning.[7,11] A framework will also give your
reflection greater direction. One model that is frequently used in nursing and
midwifery is Gibbs' reflective cycle[17] (see Figure 17.2). This is a straightforward model
for the beginning practitioner to use, but may not encourage the depth of reflection

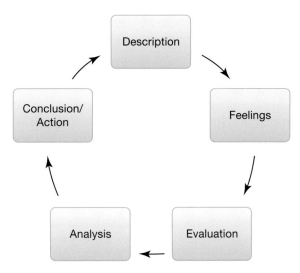

Figure 17.2
Gibbs' reflection model

Source: *G Gibbs,* Learning by doing: a guide to teaching and learning methods. *Oxford, UK: Oxford Brookes University; 1988.*

EXERCISE 17.2

Select a recent significant event that has scope for deep reflection. Using the Gibbs cycle, reflect on the event. You may find it helpful to ask additional questions at each stage. For example, under the analysis stage, you might ask: What are some explanations for what happened? How might others perceive this event? Having researched this topic, what are some alternative explanations for what happened?

associated with other more complex models such as those developed by Johns or Stephenson.[8] Techniques that might be used in reflection include journalling[18] and peer or group debriefing, the latter often occurring following critical incidents.[7]

MAINTAINING LIFELONG LEARNING THROUGHOUT YOUR NURSING OR MIDWIFERY CAREER

Lifelong learning is an important component of all professional disciplines.[11,19] Lifelong learners have been described as individuals who accept responsibility for their own learning and are enthusiastic about making the effort and finding the time to immerse themselves in learning on a continuing basis. They are persistent and diligent practitioners who reflect, question, enjoy learning, understand the dynamic nature of knowledge and engage in learning by actively seeking learning opportunities.[11,19] As a new graduate, you have experienced a unique learning journey incorporating learning experiences prior to your nursing or midwifery studies, as well as the diverse classroom and clinical practicum experiences throughout the program.[16] Upon entering a profession, you need to embrace opportunities to maintain and enhance your graduate-entry knowledge and competencies as you progress on the continuum from novice to expert practitioner. Indeed, Queensland Health[20] states: 'Nurses/midwives take a proactive role in the enhancement of nursing knowledge and engage in current and emerging professional practice' (p 6).

The technological imperative in contemporary healthcare poses both opportunities and challenges for health professionals and the people for whom they care. The challenges arise through the rapidly changing technologies and the increasing complexity of interventions and acuity of patients.[20] At the same time, however, rapid developments provide opportunities to collaborate with patients to maximise their outcomes. Similarly, the rapid increase in the accessibility and availability of health information has resulted in greater health literacy among health consumers. Again, this development is both an opportunity and a challenge for health professionals. Meeting the challenges identified here, and many of the challenges that you will encounter in your career, will require expert command of professional attributes including lifelong learning, communication, ethical practice and accountability.

Benner[21] has written extensively on the evolution of nurses, from novice to expert practitioner. You will experience this evolution first-hand as you transition from student to registered nurse, undergoing an intense period of on-the-job learning as you move from the formal learning processes associated with a novice practitioner to the more self-directed informal approach of the confident expert practitioner. During this time, you will find yourself relying more on your developing intuitive knowledge and confidence in your own practice while becoming less rigid about the need to seek reassurance for your actions.[21] Transition is an exciting and invigorating time for most graduates, but it should also be a time of critical reflection when your own ideas about nursing or midwifery may be significantly challenged. All of the theoretical and experiential learning you undertake will assist you to develop your intuitive knowledge as you progress towards becoming an expert nurse.[21] All of these learning opportunities should be recorded and reflected upon in your professional portfolio.

Strategies for Achieving Lifelong Learning

As a registered nurse, there will be many opportunities to develop personal and professional skills to enhance your career progression and develop expertise in patient care. Table 17.2 outlines key indicators and strategies to facilitate this process in your career.

Lifelong Learning Resources in the Workplace

Health workplaces provide numerous opportunities for practitioners to engage in lifelong learning and professional development. They may include access to online literature and other resources to assist staff to build capacity and support evidence-based practice. Engaging with these resources will advance the development of your professional identity as you maintain currency with professional issues and research. Other education opportunities include those at the ward level, formal in-service, conferences and seminars, as well as post-registration education such as graduate certificates, graduate diplomas, or masters and doctoral degrees.

TABLE 17.2

Resources for lifelong learning

Descriptor	Strategy	Rationale
Maintaining contemporary knowledge in nursing and midwifery	Postgraduate studies, whether university-, college- or industry-based Professional development opportunities in your workplace Regular reading of peer-reviewed journal articles Maintaining currency with policies and procedures at industry, state and national level	Although the major motivation for completing these postgraduate courses may be practice-based to develop higher-level clinical skills, academic scholarship is often enhanced. As a graduate, you need to be well informed regarding courses on offer to ensure that the targeted course addresses your learning needs, assists with the development of your chosen career path and maintains the continued professional development requirements of the NMBA[12] or the Nursing Council of New Zealand.[13] Currently, it is an expectation that graduates enter the healthcare domain with the ability to demonstrate self-reliance and self-directed learning capacity[12,13]
Membership of professional organisations	Joining special-interest groups, reflective of your clinical interest/s – specialty interest groups affiliated with larger organisations such as the Coalition of National Nursing Organisations (CoNNO)[21] Joining national and international nursing and midwifery organisations; for example, Australian College of Nursing, (ACN), Australian College of Midwives (ACM), College of Nurses Aotearoa (NZ), New Zealand College of Midwives Inc. (NZCOM), Sigma Theta Tau International (STTI)	Access to peer-reviewed journals and bulletins, as well as opportunities to attend seminars, professional days and conferences that enable clinicians to enhance lifelong learning, network, develop collegial relationships (including mentoring), debate professional issues, and keep up to date with current practice and research. Professional organisations continue to support nurses and midwives in their pursuit of lifelong learning by offering scholarships for postgraduate study, conference attendance and research
Membership of an industrial organisation	Engaging with industrial media bulletins, press releases and journals Attending workplace meetings of the organisation Participating as delegate in the organisation – for example, Australian Nursing and Midwifery Federation, New Zealand Nurses Organisation	Industrial organisations are the nurses' advocate, negotiating on our behalf with employers and governments for provision of professional development opportunities when negotiating industrial awards. Industrial organisations also arrange workplace-related seminars and workshops to keep members informed of safe work practices and other workplace issues. These organisations offer professional seminars, online learning opportunities, and access to databases and other literature. Professionally moderated social media discussion sites may also enhance professional development through collaboration and networking

Source: *Adapted from Nursing & Midwifery Board of Australia.*

APPLYING FOR NURSING OR MIDWIFERY POSITIONS

Whenever you apply for a position, you will almost always be competing against other applicants with impressive qualifications and relevant experience. Therefore, it is of the utmost importance that your application is of the highest standard, eye-catching and tailored specifically for the position for which you are applying. This is one of the occasions when your up-to-date professional portfolio will be of great benefit to you.

A clear understanding of the process of staff selection and the requirements of the position will maximise your chance of success. Prior to preparing your application, review the provided documents carefully and ensure that you have the requisite capabilities. It is also a good idea to seek information from the contact person specified in the position announcement. This person is likely to be a senior person who is knowledgeable about the position, its associated responsibilities and the area in which the successful applicant will be practising.

Leave yourself plenty of time to prepare a professional application; otherwise, you run the risk of submitting a sub-standard application or missing the deadline altogether. Even with a portfolio, the preparation of a professional application will require many hours of work. Begin your application by addressing the selection criteria (Box 17.2). This will give you an indication of the essential and desirable attributes of the person being sought for the position. As your chances of being selected for interview are highly dependent on your statement addressing the criteria, it is

---

BOX 17.2 Sample selection criteria

Registered nurse/midwife (reference number 15/2014)

Neonatal Unit, Lansdowne Hospital

The Division of Nursing and Midwifery, Lansdowne Hospital, invites registered nurses or midwives to apply for a full-time position in the neonatal unit.

Essential

1. Current registration with the Australian Health Practitioner Registration Agency.
2. Recent clinical experience in an acute care setting.
3. Demonstrated ability to organise and prioritise work.
4. Demonstrated ability to work effectively within an interdisciplinary team.
5. Demonstrated effective written and oral communication skills.
6. Commitment to and documented evidence of professional development.
7. Proficiency in information technology.

Desirable

1. Previous experience in a neonatal unit.
2. Appropriate postgraduate qualifications.

Closing date: 31 December 2014.

Enquiries to Sally Yu at sallyyu@lansdowne.gov.au

Applications to be submitted online through the hospital's recruitment portal recruitment@lansdowne.gov.au

imperative that you commit the time and attention to detail required to produce a quality response. Rather than just stating that you can undertake whatever is outlined in the selection criteria, it is important that you provide actual examples that demonstrate your capabilities in relation to the criteria. Consider using frameworks such as STAR (situation, task, action and result) or CARL (context, action, response and learning) to guide you in addressing the selection criteria. Use action verbs such as 'develops', 'creates', 'delegates', 'formulates', 'coordinates' or 'collaborates'. Be honest when addressing selection criteria, but do not understate your achievements. It is also vital to adhere to the recruitment requirements outlined in the announcement, such as attachment of all requested documents. This is another occasion where it will be judicious to seek guidance from mentors or others who may be experienced in contemporary employment application procedures. Failure to showcase your ability to meet all essential criteria will usually result in your being culled from the interview process. Therefore, if you wish to be successful, it is important to present yourself in writing in a manner that enhances your appeal to prospective employers. This requirement will include careful proofreading of your application to check for mistakes and to ensure that formatting is correct prior to submission.[4]

The application will most likely be lodged electronically, requiring supporting information to be submitted via a password-protected portal. The submission will include your CV and a selection of other relevant information from your portfolio. As part of the submission process, you will be required to indicate your consent to mandatory screening processes as part of the terms of employment.

PREPARING FOR THE PROFESSIONAL INTERVIEW

Being invited to an interview means your application has convinced a selection panel that your qualifications, experience, knowledge and competencies match the selection criteria and that you may be a suitable person for the position. It represents the successful completion of another step in the process of obtaining the position. As such, the prospect of an interview typically engenders feelings of excitement, tempered somewhat by nervousness and anxiety.[22] Adequate and strategic preparation for the interview can help you overcome some of these feelings. It is important to begin this preparation process immediately you are informed that you have been selected for interview. An ideal beginning for your interview preparation is to review your application. Focusing on your strengths will give you the confidence to expound how your strengths, qualities and expertise make you the right person for the position. Other steps in the preparation process may include:

1. Research the healthcare facility or organisation. Relevant websites will be a valuable source of information about the organisation.
2. Learn as much as possible about the position and what it entails.
3. Be clear about why you are interested in the position and why you applied. Think about how it matches your professional interests. Will it provide you with the opportunity to practise in an area you find stimulating and satisfying?
4. Think about the interview process. Anticipate the questions that may be asked for each of the selection criteria and rehearse your answers. You may consider undergoing a 'mock' interview with mentors, colleagues or another experienced person.

5. Ensure that the date, time and location of the interview are in your diary. Consider a visit to the venue prior to the interview to familiarise yourself with logistics and to reduce anxiety.

Research the Healthcare Facility or Organisation

Research the organisation's website.[4] Find out as much as you can about the values and vision statements of the organisation. Reflect on your own values and interests, and consider how they would enhance the organisation. You may know people who already work there who would be an invaluable source of information about the structure of the organisation.

Review the Position Specifications

Learn as much as you can about the position for which you are being interviewed. Start with a detailed review of the position description and the essential and desirable criteria. It may also be useful to undertake background reading to enhance your knowledge about specific aspects of the position.

Know Why You Are Interested in the Position

It is usual for a selection panel to ask you why you have applied for the position. This is a question that can be difficult to answer if you have not thought about it in advance. It will require you to articulate the qualities you bring to the position and how you think you can make a difference. Consider expressing your passion for the specialty area of nursing or midwifery, and your commitment to quality and to maximising outcomes for patients.

Think about the Interview Process

The composition of selection panels is usually advised to interviewees in advance, and may comprise as many as five panel members. Although the chairperson of the selection panel will usually try to put you at ease, responding to multiple panel members can be anxiety-provoking. It is worth taking some time to prepare yourself psychologically. So that you are not surprised and overwhelmed on the day, anticipate that the venue may be large and appear impersonal.

The standard format for the interview is for each member of the selection panel to ask one or two questions. The questions are identical for each person being interviewed. Time is usually available at the end of the interview for you to ask questions of the panel, if you wish. This juncture is a valuable opportunity to ask an impressive question that will leave the panel with a lasting impression of your level of confidence, interpersonal and other skills, and your overall suitability for the position.

Anticipate the Questions that May Be Asked

Interview questions are based on the position description and the selection criteria. Being very familiar with these will enable you to anticipate the topics that will be included in the interview questions and to give appropriate responses. Review the main aspects of each of the criteria and write questions that you think may be asked to evaluate your knowledge and experience. The panel may ask you to give examples to support the claims that you make about your ability. The interview format may include a request to pre-prepare a response to a given scenario, or you may be given a scenario during the interview, to which you will need to respond spontaneously.

The selection panel will pose questions to determine your ability to communicate effectively, to work independently and/or collaboratively, to problem solve, and to set short-and long-term goals. In addition, the panel will assess your ability to identify and articulate your strengths, weaknesses and capacity for managing challenging situations, as well as your familiarity with workplace health and safety and equal employment opportunity legislation. The panel may wish to ascertain your strategies for practising critical self-reflection when evaluating your practice. Think about what evidence you may need to provide to the selection panel to convince members that you have detailed knowledge of all aspects of the role and that you are the right person for the position. Reference to the contents of your portfolio will assist you to answer these questions.

EXERCISE 17.3

Locate an announcement for a registered nurse or midwife position, either from a newspaper or on the internet. Note the essential and desirable criteria listed in the announcement, then compose at least five questions that could be asked at an interview. Develop written responses to these questions.

Rehearse Answers

Once you have considered what questions are likely to be asked, prepare answers that are focused on the question, and that are always succinct. Be disciplined in your thinking and do background reading if you cannot explain concepts in sufficient detail. Ask friends and work colleagues to review the questions with you and to give you honest feedback about your answers. Despite your best efforts, it is always possible that questions for which you have not rehearsed will be asked on the day. However, you can prepare for this eventuality. Panel members will give you some time to compile your responses to spontaneous questions; so recall your reasons for applying for the position, and the match between your own personal and professional strengths and the position. Reviewing your strengths will assist you during this stage of the interview.

Write the Date, Time and Venue of the Interview in Your Diary

Ensure that the interview date, time and venue are noted in your diary. Leave nothing to chance. If you are not familiar with the address or the venue, visit the location before your interview and research the availability of parking or public transport.

Interview Day

There are some golden rules that you should follow on the day of the interview. Attention to grooming will help you to project a professional image that will impress the panel. Remember that first impressions are important. Minimise body adornments.

Give yourself sufficient time for travel so that you arrive at the interview with time to spare. Be courteous when introduced to the panel, maintain good eye contact, and respond to questions with interest and enthusiasm. Be thoughtful when responding, but get to the point of your answer quickly. At every opportunity, illustrate the point you are making with an example. If you are unsure about what is meant by a question, ask the panel to clarify what they are asking. Take care not to ask questions that may indicate a lack of preparation on your part or a lack of knowledge about the position. The chair of the panel will inform you of the next stage in the selection process, and when you are likely to hear the outcome of the interview.

After the Interview

Irrespective of your success in gaining the position, critical self-reflection about your performance at interview can help you to develop your interview skills. Journal how you felt on the day, what questions were asked and your evaluation of your responses. Inevitably, you will think of things you wish you had said. Write these down, too, so that they can inform your preparation for any subsequent interviews. Seek feedback from the panel, through the chairperson. Compare the panel's feedback with your own reflections and, above all, learn from the experience. Doing so will enable you to develop interview-related skills and strategies that will be useful throughout your career.

CONCLUSION

As a registered nurse or midwife, you will find that nursing and midwifery present you with many opportunities for career development. In this chapter, we have provided information about establishing your professional portfolio, which includes the development of a professional profile to promote your attributes. Your portfolio should also include your CV, record of CPD, and reflection on education and experiential activities. The discussion of lifelong learning highlighted its contribution to your development as a safe and professional practitioner, capable of providing the highest level of person-centred care. This chapter has also provided strategies for preparing position applications and presenting yourself confidently at employment interviews. Showcasing your career development through a professional portfolio will enable you to reflect on your career strengths, identify and address your weaknesses, and assist you with career planning to achieve your goals.

The authors would like to thank and acknowledge Debra Jackson, Nikki Brown, Ana Smith and Judy Mannix for their contribution to this chapter in previous editions of the text.

CASE STUDY 17.1

Joseph, a final-year student, has been placed in an outer metropolitan community health setting for his clinical practicum. Joseph is required to attend an orientation day and complete a series of learning modules to prepare for this clinical practicum. He has been assigned to a Clinical Nurse Specialist (Community Care) who will facilitate his introduction to the environment and guide his learning experience within a community setting.

REFLECTIVE QUESTIONS

1. How should Joseph record this experience in an insightful manner for documentation in his professional portfolio to reflect both theoretical and clinical learning?
2. How will Joseph demonstrate achievement of the competency standards for the registered nurse or midwife in the portfolio?
3. What are the important elements of reflection on practice that Joseph should be undertaking during this placement?

CASE STUDY 17.2

Rosie, a registered midwife (RM), is undertaking her second rotation in her graduate year in a 28-bed acute midwifery care unit in a large tertiary referral healthcare facility. On arrival for an evening duty, Rosie was informed the experienced midwife rostered as team leader is on sick leave at short notice and is being replaced by an agency midwife. The Midwifery Unit Manager has allocated Rosie into the team leader position for the 8-hour shift. The staff mix is now: team leader RM (Rosie), agency RM, endorsed enrolled nurse (EEN), undergraduate assistant in nursing (AIN).

REFLECTIVE QUESTIONS

1. Reflect on a similar experience or visualise this scenario.
2. How might Rosie prepare for this challenge?
3. What strategies and resources may assist Rosie to coordinate the staff to maximise patient safety?
4. Which model of care will be most appropriate to minimise risk and optimise patient outcomes in this situation?

RECOMMENDED READING

Andre K, Heartfield M. *Nursing and midwifery portfolios: evidence of continuing competence.* 2nd ed. Sydney: Elsevier; 2011.

Dempsey J. Thoughtful practice: self-awareness and reflection. In: Dempsey J, Hillege S, Hill R, editors. *Fundamentals of nursing and midwifery.* 2nd ed. Sydney: Lippincott Williams & Wilkins; 2014. pp 238–52.

Howatson-Jones L. *Reflective practice in nursing.* Los Angeles: Learning Matters; 2013.

Reed S. *Successful professional portfolios for nursing students.* Exeter, UK: Learning Matters; 2011.

Timmins F, Duffy A. *Writing your nursing portfolio: a step-by-step guide.* Maidenhead, UK: Open University Press; 2011.

REFERENCES

1. Laker DR, Laker R. The five-year resume: a career planning exercise. *Journal of Management Education* 2007;**31**:128–41. doi:10.1177/1052562906290525.
2. Andre K. E-portfolios for the aspiring professional. *Collegian (Royal College of Nursing, Australia)* 2010;**17**:119–24. doi:10.1016/j.colegn.2009.10.005.

3. Capan ML, Ambrose HL, Burkett M, Evangelista TR, Flook DM, Straka KL. Nursing portfolio study. *Journal for Nurses in Professional Development* 2013;**29**(4):182–5. doi:10.1097/NND.0b013e31829aecof.

4. Richardson J. Career pathways. In: Birchenall P, Adams N, editors. *The nursing companion.* Houndmills, UK: Palgrave Macmillan; 2011.

5. Timmins F, Duffy A. *Writing your nursing portfolio: a step-by-step guide.* Maidenhead, UK: Open University Press; 2011.

6. Reed S. *Successful professional portfolios for nursing students.* Exeter, UK: Learning Matters; 2011.

7. Andre K, Heartfield M. *Nursing and midwifery portfolios: evidence of continuing competence.* 2nd ed. Sydney: Elsevier; 2011.

8. Dempsey J. Thoughtful practice: self-awareness and reflection. In: Dempsey J, Hillege S, Hill R, editors. *Fundamentals of nursing and midwifery.* 2nd ed. Sydney: Lippincott Williams & Wilkins; 2014. pp 238–52.

9. Johnson JA. The professional portfolio – a tool to document nursing competency. *Journal for Nurses in Staff Development* 2012;**Mar/Apr**:91–2. doi:10.1097/NND.0b013e31824c028d.

10. Mannix J, Stewart L. Establishing and maintaining a professional profile: issues in the first year of practice. In: Chang E, Daly J, editors. *Transitions in nursing: preparing for professional practice.* 3rd ed. Sydney: Elsevier; 2012.

11. Howatson-Jones L. *Reflective practice in nursing.* Los Angeles: Learning Matters; 2013.

12. Nursing and Midwifery Board of Australia. *Continuing professional development registration standard.* Available: <www.nursingmidwiferyboard.gov.au/Search.aspx?q=continuing%20professional%20development>.

13. Te Kaunihera Tapuhi o Aotearoa Nursing Council of New Zealand. Available: <www.nursingcouncil.org.nz/>.

14. Nursing and Midwifery Board of Australia. *Code of professional conduct for nurses in Australia. Available*: <www.nursingmidwiferyboard.gov.au/Search.aspx?q=continuing%20professional%20development>.

15. Nursing and Midwifery Board of Australia. *National competency standards for the registered nurse.* Available: <www.nursingmidwiferyboard.gov.au/Codes-Guidelines-Statements/Codes-Guidelines.aspx#competencystandards>.

16. Green J, Wyllie A, Jackson D. Electronic portfolios in nursing education: a review of the literature. *Nurse Education in Practice* 2014;**14**:4–8. doi:10.1016/j.nepr.2013.08.011.

17. Gibbs G. *Learning by doing: a guide to teaching and learning methods.* Oxford: Oxford Brookes University; 1988.

18. Levett-Jones T, Bourgeois S. *The clinical placement.* Sydney: Elsevier; 2011.

19. Davis L, Taylor H, Reyes H. Lifelong learning in nursing: a Delphi study. *Nurse Education Today* 2014;**34**(3):441–5. doi:10.1016/j.nedt.2013.04.014.

20. Queensland Health. *Building blocks of lifelong learning: a framework for nurses and midwives in Queensland.* Available: <www.health.qld.gov.au/nmoq/documents/qhnmsdf.pdf>.

21. Benner P. *From novice to expert: excellence and power in clinical nursing.* Menlo-Park, CA: Addison-Wesley; 1984.

22. Sieverding M. 'Be cool!' Emotional costs of hiding feelings in a job interview. *International Journal of Selection and Assessment* 2009;**17**:391–401.

CHAPTER 18

Reflective practice for the graduate

Kim Usher and Kim Foster

LEARNING OBJECTIVES

When you have completed this chapter you will be able to:

▲ understand the benefits of reflection and identify its importance to nursing practice, research and leadership
▲ appreciate the link between reflection, self-monitoring and improved client outcomes
▲ understand how reflection is linked to an effective and fulfilling career
▲ recognise the usefulness of using a reflective framework to assist in the development of your reflective processes
▲ apply the key elements of reflection to your practice.

KEYWORDS: reflection, nursing practice, self-monitoring, leadership, research

INTRODUCTION

Nursing has embraced the idea of reflective practice to varying degrees and applied it across the areas of nursing practice, education, research and leadership with the intent of achieving best outcomes for clients. Reflection has been described as a process of going back over something after it has occurred with the aim of making sense of the situation so that necessary decisions can be made and opportunities for changes can be identified.[1,2] In other words, the purpose of reflection is that it leads to action that is better informed. This occurs via a process of learning through experience in a way that aids in the development of new insights about self and practice.[3] Reflection is also closely linked to critical thinking.[4] While not identical, it is paramount that reflection has a critical intent,[5] as being a critical thinker involves questioning the world and challenging assumptions that are taken for granted. In this chapter we have chosen to use the word *reflection*, but our intent is to convey the link between critical thinking and reflection at all times.

Reflection has also been linked to self-awareness or self-development. Johns[6] terms this as being 'mindful' of self. In this way he believes a practitioner can use reflection with the aim of confronting and resolving the contradiction between one's vision and actual practice. Through the development of this notion of contradiction, Johns[6] would say, we come to understand why things are the way they are, which allows us to develop new insights that assist us to respond more effectively in the future. The outcome is thus a process of continuous monitoring that leads to improvement of practice (pp 117–36).[7] We assume that as a graduate nurse you are interested in knowing and realising desirable and effective practice, but as Johns[6] reminds us, we sometimes work in conditions where such a realisation may be difficult or even impossible. In these cases, reflection takes on an even more important role in the goal of professional development. We hope this chapter will help you, as a new graduate, to recognise the importance of the ability to self-monitor and self-regulate and come to understand the benefits and rewards reflective practice can bring to your role in the years ahead.

This chapter assumes you already have a basic understanding of reflective practice and have utilised many of the processes suggested as ways of enhancing reflection, such as keeping a journal and exploring critical incidents, during your undergraduate years.[7] Hence, we will not be offering a comprehensive theoretical overview of reflection here but will instead focus on what we believe to be of most importance to the graduate nurse from a practical perspective: the impact of reflection on practice, leadership and management, and research. We have focused on these areas because we believe reflection can help the new graduate to assimilate to the new practice environment and manage effectively the challenges of daily practice. It will also be important for you as you move on in your career and start to take on management and leadership roles, and likewise as you begin to become involved in research within the clinical arena. The first section of the chapter addresses reflection and how it can benefit your practice; the second section applies the usefulness of reflection to the areas of management and leadership; and the last section connects reflection to the research process.

If you feel your understanding of the theoretical underpinnings of reflective practice is not sufficient to appreciate this chapter fully, please read an introduction to the material, such as the chapter by Usher and Holmes.[7] In that chapter, the framework developed by Rolfe and colleagues[5] was used as an example of a framework to guide reflection. We have also referred to that framework throughout this chapter and have included it as Figure 18.1 for your reference. While we do not propose that frameworks are necessary for reflection to occur, many novice practitioners find them a useful starting point.[8] There are a number of other frameworks or models of reflection that may be more suitable to your use, including those of Burrows[9] and Smith and Russell.[10] You will find helpful texts in the recommended reading at the end of this chapter.

NURSING PRACTICE IN THE GRADUATE YEAR AND BEYOND

This section addresses the usefulness of reflective practice for the graduate nurse during the transition year and beyond. Criticisms of reflection, as Usher and Holmes[7] remind us, include the notion that the reflective process is often viewed as simply an

Descriptive level of reflection	Theory- and knowledge-building level of reflection	Action-oriented (reflexive) level of reflection

What . . .	So what . . .	Now what . . .

. . . is the problem/difficulty/reason for being stuck/reason for feeling bad/reason we don't get on?

. . . was my role in the situation?

. . . was I trying to achieve?

. . . actions did I take?

. . . was the response of others?

. . . were the consequences
• for the patient?
• for myself?
• for others?

. . . feelings did it evoke
• in the patient?
• in myself?
• in others?

. . . was good/bad about the experience?

. . . does this tell me/teach me/imply/ mean about me/my patient/others/our relationship/my patient's care/the model of care I am using/my attitudes/my patient's attitudes?

. . . was going through my mind as I acted?

. . . did I base my actions on?

. . . other knowledge can I bring to the situation?
• experiential?
• personal?
• scientific?

. . . could/should I have done to make it better?

. . . is my new understanding of the situation?

. . . broader issues arise from the situation?

. . . do I need to do in order to make things better/stop being stuck/improve my patient's care/resolve the situation/feel better/get on better?

. . . broader issues need to be considered if this action is to be successful?

. . . might be the consequences of this action?

Figure 18.1

Framework for reflection

Source: G Rolfe, D Freshwater, M Jasper. Critical reflection for nursing and the helping professions: a user's guide. New York: Palgrave; 2001. p 35.

academic exercise. Graduate nurses may have memories of keeping a reflective journal as a tedious classroom assignment, but may consider that 'it does not happen in the real world'. We know you will have spent some time during your undergraduate or preregistration course completing classroom exercises and assessments of a reflective practice nature, and you may have found these activities more or less helpful. However, we remain committed to the ideal of registered nurses who continue to think critically and to reflect upon their practice so that they become the best practitioners possible. We hope that registered nurses will not only see the usefulness of reflection in their early years but consider it an important skill for the future where they will continue to reflect and mentor others, and that they retire from the profession with the knowledge of that contribution to nursing practice and to the care of their communities.

Consider your own situation now as a new graduate. Imagine that you have incorporated Rolfe and colleagues'[5] framework into your practice so that it is almost second nature to what you do – it is part of your practice. An event occurs at work and you ask yourself:

- What is the problem here?
- What is my role in this situation – how have I contributed to what happened?
- What does this teach me?
- Now what do I need to do to make things better next time?

Using this framework to unpack everyday experiences allows us to describe events to ourselves more clearly, to build more knowledge from that description, and to take action ourselves to improve situations. This is where we can truly become empowered as nurses: where we have the opportunity to use a reflective approach to unravel a complex situation, see it for what it is, identify ways to ensure it does not happen again, or identify strategies to improve the outcomes in the future. The alternative is to leave things as they are and go on as if nothing has happened. This usually means we go away, justify our actions in an uncritical or unreflective way, and then find it difficult to move on. The practice arena may not always turn out to be what it first seemed and, as a result, nurses may struggle to hold on to the ideals of why they wanted to be a nurse in the first place, leading to people leaving the profession. Reflection offers stability in this situation, something to which health professionals can turn to help make sense of the world, re-evaluate their practice, develop self-confidence, and affirm as well as change thinking and action.[11,12] In other words, the reflective approach helps us habitually to self-correct, and to assist others to do the same, so that the whole notion of continuous improvement becomes part of who we are as nurses. Reflection on nursing practice then becomes 'a way of being, an active way of engaging practice towards realising desirable practice in whatever way it is known and understood'.[6]

This sort of knowledge – learning from practice, or practice wisdom[13] – began to an extent during your first clinical placement, and can become a habit (or not!) during your first year of practice and beyond. It is important that you realise the benefits, both personal and professional, of being a reflective practitioner from the outset of your career. We cannot persuade you to do this with what we might consider to be the power of the good logical argument. You are the one who will make that decision for yourself – we can simply provide you with guidance to arrive at that decision.

A key component of reflection is to remember what happened. Burton (cited in Usher and Holmes, p 130)[7] calls this 'a type of cognitive "postmortem" or an act of looking back at practice'. This is what is also termed *reflection on action*, which occurs after the event has taken place. This type of reflection can be extremely powerful and will contribute greatly to your effectiveness as a practitioner. Reflecting *in* action is also possible, and this implies pausing within a particular situation with the intent of trying to make sense of or reframe a situation to enable a better outcome.[14] We know that this is about persistently cycling through the testing of theories and hypotheses while you are actually engaged in practice.[15,16] Sound difficult? Of course it can be, and the challenge is to attempt this more advanced form of reflection so that it becomes habitual, rather than being just another difficult task you have to turn your mind to in the midst of a busy working day. The issue here is that habitual unconscious action is largely replaced by habitual reflection by the self-aware nurse who, with customary self-monitoring, delivers the sort of nursing care that leads to improved client outcomes.

You may be familiar with the term *clinical supervision*, for which there are varying definitions and models in practice. While we recognise the lack of agreement as to the term, one way of understanding clinical supervision is that it is a formal, structured and systematic process of engaging in learning and reflection on action (practice) that occurs within the context of a supportive professional relationship between a supervisor and supervisee. The process seeks to enhance practice through supporting and developing the nurse's job identity, competence, knowledge, ethics and skills.[17] Clinical supervision is therefore one of a number of ways in which nurses can engage in reflective practice.[18] It is important to note, though, that the term *supervisor* does not refer to the nurse's direct line manager or nursing supervisor (although it is possible the clinical supervisor role may be performed by this person); rather, it refers to the role of an experienced and competent health professional (often a nurse) with whom the supervisee works, either individually or in a group.

While it is most often associated with mental health nursing, clinical supervision has also been reported as an important facet of practice in midwifery, and for nurses working in settings such as hospices and palliative care, the community and medical/surgical areas.[19] Clinical supervision can also offer a particularly helpful form of professional support for nurses working in isolated and/or rural and remote settings.[6,20,21] In this process, nurses meet with their supervisor on a regular basis to discuss various aspects of their practice (a form of dialogical reflection), which includes nurses' self-assessment of their performance in order to develop and sustain further competence in their work through transforming their knowledge.[22] While this may appear to be a rather daunting process, when managed in a constructive and supportive way, many nurses find that having an opportunity to reflect on their practice with a clinical supervisor brings significant benefits. Indeed, you might be aware that clinical supervision is viewed increasingly as an integral form of professional support for nurses that can assist in recruitment and retention and that some health services provide it for staff as a part of their employment package.

So, like many other nurses, reflecting on action and using clinical supervision in your practice may help to deepen your self-awareness and self-understanding, balance work and the rest of your life, reduce uncomfortable feelings of distress related to your work, and explore problematic issues related to your practice.[23] The benefits extend to your clients through the enhanced nursing knowledge, skills and strategies you bring from engaging in this process, and researchers are seeking to illuminate client and other outcomes associated with nurses participating in clinical supervision.[24] Clinical supervision is not limited to clinical practice, however, and can also be a valuable aspect of nursing management and leadership, where it has been found to assist in the development of communication, coping and leadership skills.[22]

THE NURSE LEADER AND MANAGER

Remember, reflection is essentially concerned with thinking about what you do so that you can learn to do it better. This is not something we tend to do naturally. Instead, as Johns[25] reminds us, 'as we go about our everyday business we take the world largely for granted and respond habitually' (p 1). We have already discussed the importance of reflection to the novice practitioner. This section explores how reflective practice may benefit you now in your work as a graduate nurse and in your future career as you take on management and leadership roles.

Taylor[2] has suggested that reflection can be emancipatory. Emancipation means freedom from your own and from other people's expectations and roles in order to adopt other ways of being.[2] Emancipation involves the processes of critiquing, imagining and analysing the situation in order to explore possibilities that would make a situation more equitable and just.[26] This type of reflection is linked to empowerment, which is the process of giving and accepting power[1] and helps the practitioner take actions that are based on insights.[5] The aim of reflection can therefore be to 'free practitioners from the taken-for-granted assumptions and oppressive forces which limit them and their practice' (p 12).[27] This is particularly important when thinking about nursing leaders and managers, as they have an important role in change.[2] Think about how nurse leaders and managers shape the organisation and how they go about improving patient or client care. Also consider how they influence you as a graduate nurse. Finally, think about the sort of nurse leader and manager you are going to be. Johns proposes that 'the Buddhist perspective would view reflection as a way to nurture and realise wise and compassionate practice within a strong ethic of doing good in the world' (p 7).[25] Sounds like something to aspire to, does it not? Likewise, reflection for nursing leaders and managers could assist them to realise why they do not always 'do good in the world' and would help them to explore how they could do more good.

Reflection requires that nursing leaders and managers take a critical approach to their practice. Essentially:

> Critical theorising ... looks at the way life is and asks how it might be different and better for the majority of people, not just for the privileged few who hold and use power (p 144).[27]

Emancipatory and empowering reflection is important for nurses in leadership and management positions in healthcare. Think for a moment about your own life and how you live it, going about your everyday business with family, friends and work colleagues, perhaps not reflecting a great deal on the things that happen and why they happen – you just live. You do the sort of things that most other people do in your environment – you eat, sleep, talk with people, have disagreements, make up, fall in love, fall out of love, attend classes, study, work, party, go shopping, watch TV, go to the movies. Think of this as your 'everyday life'. That is, 'we just do stuff', and that 'stuff' of everyday life is nevertheless strongly influenced by elements such as the culture within which we live, family background, school education systems, and so on.

Now think about what happens, for example, in a hospital (or a school, or a university). Have you ever attended a formal meeting in one of these settings? If so, you will have noticed that 'everyday life' looks a bit different. There are rules for behaviour that seem to apply, and most people follow these rules. The rules will be about things such as what is said, what is permitted to be said, who speaks, whose voice is heard, who is not permitted to speak, maybe whose voice is not heard. From a critical perspective we would say that people in such a meeting are engaged in 'discourse', this being 'an unusual form of communication in which the participants subject themselves to the force of the better argument, with the view to coming to an agreement about the validity or invalidity of problematic claims'.[28] This sounds wonderful; that people might be able to get together and talk carefully, openly and freely about problems, and arrive together at good solutions to those problems. Remember those rules, however – does everyone get to speak in the same way? Obviously not, and that is the problem. Discourses like this become institutionalised;[28] that is, we make rules for what is allowed to be said, and these rules tend to govern the sort of decisions (sometimes very bad ones) that are allowed to be made to solve problems. We ask ourselves questions in these meetings about what is going on, questions such as, 'why aren't there enough beds for patients in our public hospitals?', but the answers to those questions are not always arrived at from free and open discussion; instead, they are governed by the institutionalised rules that are in play. This is where it becomes interesting. Unless healthcare leaders and managers – in our case, nursing leaders and managers – reflect upon how power is used or misused in this way, this tendency to control people and processes, so much of the creative thinking that happens in everyday life is lost. This is what reflection is all about – it is about nursing leaders and managers reflecting upon these social circumstances, and moving forward with this understanding. It is about encouraging those disparate voices at the level of discourse – for example, in formal meetings – rather than leaving people whispering in corridors.

Obviously, in healthcare organisations or universities, the nursing leaders and managers do not 'hold all the power'. They do have their share, though. How do they use or misuse this power? Power can be power with others or power over others. The goal for the effective nursing leader and manager would be that of power *with* rather than *over*: the notion of empowerment of everyone – themselves, nurses, students, clients or patients, other members of the healthcare team. 'When leaders share power with others, they're demonstrating profound trust in and respect for others' abilities.'[29] In order to understand this good use of power, nursing leaders and managers need knowledge about how they themselves behave – that is, how they use or misuse their power.

Effective leadership and management always seem to start with self-knowledge,[30,31] and self-knowledge comes from reflection upon our thinking and behaviours. Knowing ourselves does not come from wandering rather sleepily through life, behaving in habitual ways that are often culturally determined and socially constructed. We need to be awake to the effects of these social and cultural factors, so we can change our responses when we need to. Kouzes and Posner[29] describe 'exploring your inner territory' as a key to effective leadership. Think about the nursing leader and manager who has clarified his or her values, figured out where she or he wants his or her organisation to go, what she or he wants for his or her clients or patients, what she or he wants for the nursing team. Compare this person with the nursing leader and manager who has never done this, never 'explored their inner territory', but rather, simply reacts to what happens on a daily, weekly, monthly, yearly basis. Can you begin to see the difference between the reflective and the non-reflective life? Ask yourself which of these lives you want. It is crucial at this stage to note that reflection itself is not simply another imposition by others on your precious time:

> ... it is not an artificial technique that is imposed by regulatory authorities or universities; rather, it is the refinement of a natural process that is part of being human, and which needs to be nurtured and encouraged.[7]

Think about emancipatory reflection for a moment now in relation to your own nursing practice. How do nursing leaders and managers (and others) either empower you or disempower you in relation to your practice? It has been claimed that 'emancipatory reflection leads to "transformative action" which seeks to free nurses and midwives from taken-for-granted assumptions and oppressive forces which limit them and their practice'.[32] It may be that through the role of the nursing leader and/or manager you will use reflection as means to attain a higher level of self-awareness in order to be a more effective leader/manager.

So, how can this help you now in your role as a new graduate? Perhaps it is first of all worth considering the idea that it is important for new graduates to accept that others will be their leaders. It is not always easy to follow others, but at times we need to be able to accept leadership and learn from those with more experience, particularly when we begin our career. Imagine a graduate nurse who experiences a crisis at work, perhaps makes a mistake or becomes stressed due to workloads. This experience, this crisis, with the guidance of a reflective, wise and supportive nursing leader and manager, could be a means of developing higher levels of skill and better coping mechanisms for use in the future.

The nursing leader and manager could utilise a framework such as that developed by Rolfe and colleagues[5] and guide you, through asking questions such as:

- What is the reason for this mistake that was made?
- What was my role in this?
- What was going through my mind when I did this thing?
- What is my new understanding of this situation?
- Now what do I need to do in order to make it better the next time?

This provides a nurturing environment where you can learn, and where the organisation also learns.[5] In essence, where members of the healthcare facility have ongoing experiences like this with their leaders and managers, then this becomes part of the culture of the organisation.

Reflective nursing leaders and managers are transformational in the way that they practise,[5] and transformational leadership cultures are reflective cultures. Getting better at what we do comes from reflecting upon what we do and making necessary adjustments to our thinking and behaviours for future situations. Emancipatory reflection is about, as Taylor[27] explains, daring, imagining, planning and acting 'in ways that are capable of transforming your world'. You may be thinking that becoming a leader or manager is far in your future. However, nurses in their graduate year are being socialised by those with whom they work. The culture of a ward, department or community health service is largely shaped by the leadership on offer in that particular environment, and it is the people in that environment who will be shaping the graduate's practice. That leadership, culture and nursing practice has an impact upon the type of care that clients are receiving. An environment of reflective practitioners is one resulting in better client outcomes, whether this be through the graduate nurse administering medications safely, or the nurse manager embedding reflection on action into the culture of the environment.

So far, we have been focusing on the importance of reflection to your practice as a manager and leader. Research and the need to base our practice on valid evidence are also important to the role of the nurse in practice, management and leadership, so let us now move to consider the link between reflective practice and research.

RESEARCH

As a graduate nurse working in a practice profession, it is important that you maintain your professional development throughout your career in order to remain up to date with advances in healthcare and nursing practice. Part of this development will include involvement with research. Most often, this will be through use of evidence from empirical or scientific research that informs your practice – evidence-based practice. You may also conduct research as part of your nursing role; through undertaking postgraduate study; and/or through an interest in exploring a particular clinical issue that arises in your practice. While you may not have considered that you would be conducting research as part of your work, it is increasingly common for registered nurses to be involved in research through practice development projects and collaborative research with experienced researchers. In this section, we explore how reflective practice may be useful in both conducting and using research for practice, for, as Taylor[27] suggests, the processes and thinking required in reflective practice are those required in any kind of practice, including research.

A reflective approach privileges subjective or personal experience and interrelated ways of knowing, and can be seen to blur the distinctions between knowing and doing, art and science, theory and practice.[27] In addition, if reflection can be considered a paradigm or framework for collecting, evaluating, understanding and applying knowledge, then it can also be seen as the standard for generating and judging knowledge for reflective practice. From this perspective, reflective practice and evidence-based practice may be viewed as complementary philosophies from which to examine nursing practice.[33] Reflective methods can therefore not only guide nursing practice, education and leadership; they can also provide evidence for supporting developments and changes in practice. Reflective processes may be used as the framework for a research project; they can be incorporated with other research approaches; and/or they can be the focus of research itself.[34] As a framework for research, the processes of reflective practice can be used to develop a research project. The framework of reflection proposed by Rolfe and colleagues,[5] for instance, could be applied to a clinical problem and used to facilitate the development of a clinical research project.

Reflective practice has also been incorporated with other research approaches such as qualitative, quantitative or mixed methods studies, and used to inform nursing practice.[34] While we will not be exploring the types of research in detail here, a brief review of the major types of research approaches is useful. In qualitative research, the focus is on lived subjective (personal) experience and people's use of language to share their experiences. Qualitative researchers therefore focus on participants' experiences of events, situations and relationships, and seek to interpret or uncover meanings they may have made of them. This is in contrast to quantitative research, which investigates objective (observable) data and seeks to quantify it through use of statistical methods. In mixed methods research, both qualitative and quantitative research methods are used in combination, or sequentially, to enrich the exploration of a specific issue.

Action research and reflection are a particularly effective combination. Reflection forms part of the action research method which involves cyclical stages of planning, acting, observing and reflecting.[35] The combination of reflective practice and action research can be a valuable tool for developing knowledge in nursing and reducing the theory–practice gap.[36] An illustration of this combination can be seen in a study by Taylor,[36] who used these methods to facilitate reflective practice processes in 12 registered nurses. In the study, the nurses worked collaboratively with the researcher to explore dysfunctional nurse–nurse relationships such as workplace bullying and violence. In a series of action cycles, they critically reflected on practice issues and their stories of these, and looked for particular themes and issues. The thematic concern of dysfunctional nurse–nurse relationships was explored through a plan of action containing skills and strategies implemented to address this issue. As might be expected, the nurses encountered difficulties in addressing workplace relationships and in implementing the action plan, but also found significant benefits through engaging in this process, such as more effective personal communication, the use of leadership skills, and recognising the complexities that can exist in workplace relationships.

In another example of how reflective practice may be included in research, Kim[37] developed a method of critical reflective inquiry that can be used to develop nursing knowledge and practice. This research method incorporates notions from reflective practice, action science and critical philosophy and involves three phases: (1) descriptive, (2) reflective, and (3) critical/emancipatory. In the descriptive phase, nurses provide narratives of their practice which describe their thoughts and feelings, actions and circumstances of the particular situation/s. In the reflective phase, these narratives are analysed in the context of the nurse's personal beliefs, assumptions and knowledge. In this phase, models of 'good' practice and knowledge may be developed from reflective analysis and exploration of the nurse's practice. In the critical/emancipatory phase, the focus is on the correction and change of less desirable or ineffective practice, and/or moving on to new innovations that may have emerged from practice. Kim[37] suggested that this process can be used as a research method; it can be adopted in practice and nursing education as a way of improving practice; and/or it can be the basis for shared learning, where clinicians hold regular case conferences to explore issues.

Reflective practice has itself been the focus of research.[38,39,40] Dube and Ducharme,[39] for example, developed a reflective practice intervention of eight workshops which included structured reflection, reflective journalling and best practices for aspects of nursing care, for nurses caring for older persons in a hospital setting. In this action research study, using qualitative data, 22 nurses reported developing a range of knowledge and reflective practice skills, including critical analysis, and being open-minded and more introspective. Importantly, nurses found their communication skills had improved and they were able to analyse their daily practice more effectively. In another study,[41] the innovative use of technology to support staff's reflective learning was explored over a 2-year period. Software applications – apps – were introduced to support aspects of staff's personal and collaborative reflection practices. In surveys, staff reported that the use of apps helped them to discuss issues with colleagues and supervisors, and increased their job satisfaction.

Reflection and Reflexivity in Research

As we have seen, reflective processes can frame the research process and/or be a valuable part of the research process, as well as being integral to the development of nursing practices. In research, particularly qualitative research, reflection is an important aspect of reflexivity. Although there are various definitions of reflexivity, it can be understood as being based in the notion of researcher self-awareness and self-reflection on their role in the research they are conducting. A reflexive orientation includes being conscious of the role the researcher plays in constructing meaning in the research.[42] Reflexivity requires that, for the duration of the study, researchers critically examine their actions through each stage of the research process. This includes issues such as the participants' responses to the researchers, how researchers are collecting their data or field text, what they are seeing and hearing, and how they are making their interpretations of the data. It may lead to alterations to aspects of the design and/or implementation of the research. The resulting reflections are then written up as part of the research report in order to make reader evaluation of the research possible through the process of transparent and auditable documentation.[43] You may notice that this process bears a number of similarities to the reflective methods for practice discussed earlier in the chapter. Similarly to reflective processes used to reflect upon practice, reflexivity in research is a creative as well as analytical method which may include the keeping of written and/or audiotaped research diaries, journals or field notes while conducting research, and/or the writing of reflective narratives and poetry.

Research methods in nursing that have been particularly associated with reflective practice and reflexivity include narrative inquiry and autoethnography. As you will have seen throughout this section, narratives are often used in reflective processes as people can be seen to share the meanings they have made from their experiences through the stories they tell of them. While narratives can be found in many qualitative research studies, this is often in the form of data rather than as a research method. Narrative inquiry, however, is a specific research methodology that seeks to understand personal experiences by focusing on the stories that structure and recall those experiences and using narrative analytic methods to interpret them.

Narrative research can be considered particularly pertinent to nursing, as nursing is an oral culture and stories may resonate as research that is meaningful and relevant to nurses. The stories derived from research into nurses' practices can shed light not only on what nurses do in practice, but also on why they have practised in a particular way.[44] Reflexive narratives of nursing practice, for example, are a form of self-inquiry which can assist in transforming practice through exploring and reflecting upon particular patients and situations. Jarrett[45] explains how her reflexive exploration of two narratives of patients she cared for assisted her to make changes to her nursing of people with a disability:

> Both experiences help[ed] me to focus on an important aspect of my role and development of skills: easing the path for people with complex disabilities to come in, through and out of hospital. Predominantly this was triggered by recognising that people with complex needs fear being admitted to hospital ... Coming into hospital, a large disruption for most people can become an even bigger deal if you have complex needs. Often the impact is as big for the carer who may take the lead in trying to negotiate care rather than doing it.

Another form of narrative research which relies on reflexivity is autoethnography, also referred to as personal narratives or narratives of the self. Autoethnography is a form of critical inquiry about personal or professional issues where researchers focus on their own experience for narrative data collection and analysis.[46] The researcher's personal experience is important primarily in terms of how it sheds light on the issue that is being studied. Autoethnography can range from starting research from one's own experience, to studies where the researcher's experience is explored alongside those of the participants, through to stories where the researcher's experiences of conducting the research become the actual focus of investigation.[47] Although it has been used by a number of professional disciplines, autoethnography is considered an emergent method in nursing research, with relatively few studies conducted by nurses.[42] Foster, however, included her own story and experience for analysis alongside those of her participants when she explored what it was like to grow up with a parent with serious mental illness. She reflects on her experience and the benefit of using autoethnography as a research method:

> ... having a parent with a mental illness sometimes places me in tension with my identity as a psychiatric mental health nurse. Identity is clearly not fixed. Thus, wounds and difficulties received in childhood can be transmuted into opportunities for insight and growth. As I have prepared for the field text [data] collection and analysis phase of this research inquiry, I have come to see that experiences are diverse, and meaning is shaped by many things, including the experience, reflection on that experience, and conversing about it with those who might share points of similarity and those who do not.[48]

CONCLUSION

In summary, we have suggested that, as a practice-based profession, nursing requires reflection on practice so as to enhance and develop nurses' knowledge, skills and practice. Reflection, as described in this chapter, not only helps us to identify and question poor practices, but also allows us to identify strategies for improvement. In this way we can provide the most effective care for our patients. The chapter also outlined how reflective practice can help you to develop a higher level of self-awareness. The development of this awareness helps us to become more aware of the needs of others and more aware of the impact of our behaviour on those around us. Yet, reflective practice is useful not only for practice and leadership, but also as a method for research into nursing issues and practice, and/or to be used in combination with other research methods. As a graduate nurse, you can therefore use reflective practice to undertake a research project on an issue of clinical significance for you; to reflect on your experiences in practice and leadership; and to reflect upon and implement findings from research that enhance your nursing of the patients in your care.

CASE STUDY 18.1

Hemlata's second rotation during her graduate year is to an operating theatre in a large tertiary hospital. When acting as 'scout' in the orthopaedic theatre, she accidentally leans on and unsterilises the instrument tray. The orthopaedic surgeon shouts at her; the instrument nurse asks him to calm down and immediately sets about organising a replacement instrument tray with Hemlata's assistance. Afterwards, she sits down privately with Hemlata and gently takes her through a reflection on the situation.

REFLECTIVE QUESTIONS

1. What is Hemlata learning about the different approaches to leadership in this situation?
2. What impact might this reflection process have on her own attitudes to communicating with less experienced staff?

CASE STUDY 18.2

Sue is working in a mental health unit. A client is removed from the activity area and put into a secure room alone because of abusive behaviour. Sue is very upset by the removal of the client and the approach the nurses used when placing him in isolation.

REFLECTIVE QUESTION

How can Johns'[6] notion of contradiction between vision and actual practice help Sue to resolve her feelings?

CASE STUDY 18.3

Jo has just started working on a busy medical unit. In the unit, a small group of nurses have been developing an action research project on nurses' and patients' perspectives of handover practices. Jo has been invited by the clinical nurse consultant, the project leader, to join the team. Jo is interested in the issue of handover and is keen to learn about research but feels anxious about being involved because she does not think she has a good understanding of the research process. As part of the initial phase of the project the team meets to plan and discuss the phases of the project and the respective roles they will take. Jo notices that, although there are some very senior nurses in the team, all the team members join in the discussion and everyone's opinion is valued.

REFLECTIVE QUESTIONS

1. Think of a particular situation with a patient or family which you found challenging and/or where you felt troubled or concerned by their behaviour and/or your responses to it. How might engaging in clinical supervision have been helpful in addressing this situation/issue and in developing your knowledge and skills for the future?

2. When you attend your next work unit meeting, take careful note of the 'rules' for behaviour that seem to apply. Notice who gets listened to respectfully by the person who is the leader and manager of your work unit, whose opinion the leader takes seriously and acts upon. Notice any team members who give an opinion, but whose opinion does not seem to be taken seriously by the nursing leader and manager. If you feel comfortable in doing so, ask the nursing leader and manager later in private about what causes that person to listen to some people, and not to others. Reflect later upon the 'rules' in your work unit, and ask yourself how you can function in transformational ways to improve your unit's culture.

3. Think again about the connection between reflection and research. How do you think reflection could be useful in a clinical research project? Think in particular about how reflection and reflexivity might help you to identify things about you that you bring to the research endeavour and the decisions that are made throughout the project.

RECOMMENDED READING

Bulman C, Schutz S. *Reflective practice in nursing.* 4th ed. Oxford, UK: John Wiley & Sons; 2013.

Johns C. *Becoming a reflective practitioner.* 4th ed. Oxford, UK: John Wiley & Sons; 2013.

Kinsella EA. Professional knowledge and the epistemology of reflective practice. *Nursing Philosophy* 2009;**11**:3–14.

Rolfe G, Freshwater D, Jasper M. *Critical reflection for nursing and the helping professions: a user's guide.* New York: Palgrave; 2001.

Usher K, Holmes C. Reflective practice: what, why and how. In: Daly J, Speedy S, Jackson D, editors. *Contexts of nursing.* 4th ed. Sydney: Churchill Livingstone; 2014. pp 117–36.

REFERENCES

1. Jasper M, Rosser M, Mooney G. *Professional development, reflection and decision-making in nursing and healthcare.* 2nd ed. Oxford, UK: John Wiley & Sons; 2013.

2. Taylor BJ. *Reflective practice: a guide for healthcare professionals.* 3rd ed. Maidenhead, UK: Open University Press; 2010.

3. Bulman C, Schutz S. *Reflective practice in nursing.* 4th ed. Oxford, UK: John Wiley & Sons; 2013.

4. Naber JL, Hall J, Schadler CM. Narrative thematic analysis of baccalaureate nursing students' reflections: critical thinking in the clinical education context. *Journal of Nursing Education* 2014.

5. Rolfe G, Freshwater D, Jasper M. *Critical reflection for nursing and the helping professions: a user's guide.* New York: Palgrave; 2001. p 35.

6. Johns C. *Becoming a reflective practitioner.* 4th ed. Oxford, UK: John Wiley & Sons; 2013.

7. Usher K, Holmes C. Reflective practice: what, why and how. In: Daly J, Speedy S, Jackson D, editors. *Contexts of nursing.* 4th ed. Sydney: Churchill Livingstone; 2014.

8. Asselin ME, Fain JA. Effect of reflective practice education on self-reflection, insight, and reflective thinking among experienced nurses: a pilot study. *Journal of Nurses' Professional Development* 2013;**29**(3):111–19.

9. Burrows DE. The nurse teacher's role in the promotion of reflective practice. *Nurse Education Today* 1995;**15**(5):346–50.

10. Smith A, Russell J. Using critical incidents in nurse education. *Nurse Education Today* 1991;**11**(4):284–91.

11. Pfaff K, Baxter P, Jack S, Ploeg J. An integrative review of the factors influencing new graduate nurse engagement in interprofessional collaboration. *Journal of Advanced Nursing* 2014;**70**(1):4–20.

12. Howatson-Jones L. *Transforming nursing practice: reflective practice in nursing.* 2nd ed. London: Learning Matters, SAGE Publications; 2013. p 12.

13. White J. Becoming a competent, confident registered nurse. In: Chang E, Daly J, editors. *Transitions in nursing: preparing for professional practice.* 3rd ed. Sydney: Elsevier; 2012. pp 17–30.

14. Schon DA. *The reflective practitioner.* New York: Basic Books; 1983.

15. Rolfe G. Rethinking reflective education: what would Dewey have done? *Nurse Education Today* 2014;**34**(8):1179–83.

16. Yuan HB, Williams BA, Man CY. Nursing students' clinical judgment in high-fidelity simulation based learning: a quasi-experimental study. *Journal of Nursing Education and Practice* 2014;**4**(5):7.

17. Berggren I, da Silva A, Severinsson E. Core ethical issues of clinical nursing supervision. *Nursing and Health Sciences* 2005;**7**:21–8.

18. Clouder L, Sellars J. Reflective practice and clinical supervision: an interprofessional perspective. *Journal of Advanced Nursing* 2004;**46**:262–9.

19. Dilworth S, Higgins I, Parker V, Kelly B, Turner J. Finding a way forward: a literature review on the current debates around clinical supervision. *Contemporary Nurse* 2013;**45**(1):22–32.

20. Kenny A, Allenby A. Implementing clinical supervision for Australian rural nurses. *Nurse Education in Practice* 2013;**13**(3):165–9.

21. Mbemba G, Gagnon MP, Paré G, Côté J. Interventions for supporting nurse retention in rural and remote areas: an umbrella review. *Human Resources for Health* 2013;**11**(1):44.

22. Long CG, Harding S, Payne K, Collins L. Nursing and health-care assistant experience of supervision in a medium secure psychiatric service for women: implications for service development. *Journal of Psychiatric and Mental Health Nursing* 2014;**21**(2):154–62.

23. Cross W, Moore A, Ockerby S. Clinical supervision of general nurses in a busy medical ward of a teaching hospital. *Contemporary Nurse* 2010;**35**(2):245–53.

24. Pearce P, Phillips B, Dawson M, Leggat SG. Content of clinical supervision sessions for nurses and allied health professionals: a systematic review. *Clinical Governance: An International Journal* 2013;**18**(2):139–54.

25. Johns C. Expanding the gates of perception. In: Johns C, Freshwater D, editors. *Transforming nursing through reflective practice.* 2nd ed. Oxford, UK: Blackwell; 2005.

26. Chinn PL, Kramer MK. *Integrated theory and knowledge development in nursing.* 8th ed. St Louis, MO: Elsevier Inc; 2011.

27. Taylor BJ. *Reflective practice: a guide for healthcare professionals.* 3rd ed. Maidenhead, UK: Open University Press; 2010.

28. Crotty M. *The foundations of social research.* Sydney: Allen & Unwin; 1998.

29. Kouzes JM, Posner BZ. *The leadership challenge: how to make extraordinary things happen in organizations.* 5th ed. San Francisco: John Wiley; 2012.

30. Covey SR. *Principle-centered leadership.* New York: Simon & Schuster; 1990.

31. Goleman D, Boyatzis R, McKee A. *The new leaders: transforming the art of leadership into the science of results.* 2nd ed. London: Little Brown; 2003.

32. Beam RJ, O'Brien RA, Neal M. Reflective practice enhances public health nurse implementation of nurse–family partnership. *Public Health Nursing* 2010;**27**(2):131–9.
33. Bannigan K, Moores A. A model of professional thinking: integrating reflective practice and evidence based practice. *Canadian Journal of Occupational Therapy* 2009;**76**(5):342–50.
34. Rolfe G. Evidence, memory and truth: towards a deconstructive validation of reflective practice. In: Johns C, Freshwater D, editors. *Transforming nursing through reflective practice*. 2nd ed. Oxford, UK: Blackwell; 2005. pp 13–26.
35. Sigma Theta Tau International. The scholarship of reflective practice position paper, 2005. Online. Available: <www.nursingsociety.org/about/resource_reflective.doc> [Viewed 26 December 2006].
36. Taylor B. Identifying and transforming dysfunctional nurse–nurse relationships through reflective practice and action research. *International Journal of Nursing Practice* 2001;**7**:406–11.
37. Kim HS. Critical reflective inquiry for knowledge development in nursing practice. *Journal of Advanced Nursing* 1999;**29**(5):1205–12.
38. Gustafsson C, Fagerberg I. Reflection, the way to professional development? *Journal of Clinical Nursing* 2004;**3**:271–80.
39. Dube V, Ducharme F. Reflective practice among nurses working in a teaching hospital: an action research with promising benefits for professional development. *Journal of Nursing Education and Practice* 2014;**4**:9–19.
40. Peden-McAlpine C, Tomlinson PS, Forneris SG, et al. Evaluation of a reflective practice intervention to enhance family care. *Journal of Advanced Nursing* 2005;**49**:494–501.
41. Renner B, Kimmerle J, Cavael D, Ziegler V, Reinmann L, Cress U. Web-based apps for reflection: a longitudinal study with hospital staff. *Journal of Medical Internet Research* 2014;**16**:e85. doi:10.2196/jmir.3040.
42. Foster K, McAllister M, O'Brien L. Extending the boundaries: autoethnography as an emergent method in mental health nursing research. *International Journal of Mental Health Nursing* 2006;**15**:44–53.
43. Finlay L. 'Outing' the researcher: the provenance, process, and practice of reflexivity. *Qualitative Health Research* 2002;**12**:531–45.
44. Kucera K, Higgins I, McMillan M. Advanced nursing practice: a futures model derived from narrative analysis of nurses' stories. *Australian Journal of Advanced Nursing* 2010;**27**:43–53.
45. Jarrett L, Johns C. Constructing the reflexive narrative. In: Johns C, Freshwater D, editors. *Transforming nursing through reflective practice*. 2nd ed. Oxford, UK: Blackwell; 2005. p 147.
46. McIlveen P. Autoethnography as a method for reflexive research and practice in vocational psychology. *Australian Journal of Career Development* 2008;**17**:13–20.
47. Ellis C. *The ethnographic I: a methodological novel about autoethnography*. Walnut Creek, CA: Altamira Press; 2004.
48. Foster K, McAllister M, O'Brien L. Coming to autoethnography: a mental health nurse's experience. *International Journal of Qualitative Methods* 2005;**4**:Article 1. Online. Available: <www.ualberta.ca/˜ijqm/backissues/4_4/html/foster.pdf> [Viewed 20 January 2006].

CHAPTER 19

Mentoring for new graduates

Stephen Neville and Denise Wilson

INTRODUCTION AND BACKGROUND

The role of student nurse is one of being nurtured and supervised, contrasting with the role of registered nurse, which demands a role reversal to become the nurturer, supervisor and mentor of others. Embarking on this journey to become a full-fledged functioning registered nurse involves opportunities and challenges – some are exciting, others are daunting. Often, making the transition from student to registered nurse occurs within practice environments that are busy and complex, with minimal support readily available. Mentoring as a new graduate can be overwhelming, especially when the demands of the practice environment encroach, a crisis of confidence ensues and an all-consuming desire to continue being nurtured surfaces.

The role and responsibilities of being a registered nurse include mentoring other nurses and health professionals, such as health and nursing assistants – it is a role that cannot be escaped. It is useful to have some knowledge about mentoring and developing strategies and processes to assist in undertaking this role, although time and experience will enrich knowledge and skills around mentoring. Nevertheless, new registered nurses who are mentoring more junior staff cannot realistically be expected to know everything. In this chapter, we stress the importance of mentoring in nursing and explain the differences between mentoring, preceptoring and clinical supervision. Various approaches to mentoring are described, and the skills and attributes necessary for successful mentoring are outlined, so that as a new registered nurse you will feel better prepared to participate in a mentoring relationship. We begin by exploring the reality of making the transition from student to registered nurse.

THE TRANSITION TO PRACTICE

The transition from student nurse to registered nurse is a time of great anticipation and excitement, but it is also one that is rather scary as the notion of autonomous practice becomes a reality. It is also a time of being faced with self-doubt and questions about our readiness: Do I have the necessary abilities and capabilities to be a registered nurse? What will others expect of me? Will I be able to do what is expected of me? How will I be able to juggle a full patient load? How will I manage emergencies? Will I get the help that I need when I need it? Will people treat me kindly? Will other nurses recognise my need for help? How will I mentor and support others while I am learning? It is usual to question your ability, readiness and fitness to practise and to do what is expected without the protection associated with student status. This conflicting concoction of feelings and emotions is quite normal, as at last the doing, thinking and being a nurse become a reality.

The process of becoming a professional registered nurse is influenced by a number of contextual factors in the workplace that include the expectations of self and others, the perception of status by others, being accepted, and being assisted and advocated for by others. Unfortunately, the practice reality is not always as it should be. Socialisation into the profession may not be a smooth path, and can be a stressful time as the experience of being a student differs markedly from the role of being a registered nurse.[1] During the transition to practice, the experience is discernible by any or all of the following:

- the effort of being a professional functioning registered nurse
- a practice environment that is busy, complex and unpredictable, making it difficult to reflect and learn from experiences as the new registered nurse aims to get from the beginning to the end of the shift
- unrealistic workloads to manage with little support
- working with less than helpful colleagues who at times may seem obstructive – this is often described as lateral or horizontal violence[2]
- the dissonance that occurs with trying to apply theoretical knowledge and skills to practice reality
- an inability to use acquired knowledge and evidence because of the barriers created by any of the above points
- not having beginning status recognised, as evident by the unrealistic expectation that new registered nurses 'hit the floor running' and function to the level of experienced registered nurses
- the expectation to mentor another registered nurse, enrolled nurse or healthcare assistant without the necessary knowledge, experience or mentorship.

Research into lateral or horizontal violence in nursing has identified that this phenomenon is manifest in the form of bullying behaviours, being undermined, intimidating behaviours, whether verbal or non-verbal, and withholding information.[2] All of these factors are a source of stress and anxiety experienced by many new registered nurses that may result in not achieving one's own practice expectations, especially when factors outside your control contribute to an inability to make appropriate choices and sound decisions. Although conflict is inevitable when working with people, if ongoing and unresolved it can lead to horizontal violence resulting in increased stress levels and negatively impacting on health and wellbeing.[3] Moral distress is an example of the stresses that may occur, especially when a conflict with personal values is experienced in some situations that can lead to a plethora of negative feelings and behaviours if not managed.[4] This is an example of a situation where a mentor can assist to explore sources of moral distress or conflict and develop strategies to help move forward, particularly when required to mentor others.

The self-confidence and self-worth of beginning registered nurses are potentially fragile, and are at risk in response to some practice situations. Understanding your self-concept is important for job satisfaction and managing the stresses experienced from being a new registered nurse.[5] Angel, Craven and Denson[6] claim the following dimensions assist in understanding one's self-concept: nurse general self-concept, care, staff relations, communication, knowledge and leadership. Such self-reflection can be difficult when adapting to a new environment, learning a new role and functioning in a practice setting, especially when at times it is difficult to ascertain what is right and wrong. Participating in the mentoring process has the potential to support newly registered nurses through difficult situations. In addition, mentoring can assist with the identification of individual developmental needs as a newly graduated nurse, and is especially important when you are required to mentor others in clinical practice.

With the reality of becoming a registered nurse, the illusion of safety and security experienced as a student nurse increasingly fades. An expectation of being a registered nurse includes the requirement to mentor and supervise health assistants, enrolled nurses and other registered nurses. Despite having registered nurse status, mentoring involves yet another new journey as a 'beginning' registered nurse. Mentoring requires confidence that comes with experience and developing professional practice, yet the practice environment does not always afford this luxury. Understanding the acquirement of practice experience and wisdom can be helpful.

It is important to remember that, as a new registered nurse, the preparation you have undergone as a student nurse leads you to the status of beginning registered nurse, not an experienced one, despite the expectations of others within the workplace. This is an important reality to remember when the expectations from yourself, your colleagues, and/or patients and their families are beyond what seems to be fair and reasonable. Recognising your beginning status and not being afraid to ask questions are not always luxuries afforded to beginning practitioners. This is when having an experienced, respected registered nurse with wisdom and expertise to assist you in the mentoring role is helpful. Positive outcomes of mentoring for the mentor include: the development of collegial relationships, networking, sharing of ideas, reflection, personal fulfilment and growth; and for the mentee: support, understanding, encouragement, analysis and friendship.[7] The transition to registered nurse status can be a daunting prospect, especially when required to mentor. However, the value of mentoring others cannot be underestimated, especially the contribution it can make to improving client outcomes.[8]

EXERCISE 19.1

Think about being a mentor. Fold a piece of paper into quarters. In each quarter write the following headings:

1. Expectations I have of myself
2. Expectations others may have of me (such as other registered nurses, patients, patients' families, doctors, other health professionals)
3. My readiness to be a mentor and the supports I have in place
4. My fears about being a mentor.

Identify the strengths that you have to support your development as a mentor, and the areas for development.

Undertaking this exercise may help you to develop some of the skills and attributes necessary to participate in a mentoring role successfully, and to identify your future learning needs regarding being a mentor.

WHAT IS 'MENTORING'?

Even though the term *mentoring* has been in use for a considerable period of time, it remains difficult to define. For example, in nursing there appears to be some confusion regarding the difference between mentorship, preceptorship and clinical supervision. While there are some similarities between the three concepts, the differences are important and should therefore be teased out to ensure they are better understood.

A preceptor is someone who is well versed in the skills and attitudes needed to be clinically successful, as well as being esteemed as an expert practitioner. A preceptor is frequently involved in teaching a preceptee new or different clinical skills, usually within a structure focused on meeting specific learning objectives within a specified period of time.[9] The preceptor–preceptee model is frequently utilised to foster student learning in undergraduate nursing programs, enrolled nurses and other healthcare personnel (healthcare assistants) new to working in a particular healthcare organisation, as well as new graduates as they transition from student to registered nurse.

The preceptor–preceptee relationship not only offers a supportive role for those facing the challenges associated with providing a healthcare service, but also protects the general public from relatively inexperienced new practitioners. Formal evaluation of the preceptored person's performance is frequently a component associated with the preceptor role to ensure that preceptees have the appropriate knowledge and skills to be safe to practise. Therefore, preceptorship is both pragmatic and functional and can best be described as providing transitional support.[9]

Within nursing, the concept of clinical supervision has largely been associated with mental health nurses for some time now.[10] Clinical supervision has been defined as regular, protected time for facilitated, in-depth reflection on clinical practice.[11,12] The aims of clinical supervision include enabling the supervisee to achieve, sustain and continue to develop high-quality practice. Clinical supervision may include aspects of both mentoring and preceptorship at differing times, but is largely based on the specific encounters that take place between the nurse and the client or the nurse and co-workers. It is the encounter or interaction that is the focus of the supervisory session.

Butterworth and colleagues,[13] who are key writers on clinical supervision and mentoring, differentiate clinical supervision from mentoring by identifying mentoring as 'an experienced professional nurturing and guiding the novitiate', and clinical supervision as 'an exchange between practising professionals to enable the development of professional skills' (p 12). At the same time, a mentor relationship differs from preceptorship in that there is no formal evaluation process involved in the mentor–mentee relationship. Because of the similarities between preceptorship, clinical supervision and mentoring, it appears there is no one, definitive, definition of mentoring.

The concept of mentoring can be traced back to Ancient Greek times. The traditional term *mentor* has its origins in the Ancient Greek classic, Homer's *Odyssey*. In this story, Odysseus, who is about to fight in the Trojan War, asks Mentor, his best friend, to tutor and care for his son Telemachus. Mentor subsequently becomes Telemachus's trusted counsellor, advisor and friend, teaching him about life and the world as he transitions into adulthood. In keeping with Greek mythology, mentoring relationships continued to be utilised in academic institutions such as universities. Here, postgraduate students were attached to a more senior and wise person, whose role was to support and guide their academic development.

Both of the above examples identify that a mentor is an older, trusted and wiser person who protects and encourages a younger person in a relationship that occurs over a period of time. In contemporary nursing practice, mentoring can be defined as an enduring relationship where an experienced practitioner acts as an advisor for a less experienced practitioner to assist with the development of their clinical knowledge and skills.[14] Due to the nature of their relationship, both the mentor and mentee share in the personal, as well as professional, growth and development that occur as a consequence of this relationship and subsequent interactions.[7]

HOW MENTORING BENEFITS NURSING PRACTICE

Mentorship has many benefits that not only positively influence nursing practice but also have an impact on today's healthcare market. Mariani[15] identifies mentoring as necessary to support career development and career satisfaction for any registered nurse, whether newly registered or experienced. It has also been suggested that healthcare organisations should implement mentoring programs as a means of enhancing nursing satisfaction and the retention of staff, as well as positively impacting on patient health outcomes.[16] Successful mentorship can improve corporate knowledge within an organisation and make employees feel valued, as well as forming the foundations for the development of future nurse leaders.[15]

Characteristics of Mentors/Mentees

Although not essential, a mentor is usually someone who has professional and/or academic standing within his or her field who may or may not be a nurse. As nursing evolves and recognises its full potential, more nurses are now willing to become mentors and more nurses seeking mentorship choose nurses to fulfil this important role. However, the mentor–mentee relationship is both dynamic and dyadic. Not only do mentees seek support and guidance from a mentor, but equally mentors actively seek nurses to mentor. Barker[17] claims that often mentors seek potential protégés to mentor, those who may progress the nursing profession forward, change practice and ultimately improve health outcomes.

EXERCISE 19.2

Do you consider that you:

- are intelligent?
- are motivated?
- are articulate, with good communication and interpersonal skills?
- are not afraid to work hard or take risks?
- are open to new ways of doing things and seeing the world?
- have integrity and are trustworthy?
- have good professional presentation skills?
- are willing to invest in your career?
- are curious by nature?
- have vision both for yourself and for nursing?

(Adapted from Grossman and Valiga[18])

If you answer 'yes' to all of the above, then you have the qualities necessary to enter a mentoring relationship either as a mentor or a mentee.

MENTORING APPROACHES

Mentor relationships revolve around supporting, coaching, listening, challenging and encouraging the mentee, whether the relationship between the mentee and mentor is formal or informal.[19] Having an understanding of the mentoring approaches that can be used to model and develop relationships is useful. Mentoring can vary from country to country, and there are a number of approaches that can range from the more traditional concept of mentoring that is considered informal, to the structured and formalised approach. A structured or formalised approach, however, is often limited as it tends to be based on an organisation's interest in improving quality, practice outcomes for clients or the retention of staff, rather than on the nurse's or health worker's personal developmental needs.

Informal mentoring is a reciprocal and relational process that occurs naturally, where two people are attracted and develop a relationship based on mutual respect and positive role modelling by the mentor, and where both have a commitment to nurturing and mutual sharing.[20] At times, the mentoring relationship is not recognised as such, due to its unstructured nature and the development of friendships over time. Many nurses and health workers have been informally mentored by someone who is an expert whom they have professionally admired and respected as a representation of how they would like to practise. They themselves have generally been mentored by someone they have admired, who has nurtured, supported, challenged and encouraged them in their practice development. However, it should be noted that, without some structure and infrastructure for the mentoring relationship, the process of mentoring may lack focus and direction.

Formal approaches to mentoring, however, differ in intention, the context in which the mentoring relationship occurs, the duration of the relationship and the outcomes expected of the mentoring process, including the retention of staff.[21] Formal mentoring programs are either a requirement or available, depending upon the organisation's culture and aim. They are distinguishable by their structured nature and the purposeful assigning of mentee to mentor,[22] and may or may not differentiate between areas of practice. Also evident in formal approaches to mentoring is the selection of volunteers deemed appropriate to undertake training and the role of mentoring, and evaluation of the effectiveness of the program in some way.[22] Specific groups of healthcare workers are frequently targeted for mentoring of some type. For example, new graduate programs for newly registered nurses may be an example of a formalised mentoring program, where mentoring is a component of the program.

There are a number of models for mentoring.[23] The following is an overview of a selection of mentoring models.

One-to-one Mentoring

One-to-one mentoring may take one of the following forms:

- *Traditional* – characterised by a mentor–mentee relationship that is usually based on the expert mentoring of the novice.
- *Pair mentoring* – there is a horizontal relationship between the mentee and the mentor where the mentoring relationship is predicated on sharing expertise. This type of relationship values the often current knowledge and skills that the mentee brings to the practice setting, but may not be valued by others.
- *Mentoring forward* – in this model there is a vertical relationship where the mentee is mentored, and a horizontal relationship where the mentee passes on the knowledge and skills learnt from the mentoring relationship to another mentee. In this model, the mentee is also learning to become a mentor.

Cluster Mentoring

Cluster mentoring may take one of the following forms:

- *Team mentoring* – there are generally a number of mentors who are experts for a mentee, and they usually function in a vertical relationship. An example of this would be the learning of independent practice, such as community nursing, where the registered nurse needs to acquire diverse knowledge and skills that may span across specialty areas and disciplines.

- *Inclusion mentoring* – in contrast to team mentoring, inclusion mentoring involves one expert mentor for several mentees, and the mentoring activities are shared. Notably with this model, relationships may not be key.
- *Group mentoring* – this type of mentoring involves a group of like-minded people getting together to discuss their work situations. This type of approach may be helpful for new registered nurses who can share like experiences and problem solve how to manage future situations. However, the disadvantage of this approach for new registered nurses is that sometimes you 'don't know what you don't know'; you are still learning the networks and how to access sources of expertise and resources.

Distance Mentoring

This approach occurs when meeting face-to-face is difficult. Mentoring occurs via telephone, email or, more recently, using videocams on personal computers. This approach requires clear goals and sound communication skills, as it has been reported to be difficult to maintain using telephone or email.[23]

CONSIDERATIONS FOR MENTORING

Prior to embarking on an organisational mentoring program you should consider the following aspects:[7]

1. *Choice* – what choices do you have within the mentoring context offered? Are you able to choose your mentee? Do you have the freedom to meet when desired?
2. *Relationships* – is the mentoring relationship based on collegiality? Is it discipline-specific, aimed at improving professional networks and relationships, and gaining knowledge about the various structures within which you have worked?
3. *Structure* – what does the mentoring experience promote and facilitate? For example, will it enhance your networks, or ethical practice? Does it function to develop professional practice, or psychosocial aspects of practice, or both?
4. *Resources* – does the organisational culture value and promote mentoring?

No matter what type or model of mentoring you engage in, the nature of the relationship you have with your mentee and the quality of communication are crucial to its success. Successful mentoring is a reciprocal process that relies on the mentee being self-motivated and using initiative to engage in the process actively, and is important to remember when working with a mentee. The old saying that 'you get out what you put in' holds true for most mentoring relationships. If you are opting for an informal mentoring process, or have the choice of mentee in a formal mentoring program, selecting a mentee whom you respect and can relate to is vital for its success. Mentees will also be looking for a role model, someone they respect and who possesses knowledge of nursing and health practice, possibly in your specialty area of practice, who is sensitive to their needs.

In the situation where an employing organisation arranges a mentoring relationship, and a mentee is assigned, you need to ask yourself: 'Am I the best person for this role?' There is no doubt that participating in a mentoring relationship will personally influence both parties in relation to achieving career aspirations as a registered nurse, as well as positively influencing practice and professional development. Having an overview of approaches to mentoring will enable you to explore how to begin a mentoring relationship.

OPERATIONALISING THE MENTORING PROCESS

As a new graduate, you may find yourself in the position of intentionally or unintentionally being a mentor to other nurses and/or healthcare assistants. It is therefore essential that you prepare yourself to undertake this role. You may have formally or informally participated in mentoring programs either as a mentor or a mentee, or as both. However, the realities of contemporary clinical practice may mean that you bring to the mentor–mentee relationship little experience of either of these processes. Exercise 19.2, earlier, identified that you have the qualities to mentor another person. It is important to realise that your work as a mentor sits alongside your role as a registered nurse, a role that is responsible for the provision of a safe and appropriate healthcare experience to consumers of that service. Now complete Exercise 19.3, which will help you to assess your capacity to become a mentor.

EXERCISE 19.3

Make a list of the knowledge, skills and attributes you think you need to be a good mentor. Then compare your list with the one in Table 19.1. You could use this list to assess the effectiveness of your mentor during your final placement, and to assess your capacity to become a mentor.

How does a nurse become a mentor? The first step in the process is to be willing to undertake this role. Once you have decided to commit yourself to being a mentor, you then need to look out for someone who might benefit from your knowledge and skills no matter how vast or limited. You might choose a person who is new to the area where you work; or, as identified earlier, you may be formally assigned someone to mentor by your employing organisation.

As previously discussed, a definitive definition of mentoring is hard to provide. However, the essential characteristics associated with being a good mentor have been identified (Table 19.1).

Getting Started

Agreeing on and formalising a mentoring agreement is the first place to start in the mentoring process. When establishing a mentoring relationship or agreement with a mentee it is important to discuss and explore how the individuals involved anticipate the relationship will work. Formalising the mentor–mentee relationship through the utilisation of an official agreement protects both parties by potentially preventing situations from occurring where either person may feel his or her expectations are not being met. Find out if your employing organisation has an existing mentoring agreement template that you could utilise. If not, the areas to be considered when

TABLE 19.1

Essential characteristics for mentoring

Characteristic	Description
Envisioner	Gives the mentee a picture of what nursing can be like
Energiser	Is dynamic, positive and enthusiastic
Investor	Invests time and energy in the mentee
Supporter	Supports the mentee through the highs and lows of providing a healthcare service
Prodder	Pushes the mentee to achieve/provide the highest standards of professional development and care
Challenger	Opens the mentee's eyes to other possibilities and encourages critical thinking
Connections maker	Opens doors and introduces mentees to people of influence
Career counsellor	Supports and encourages the mentee to develop and work towards future career aspirations and goals

establishing a mentoring relationship and agreement should include, but are by no means limited to, the following:

- name and preferred contact details of both the mentor and mentee, including preferred postal address, mobile phone number and email address
- the frequency, venue and length of each meeting, as well as how the meetings will take place – for example, whether they will be face-to-face, or by email, chat room, videocam or phone
- a mechanism for contacting each other outside the scheduled meetings in case any issue arises that demands immediate attention
- the focus of the mentoring relationship – for example, whether it will focus on clinical practice or career development, or a combination of the two – plus a well-defined timeframe
- a statement relating to the confidentiality of any communication between the mentor and mentee
- a review date, with the review to encompass both the relationship and the process.

As this is a formal mentoring agreement, both mentor and mentee should sign and date the document.

EXERCISE 19.4

Critique the above list of suggested items that could be included in a mentoring agreement. Do you agree with the points above? Are there any more you would like to add?

Building and Developing the Mentoring Relationship

All mentors need to be able to use effective verbal and non-verbal therapeutic communication skills to ensure that they are effective in their role. All new graduates understand and utilise therapeutic communication skills, which formed the foundation of their nursing degree program, as being integral to any interactions between them as registered nurses and consumers of their health service. These verbal and non-verbal therapeutic communication skills can also be utilised throughout all mentoring interactions.

Integral to the mentoring relationship is mastering the skills necessary to build, develop and maintain a positive mentor–mentee relationship, fundamentally based on trust.[21] Although all nurses are familiar with developing these types of relationships with consumers of health services as well as their colleagues, it may be challenging in a mentor–mentee relationship. It is important that the mentor is honest with the mentee and acknowledges any feelings of nervousness about working closely with that person, in addition to any thoughts or feelings of needing to know more than the mentee, as part of the relationship. Acknowledging these thoughts and feelings will only assist with the development of trust and ensuring the success of the process for both parties.

Due to the globalisation of the nursing workforce, nurses are a multicultural entity. Not only do mentors need to communicate ensuring verbal clarity, and attending to non-verbal cues, including physical actions; it is also imperative to ensure that any interactions and interpretations between both parties are cognisant of cultural variations. Consequently, mentors need to have good communication skills, and be accessible, approachable and intuitive,[24] to ensure there is no room for misinterpretation when working with mentees from different cultural and ethnic backgrounds. All mentors should therefore communicate clearly, while carefully observing the impact the information given has on the mentee.

A particularly useful and powerful strategy for beginning the mentor–mentee relationship is encouraging the mentee to set goals. Yoder-Wise[25] identifies that the setting of long-term goals may be difficult to formulate when nurses have just begun their career. However, the setting of short- and medium-term goals will greatly assist the mentor to get to know the mentee, and additionally helps with providing structure and direction to the process.

What to Do When the Mentoring Relationship Strikes Trouble

As previously discussed, the setting of goals along with timelines is important for ensuring the success of the mentor–mentee relationship. Research studies have identified that lack of commitment and time, poor preparation of both mentor and mentee, and organisational constraints were all significant issues that contributed to the breakdown in the mentor–mentee relationship.[26,27] Due to these issues the relationship between the two parties can drift apart, with contact becoming less frequent to the point where the mentoring process ceases to exist. This situation can be both hurtful and discouraging for all concerned, with both individuals left wondering what they did wrong.

Earlier in the chapter it was suggested that, as part of the contractual arrangement between mentor and mentee, a review process is undertaken to ensure that each participant's needs are being met. In situations where there has been a breakdown in the mentor and mentee relationship, an external third party may be needed to act as a mediator to resolve any issues – ideally, such a provision should be negotiated during the contractual process. However, any potential and actual problems with the mentoring relationship should be highlighted and addressed early. An integral part of any mentoring session should include opportunities for both parties to check in with each other and acknowledge the strengths and issues that relate to the mentor–mentee relationship. Although this may be difficult to do, all nurses, as part of their education, have been taught the skills of managing conflict within professional relationships. It is important to acknowledge the possibility that one or other of the parties may wish to discontinue the relationship, and to understand from the outset that this is achievable and could be part of the process. Discussions about possible termination of the relationship should occur well in advance, preferably at the very beginning of the process. A useful time for this to happen would be when the guidelines and contract are discussed and agreed on.

Another issue that may have a negative impact on the mentoring relationship relates to confidentiality and how ethical dilemmas are to be managed. The literature recommends that guidelines should be incorporated into the contract to help manage and address instances where the mentee discloses unsafe and/or unprofessional practice.[13] Familiarity with relevant legislation or regulation (such as the *Health Practitioners' Competency Assurance Act* in New Zealand, or the *Health Practitioner Regulation National Law (Victoria) Act 2009* in Australia) is crucial as it outlines the legal obligations with regard to unsafe or incompetent practice. Inherent in, and underpinning, the mentoring relationship is the professional development of the mentee.

Challenges for the mentor therefore include deciding what issues disclosed in confidence are breaches of the law and/or the code of conduct associated with being a health worker and those where no harm has occurred but significant professional development has taken place. Ideally, when beginning a mentor relationship, limits to confidentiality should be made clear. For instance, when patients' safety is compromised by unsafe practice, such as working outside the registered nurse scope of practice, or incidents of incompetence such as making errors in drug calculations, there is a legal obligation to report such incidents so that remedial action can be instituted as soon as possible.

EXERCISE 19.5

Take time to conceptualise and then identify how you would manage moral and ethical dilemmas[28] that may arise as part of the mentoring process.

SUPPORT FOR MENTORS

Just as mentees need support and guidance from mentors, the reverse is also true. Successfully undertaking the role of mentor does not occur within a vacuum; it requires considerable financial investment on the part of the employing organisation, as well as a personal investment on the part of both mentor and mentee. Any financial investment by the organisation may not materialise as compensation to the mentor directly, but should at least include either clinical supervision or mentoring for the mentor, or both.

If formal support structures, such as clinical supervision or mentoring for the mentor, are not offered, self-mentoring could be considered.[29] Self-mentoring requires that nurses, as a starting point, be self-reliant, believe in themselves, be innately reflective and have the confidence to ask questions. Many of these skills are fostered and encouraged in undergraduate nursing programs. Although not ideal, self-mentoring could be used to 'plug a gap' until appropriate resources and/or people are available to support the mentor formally.

EXERCISE 19.6

Identify and list things that are important for your own personal, professional and clinical practice development as a nurse. For example, your list may include items that relate to being:

- a newly registered nurse
- in the position of mentoring another nurse or healthcare assistant.

From this list, write personal, professional and clinical practice development goals. For example:

- *Undertake clinical supervision in relation to mentorship development*, or
- *Complete a beginning registered nurse professional portfolio by the end of my first year of practice.*

These goals will form the basis of your future clinical supervision and/or mentoring needs.

CONCLUSION

The process of becoming a confident and professional registered nurse occurs within an often-chaotic practice environment. It is a process of moving from practising in an 'adequate' manner to becoming more confident and competent, to feeling able to contribute to the advancement of nursing. The requirement to be a mentor to others occurs during this process. Often new registered nurses may feel inadequate to assume and undertake this important role. However, having knowledge about mentoring and its various approaches can provide the basis for developing the skills and attributes to be a positive mentor.

The mentor–mentee relationship is dynamic and dyadic, and is based on the characteristics required of all registered nurses – that is, trust, effective verbal and non-verbal communication, and the ability to share information and support development. A positive mentoring relationship contributes to improvements in practice, and ultimately to health outcomes. Mentoring others can be a source of personal and professional satisfaction, derived from seeing others grow professionally in their practice. Informal mentoring approaches bring the added bonus of the development of long-term friendships that can be an ongoing source of support.

CASE STUDY 19.1

Rosie is excited to be a new registered nurse and has been assigned a mentor, Lilly, by the nurse manager in the area. Lilly is an experienced registered nurse and is enthusiastic about nursing and patient care. While Lilly has been excellent at introducing Rosie to various people of relative importance and modelling networking behaviour, Rosie is really committed to improving the standard of her nursing practice and being exposed to challenging questions to make her think critically about various aspects of her practice. She suddenly realises she should have talked to the nurse manager about her needs earlier when she had the opportunity.

REFLECTIVE QUESTIONS

1. What strategies could Rosie use to ensure that her mentoring needs are met by Lilly?
2. Why should Rosie have determined the characteristics needed in a mentor and her mentoring needs before getting into a situation where a mentor is assigned for her?
3. Who could Rosie have talked to about her mentoring needs?

CASE STUDY 19.2

Craig is a newly registered nurse who is working in an assessment, treatment and rehabilitation ward in a large metropolitan hospital. He is being mentored by a very experienced registered nurse and is very happy with the mentoring he has received. Two enrolled nurses have just been employed to work on the ward and Craig has been asked to mentor one of these people.

REFLECTIVE QUESTIONS

1. How should Craig prepare for his new role as mentor?
2. How should he now use his time with his mentor?

CASE STUDY 19.3

Cassie is new to her clinical area, which is a busy surgical ward in a medium-sized acute hospital in a small city where most people know each other. Cassie has been assigned a mentor who was reluctant to take on the role. They have been meeting irregularly and, when they have met, the mentor constantly complains about how busy she is and consequently rushes the arranged sessions. Cassie feels unsupported and dissatisfied, and would like to be mentored by a different registered nurse.

REFLECTIVE QUESTION

What steps should Cassie take to address her feelings of being unsupported and dissatisfied, taking into consideration that she is a newly registered nurse who is new to the clinical area and part of a small well-connected community, and is at risk of being isolated if she speaks out?

RECOMMENDED READING

Cross W, Moore A, Ockerby S. Clinical supervision of general nurses in a busy medical ward of a teaching hospital. *Contemporary Nurse* 2010;**35**:245–53.

Ferguson L. From the perspective of new nurses: what do effective mentors look like in practice?. *Nurse Education in Practice* 2011;**11**:119 23.

Grossman S. *Mentoring in nursing: a dynamic and collaborative process.* 2nd ed. New York: Springer Publishing Company; 2013.

Phillips J. Helping community-based students on a final consolidation placement make the transition to registered practice. *British Journal of Community Nursing* 2014;**19**(7):352–6.

Siu GP, Sivan A. Mentoring experiences of psychiatric nurses: from acquaintance to affirmation. *Nurse Education Today* 2011;**31**:797–802.

REFERENCES

1. Teoh Y, Pua L, Chan M. Review: Lost in transition – a review of qualitative literature of transition shock: the initial stage of newly qualified registered nurses' experiences in their transition to practice journey. *Nurse Education Today* 2012;**33**(2):143–7.

2. Lachman V. Ethical issues in the disruptive behaviors of incivility, bullying and horizontal/lateral violence. *Medsurg Nursing* 2014;**23**(1):56–60.

3. King-Jones M. Horizontal violence and the socialization of new nurses. *Creative Nursing* 2011;**17**(2):80–6.

4. Woods M, Rodgers V, Towers A, LaGrow S. Researching moral distress among New Zealand nurses: a national survey. *Nursing Ethics* 2014. doi:10.1177/0969733014542679.

5. Jahanbin I, Badiyepeyma Z, Sharif F. The impact of teaching professional self-concept on clinical performance perception in nursing students. *Life Science Journal* 2012; **9**(4):653–9.

6. Angel E, Craven R, Denson N. The nurses' self-concept instrument (NSCI): a comparison of domestic and international student nurses' professional self-concepts from a large Australian university. *Nurse Education Today* 2012;**32**:636–40.

7. Grossman S. *Mentoring in nursing: a dynamic and collaborative process.* 2nd ed. New York: Springer Publishing Company; 2013.

8. Funderburk A. Mentoring: the retention factor in the acute care setting. *Journal of Nursing Staff Development* 2008;**24**:1–5.

9. McCusker C. Preceptorship: professional development and support for newly registered practitioners. *Journal of Perioperative Practice* 2013;**23**(12):283–7.

10. White E, Winstanley J. A randomised controlled trial of clinical supervision: selected findings from a novel Australian attempt to establish the evidence base for causal relationships with quality of care and patient outcomes, as an informed contribution to mental health nursing practice development. *Journal of Research in Nursing* 2010;**15**(2):151–67.

11. Cross W, Moore A, Ockerby S. Clinical supervision of general nurses in a busy medical ward of a teaching hospital. *Contemporary Nurse* 2010;**35**:245–53.

12. Bond M, Holland S. *Skills of clinical supervision for nurses: a practical guide for supervisees, clinical supervisors and managers.* 2nd ed. Maidenhead, UK: Open University Press; 2010.

13. Butterworth T, Faugier J, Burnard P. *Clinical supervision and mentorship in nursing.* 2nd ed. Cheltenham, UK: Stanley Thornes; 1998.

14. Botma Y, Hurter S, Kotze R. Responsibilities of nursing schools with regard to peer mentoring. *Nurse Education Today* 2012;**33**:808–13.

15. Mariani B. The effect of mentoring on career satisfaction of registered nurses and intent to stay in the nursing profession. *Nursing Research and Practice* 2012. doi:10.1155/2012/168278.

16. Huybrecht S, Loeckx W, Quaeyhaegens Y, et al. Mentoring in nursing education: perceived characteristics of mentors and the consequences of mentorship. *Nurse Education Today* 2011;**31**:274–8.

17. Barker E. Mentoring – a complex relationship. *Journal of the American Academy of Nurse Practitioners* 2006;**18**:56–61.

18. Grossman S, Valiga T. *The new leadership challenge: creating the future of nursing.* 4th ed. Philadelphia: F.A. Davis; 2013.

19. Donner G, Wheeler M. *Taking control of your nursing career: a handbook for health professionals.* Canada: Mosby; 2009.

20. Ryan A, Goldberg L, Evans J. Wise women: mentoring as relational learning in perinatal nursing practice. *Journal of Clinical Nursing* 2010;**19**:183–91.

21. Ferguson L. From the perspective of new nurses: What do effective mentors look like in practice? *Nurse Education in Practice* 2011;**11**:119–23.

22. Phillips J. Helping community-based students on a final consolidation placement make the transition to registered practice. *British Journal of Community Nursing* 2014;**19**(7):352–6.

23. Heartfield M, Gibson T. Mentoring for nurses in general practice: national issues and challenges. *Collegian (Royal College of Nursing, Australia)* 2005;**12**:17–21.

24. Siu GP, Sivan A. Mentoring experiences of psychiatric nurses: from acquaintance to affirmation. *Nurse Education Today* 2011;**31**:797–802.

25. Yoder-Wise P. *Leading and managing in nursing.* 5th ed. St Louis, MO: Mosby; 2011.

26. Beecroft P, Santner S, Lacy M, et al. New graduate nurses' perceptions of mentoring: six-year programme evaluation. *Journal of Advanced Nursing* 2006;**55**:736–47.

27. Gilmour J, Kopeikin A, Douche J. Student nurses as peer-mentors: collegiality in practice. *Nurse Education in Practice* 2007;**7**:36–43.

28. Butts J, Rich K. *Nursing ethics across the curriculum and into practice.* 3rd ed. Burlington, MA: Jones & Bartlett Learning; 2013.

29. Cherry B, Jacob S. *Contemporary nursing: issues, trends and management.* 6th ed. Philadelphia: Mosby; 2014.

CHAPTER 20

Professional career development: development of the CAPABLE nursing professional

Jane Conway and Margaret McMillan

LEARNING OBJECTIVES

When you have completed this chapter you will be able to:

- differentiate between professional career development and career progression
- identify factors that result in changing career development opportunities for nurses
- apply the CAPABLE framework to thinking about your professional career development
- identify interrelationships among professional career development, reflective practice and lifelong learning
- identify a range of strategies for career development.

KEYWORDS: career, capability, lifelong learning, career pathway, role transition

INTRODUCTION

This chapter explores the concept of professional career development in nursing. It identifies the need to view professional career development as uniquely personal yet aligned to the directions of the nursing profession and responsive to community and organisational expectations. The chapter introduces the CAPABLE framework in order to assist those in transition to examine, reflect upon and validate their professional careers. The framework has been derived from key concepts related to career development in nursing and other literature.

DEFINING PROFESSIONAL CAREER DEVELOPMENT

A career can be defined as the lifelong process of aligning individual interests and the opportunities (or limitations) present in the external work-related environment, in order to meet both individual and environmental needs.[1] Although a single career can involve multiple work roles and positions in numerous organisations,[2] developing and self-managing a career is proposed to be closely linked to 'the adaptive, process behaviors to which it can be applied (e.g. career decision making/exploration, job searching, career advancement, negotiation of work transitions and multiple roles)'.[3]

Career planning is the process through which individuals evaluate the opportunities that exist, determine their career goals, and take advantage of employment experience, education and other developmental opportunities that will help them reach these goals.[4] Career progression involves developing through a frequently hierarchical career pathway where each new position is viewed as having greater responsibility, authority and remuneration. Historically, measures of success in a career have often valued extrinsic factors such as status, remuneration and opportunity for further promotion.[5] Career progression can be one outcome of career development. However, career development is a much broader process than achieving career progression. Career development is directed to meeting subjective as well as objective determinants of success and satisfaction. It is the process of managing life, learning and work over the lifespan and involves life planning, career exploration, career building and skill building.[6]

The view of a career as a contract between employer and employee, which is based on long-term mutual commitment and establishment of a profound relationship within which there are well-defined opportunities for hierarchical promotion, is increasingly being superseded by the view of a career as a series of shorter-term interactions between employers and employees based on exchange of services and benefits. Reasons for this include increased mobility in the workforce, increasing flexibility in patterns of work, flattened organisational structures and differing expectations among generations of workers.[7] There has been significant change in the nature of work in the 21st century,[8] with changes in the availability, distribution, retention and work patterns of workers in all industries[9] including nursing and other health professions.[10]

In addition to this global change, there has been a marked change within nursing from the model of the 1950s, in which nurses' practices were directed largely within a medically dominated paradigm, to contemporary times which have seen advancement in the roles nurses can fulfil as a result of reforms in policy, practice and education.[11] Nursing is also increasingly governed by nurses. Within a healthcare workforce that is increasingly multi- and interprofessional,[12] nursing remains informed by other disciplines but is transmitted and co-created through a range of strategies framed by a consciousness of the uniqueness of the knowledge, skills and attitudes that constitute the practice of nursing. Over the last century, nursing has continued to emerge as a profession with a philosophical and conceptual basis that emphasises nursing as a unique discipline distinguished from others[13] increasingly as a result of its focus on relationship-based care, creative inquiry and leadership.[14]

New nursing career paths and roles have emerged and evolved. 'Today, virtually every professional nurse leads, manages and follows, regardless of title or position.'[15] These new career paths and roles place emphasis on professional achievements which are inclusive of, but not limited to, educational achievements. Moreover, the dominant concept of professional career development as progression up a career ladder with hierarchical promotion, which pervades male-dominated conceptions of career development, has to coexist with more contemporary thinking which identifies professional career development, particularly for women, as fluid, zig-zag, up and down, and at times static. There is increasing emphasis placed on acknowledging the desire for work–life balance and wellbeing as part of career planning, as well as recognition that workplaces and employees are altering patterns of work to include casual, part-time and contracted work arrangements.[16] Those engaged in research related to the careers of nurses have also noted continued attention to the career trajectories of men in what continues to be a female-dominated profession.[17,18] Professional career development for new and experienced nurses is directly linked to the maintenance of high-quality care delivery. Quality care and sustainable career development are integral to health workforce development, and must be supported and sustained through educational systems and processes, career structures, and pathways that are aligned to organisational need yet are sufficiently flexible and responsive to accommodate individual goals, aspirations and circumstances. There is a need to examine the extent to which both career development and progression foster fitness for purpose within an environment of changed, and continuously changing, expectations of nurses and nursing.[19]

The outcomes of professional career development vary for individual nurses at different points in their careers; however, collectively, professional development results in enhanced capacity, competence, confidence and cohesion of nurses within the health workforce. There is acknowledgment that career opportunities are shaped at least as much by personal aspirations, expectations and confidence as they are by factors such as economics, employment opportunities and societal views about the interdependence among employers and employees.[20] A confident, competent nursing workforce that has the capacity to provide comprehensive, person-centred care and is part of a cohesive, interprofessional healthcare team is dependent upon the professional career development opportunities undertaken by nurses. In writing this chapter, we have concluded that the chapter should focus on presenting a framework for professional development that can be used to guide transition and promote excellence in current and future roles and positions.

While we do not intend to focus specifically on career progression per se, it is necessary to acknowledge that career pathways in nursing have changed, and will continue to change, in response to the changing role of nurses and other health professions within healthcare.

We concur with others that career development is an iterative, rather than a linear, process that requires nurses to take responsibility for themselves and their careers. It is important to acknowledge that every nurse's career will consist of periods of 'exploration, establishment, maintenance, and disengagement',[21] and that each of these necessitates some type of transition. Individual capacity to transition and develop in careers requires effort, self-knowledge and confidence.[22] The response to transition should be both directed towards and emerge from personal, professional and organisational strategy. According to Mintzberg,[23] strategy is a combination of:

- a direction – a guide or course of action into the future
- a pattern – consistency of behaviour over time
- positioning – examination of relative and competitive advantage
- perspective – ways of doing things.

In this chapter, we propose the CAPABLE framework as a mechanism for configuring a professional career development strategy in a way that involves examination of the dynamic interplay among personal, professional and organisational factors. In doing so, we commit to professional career development as strategic, rather than positional, and nest the CAPABLE framework within a humanistic rather than mechanistic view of career development.

THE CAPABLE FRAMEWORK: A VEHICLE FOR PROFESSIONAL CAREER DEVELOPMENT

The curriculum vitae (CV) is the formal record of career development used when applying for positions. We propose that the concept of 'curriculum' can be readily used to frame professional career development, as professional career development is both the process and culmination of a range of learning experiences.

Many readers of this chapter will be familiar with the notion of a curriculum as the overarching structure of formal courses in nursing. A curriculum determines the content of a program of learning, the outcomes to be achieved and the processes by which these should be achieved. Learning experiences are fundamental to building knowledge, developing skills and fostering professional behaviours. A curriculum is the blueprint against which learning experiences occur. Sound curriculum frameworks integrate learning experiences and the outcomes of those experiences. They are responsive to both the needs and the expectations of learners and other stakeholders such as employers, communities, professional bodies and regulatory authorities. Furthermore, in practice-oriented professions such as nursing, a curriculum provides the nexus between the expectations of the workplace and the outcomes of the learning experience. The challenge for many nurses is to continue to use what Moore[24] has termed the 'curriculum of experience' following graduation in order to create personalised and situated learning that is directed towards enhanced professional career development.

The CAPABLE framework provides a mechanism for nurses to individualise a 'curriculum of work experience' in order to identify and respond to their professional career development needs. CAPABLE is an acronym for interrelated aspects of professional career development. The aspects involve an ability to explore and align:

- Context
- Appraisal
- Personal and professional conditions
- Authenticity
- Beneficence
- Lifelong learning
- Evidence.

It has been observed that traditional approaches to career management that were based in formalised career structures embedded in industrial and regulatory frameworks will not be sustained in the future, as both workplaces and workers become 'boundaryless'.[25] This will require nurses to have strategies to respond to increased diversity and flexibility, not only in career structures but also in their professional career development. There is widespread and longstanding recognition that both the individual and the organisation have joint responsibility in career development;[26] however, there is increasing emphasis on individual ownership, control and direction of one's professional career. CAPABLE is an iterative and integrated framework that acknowledges that personal and professional contexts are the crucial moderators of professional career development and that each of these is dynamic. In the remainder of this chapter, we discuss each of the aspects of the framework and elaborate on the application of each of these to the curriculum of work experience.

Exploring Context

In a seminal work, Kanter[27] described a career as an event that is connected, in a dynamic relationship, with economic, social or political issues within a society and plays a role in outcomes for that and other societies. Thus, professional career development within nursing both directs and emerges from practice and has a need to be responsive to a range of stakeholder interests. Just as effective clinicians are aware that context is the crucial moderator in nursing practice and have developed mechanisms for managing situations contextually rather than seeking to manage all situations in the same way, those who have effective careers transfer this concept to recognition of how context has an impact on professional career development and make wise and informed decisions.

The context in which professional career development occurs can be viewed from personal and macro and micro workplace levels. In the CAPABLE framework, we discuss the impact of personal context as part of aligning personal and professional conditions. Initially, we encourage exploration of the workplace context as a first step in framing professional career development, as many people may have outmoded or unrealistic expectations of the workplace or limited understanding of how the context of the workplace shapes opportunities for professional career development.

At a macro level, access to professional development for nurses is shaped by a number of factors in the broader healthcare and social policy context.

CASE STUDY 20.1

Three student nurses were given an assignment that required each student to interview a nurse about his or her career.

Student A

The person I interviewed was a nurse with over 40 years' experience. When she was at school, she was not sure about her future and the job she wanted. Here is part of her story.

> Someone who studied science, maths and languages and stayed on to complete high school in my day was not usually encouraged to take nursing as a career option. After I left school I had a range of experiences. I worked in a factory with educated migrant workers, a delicatessen in an affluent suburb – becoming familiar with gourmet foods, demeaning clientele and a demanding boss – and had a stint in a bank. I became an assistant in nursing, caring for terminally ill cancer patients. Despite never having considered nursing as a career, I was exposed to articulate, resourceful women [registered nurses] who seemed to like what they did, to be truly engaged with the people for whom they were caring and who displayed a willingness to invest in me as a 'novice' in a fairly confronting environment. They made a difference!

Once I had decided to become a registered nurse, success in nursing studies was of utmost importance to me and has provided me with many opportunities for exciting work with the health sector. Once I had completed a Bachelor of Arts and Masters degrees I realised I had a sound set of skills.

As the first person in my immediate family to complete a degree, I identify strongly with those for whom attending university is something that is both an aspiration and motivation. Nurses and nursing have to overcome an initial sense of being an imposter in academic environments.

I entered nursing and stayed in that profession because it enabled me to really deploy my skills in problem solving, in dealing with novel situations; it provided me with a reason to pursue further studies that were relevant to my work and meaningful to me; enabled me to seek answers to the larger questions about people and societal challenges over 40 years. I was exposed to a range of cultures and situations, always learning more about myself and others. I made myself highly employable through further study. Numerous colleagues have invested in me over the years and I have learnt a great deal from a number of key people, some of whom have been my own students. As you move through your career you should reflect on the learning you have experienced as an investment, by others, in you and my challenge to you is to pass that investment on by continuing to learn and share your learning with others.

The only person who can truly direct your professional future is you. What really matters is that we cherish the people who are co-travellers on any life journey that we choose to take.

Student B

The person I interviewed was a registered nurse who had 12 years of postgraduate experience. He has been working as a clinician in the same area of practice since graduating. I asked him whether he had ever considered a career change. He told me that he had been approached by others to consider working in management or education, but didn't want to do that. He said his passion was for clinical work and that the things he really enjoyed were being able to work as part of an interdisciplinary team, and to develop and refine his clinical knowledge and help others develop theirs. He said he felt it was very important to him that I didn't make assumptions about people who had been in the same job role for a long period of time. He thought some people might see this as reflecting a lack of ambition or commitment to nursing; but, for him, the essence of nursing work is being able to provide excellent care and maintain practice standards as a role model in clinical practice. He said that, to him, knowing what he wanted to achieve and getting work–life balance were important, and that he had seen some people end up dissatisfied in either their work or personal life when they made unwise choices.

He said that he had undertaken another degree in a field other than nursing because he wanted some different intellectual stimulation and to mix with people who were from a range of backgrounds. I asked him if he felt it was important that nurses had lots of experience to be able to provide care with confidence. He thought about this and said that, while experience was important, it was how you thought about what you did in practice and your willingness to maintain and develop your knowledge and skills that were important. He told me he spent at least 5 hours each month in independent professional reading. This was very important to him because he enjoyed learning, but also because he discussed what he had learnt with others in the workplace. He told me that his proudest moments in recent times were when the wardsmen voted him the nurse in his workplace that they would most like to have provide care to them or their families, and when he had been able to support an undergraduate student gain confidence in the work unit.

Student C

The person I interviewed was a recently graduated nurse. She came to nursing because she wasn't sure what she wanted to do when she left school and thought it would provide her with a starting point and she could transfer to another degree if she wanted to. After the first 6 months of study, she came to realise that nursing was far more interesting than she had initially thought. She liked the exposure she had to a range of practice areas as an undergraduate student and used this to identify what she liked and didn't like. Since graduating 12 months ago, she has decided she will aim towards a nurse practitioner position. She told me she is in the process of finding a workplace mentor and has a 5-year career plan drafted.

REFLECTIVE QUESTIONS

1. Are there similarities between any or all of these people's stories and your own or that of other nurses? What is similar, and what is different?
2. When you read these nurses' experiences, what aspects reflect the utility of the CAPABLE framework as an approach to career development?
3. When you read these people's experiences, how do they cause you to think about:
   > the contextual and personal factors that shape your professional career development?
   > the opportunities you have for career consolidation?
   > new career opportunities developing in nursing?
   > how best to position yourself to gain access to these?
   > the extent to which the role you work in or aspire to demands knowledge, skills, attitudes and circumstances consistent with your present ones?
   > things you might need to change or learn in order to fulfil the role?
   > ways you can demonstrate your accomplishments?
   > seeking and responding to feedback you have received about your performance?
   > the enablers and barriers to professional career development?
   > strategies to make the most effective use of the enablers and reduce the barriers?

EXERCISE 20.1

Interview a nurse in the workplace and ask him or her: 'What opportunities for career development exist in nursing now that may not have been available previously? How do you think career opportunities for nurses will change over the next decade?'

Nurses are regarded as a trustworthy group of professionals. Perceptions of inherent 'good' prevail, but these must be re-examined in light of the needs of clientele in the contemporary environment. According to a report about nursing in the United Kingdom, produced almost a decade ago, the contemporary nursing workforce should:

- organise care around the needs of patients
- ensure patients have a good experience of nursing, as reputations of organisations and patient choice will rest on the quality of nursing
- work in a range of settings, crossing hospital and community care, and use telemedicine
- have the skills and competencies to care for older people and people with long-term conditions, who may have both physical and mental health needs
- be able to use preventive and health promotion interventions
- work for diverse employers, and take opportunities for self-employment where appropriate
- have sufficient numbers of nurses with advanced-level skills to meet demand
- work as leaders and members of multidisciplinary teams inside and outside hospital, and across healthcare and social care teams
- work with new forms of practitioners – for example, assistant practitioners and anaesthesia practitioners
- deliver high productivity and best value for money.[28]

Similar expectations of nursing workforces are being established in other countries, including Australia and New Zealand.

Initiatives related to professional career development in nursing are intrinsically linked to the broader societal context, and nurses have to be cognisant of factors that have an impact on policy and expectations. Nursing is a dynamic and goal-oriented activity that results from individual and group needs and the problems associated with health breakdown or a need to maintain health. It takes place within and across different societies. The organisation and delivery of nursing services, and therefore the nature of professional career development in nursing, are profoundly influenced by the community expectations of the profession. The context of nursing is as extensive as the population or communities served.

Organisational theorists have developed PEST, a schema for examining the political, economic, sociocultural and technological factors that have an impact on a given activity. Figure 20.1 indicates some of the macro-level factors that have an impact on the profession of nursing and, hence, professional career imperatives, aspirations and development.

At the more micro or local level, the 'curriculum of work experience' is shaped by the extent to which nurses are engaged and enabled to be active participants in learning and practice improvement. Engagement is influenced by the practice environment,[29] the kind of learning that people engage in during organised or productive activities, the extent to which there is organisational support for learning,[30] and personal motivation to continue to learn throughout one's career. Many nurses seek formal career development opportunities, including support to attend professional development courses within their place of employment, and undertake programs

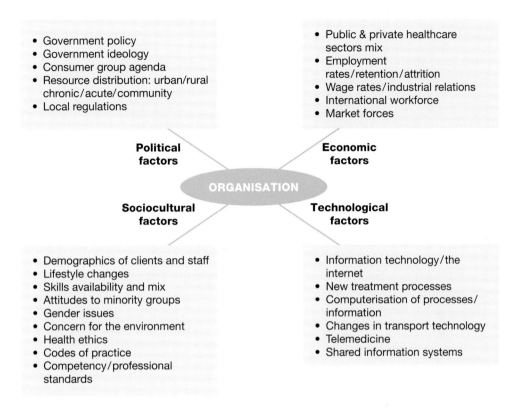

- Government policy
- Government ideology
- Consumer group agenda
- Resource distribution: urban/rural chronic/acute/community
- Local regulations

- Public & private healthcare sectors mix
- Employment rates/retention/attrition
- Wage rates/industrial relations
- International workforce
- Market forces

Political factors

Economic factors

ORGANISATION

Sociocultural factors

Technological factors

- Demographics of clients and staff
- Lifestyle changes
- Skills availability and mix
- Attitudes to minority groups
- Gender issues
- Concern for the environment
- Health ethics
- Codes of practice
- Competency/professional standards

- Information technology/the internet
- New treatment processes
- Computerisation of processes/information
- Changes in transport technology
- Telemedicine
- Shared information systems

Figure 20.1

Contextual impacts on professional change – application of the political, economic, sociocultural and technological (PEST) analysis

Source: *J Conway, M McMillan, Connecting clinical and theoretical knowledge for practice. In: J Daly, S Speedy, D Jackson, editors. Contexts of nursing. Sydney: Churchill Livingstone; 2005. pp 317–31.*

leading to further qualifications through university and other providers.[31] While this access to formal further education for nurses should be actively encouraged and supported by management, there is a renewed emphasis on the need for each individual nurse to actively participate in a range of learning activities and continuing professional development to maintain registration.[32] Selecting the most appropriate approach to professional career development requires an ability to scan the environment and determine where opportunities for consolidation of existing knowledge, skills and behaviours or creation of new career directions arise. There are a range of other professional career development opportunities in the workplace that nurses should capitalise upon, including peer supervision, mentorship, secondment, reflective practice and self-directed learning. While the ability to be conscious of the environment in which professional career development occurs is important, professional career development requires individuals to possess a range of other skills and abilities. These align with the remainder of the elements within the CAPABLE framework.

Appraisal of Conduct

The ability to examine our own performance critically and be accountable for our actions is essential to professional career development. Career transition is often marked by a process of exploration of achievements and aspirations and requires the ability to conduct a realistic self-appraisal. Appraisal is a process by which people can:

- confirm outcomes of previous experience
- identify areas of strength
- identify areas for development
- remotivate and energise
- help predict and identify personal potential
- acknowledge performance against existing standards.

Appraisal is an ongoing process that can be informed by, but is not limited to, the formalised performance development meetings that should occur between nurses and their managers. Appraisal consists of assessing accomplishments and performance to make an informed judgment about strengths and limitations in order to identify areas for improvement. It is a mechanism through which nurses can self-manage their professional career development.

It is rare that one assessment strategy provides sufficient or valid evidence for the range of knowledge, skills and behaviour that underpins professional practice. Assessment can be individual or team-based; it can focus on the products of learning or the process of learning; it can be conducted by yourself, a peer, a supervisor or another expert. Of critical importance in selecting the assessment strategies you will use to inform your appraisal is an awareness of the purpose of the appraisal and the criteria against which you wish to make your judgment. These criteria should include those that are both general to the profession of nursing and specific to your local situation.

Generic criteria against which to appraise your professional career development include codes of conduct and ethics, legislative frameworks, professional competency standards and evidence-based/best-practice standards. More detailed criteria against which to make a judgment can be found in specific position descriptions and expectations of particular roles. It is important that you ground your professional career development in the criteria for a given role or position that you seek further development in or aspire towards. If you are considering applying for a new position, it is essential that you address each of these criteria specifically in your application; too often, applications from nurses include a cover letter and a CV but no indication that the nurse has been able to link the CV to the specified criteria.

Conducting an appraisal can be a process that involves both openness and vulnerability. Feedback is considered an essential part of the appraisal process. You should seek feedback that is constructive and balanced. It should include comments both about things you have done well and about areas and suggested strategies for improvement where necessary.

Nurses should be proactive in seeking and offering feedback that is supportive and constructive. All too often, feedback is perceived as reactive and punitive. Sadly, this often has much to do with the way feedback is delivered or received rather than the feedback itself. The principles of giving feedback are that it is fair, timely, specific, accurate and supportive.

Genuine feedback is not the same as validation or unconditional positive regard; it can sometimes be painful to hear, but you should enter into receiving feedback with a mindset that the feedback is intended to assist you to develop professionally. Those who receive feedback should respond in ways that demonstrate not only a valuing of the feedback itself but also respect and valuing of the person providing the feedback and an ability to control any defensiveness to the feedback through being approachable, suspending judgment and maintaining objectivity.

The individual who is appraising strengths, limitations and aspirations through reflective practice, as well as in response to feedback from others, may need validation and support. Such support should be collegial and external to the assessment and feedback process in order to avoid blurring of boundaries.

Appraisal is not only about personal performance and ability; it is also about your capacity given personal and professional conditions. These need to be aligned in order to have realistic expectations of yourself and others, and to maximise opportunities at various times of your professional career.

EXERCISE 20.2

You are being interviewed for a position. How would you respond to an interviewer who posed the following questions?

1. What would you identify as two areas of strength, and one area for improvement, in your professional practice?
2. If I asked your peers the same question, how would they respond?
3. Imagine you are being asked to give feedback to a fellow nurse who is considering applying for another position. What would you include in that feedback?

Aligning Personal and Professional Conditions

Both personal and professional conditions impact on career development in ways that should not be underestimated. Indeed, over 20 years ago, Hall[33] noted that a career constitutes a 'bundle' of socialisation experiences as a person moves into, undertakes, and moves within and from work roles.

Individual life and work priorities influence choices about professional career development. These priorities may be determined by factors such as the criteria for career satisfaction, financial necessity, and social and familial responsibility. Work–life balance is imperative in creating and maintaining personal and career effectiveness. We encourage those who are challenged to align personal and professional conditions to engage in a simple risk–benefit analysis when making decisions about career development and progression.

In our experience, people in transition may have an expectation that a series of concessions can or ought to be made on the basis of personal conditions. While it is not unreasonable to seek to test the extent to which professional conditions can accommodate personal circumstances through processes such as flexible work practice, there are situations in which these cannot be accommodated and to do so for an individual may compromise principles of patient safety, optimal use of resources and fairness to others.

It is widely recognised in the literature related to career development that the timing and sequencing of career transitions are influenced by a person's ability and means to match decisions, commitments and context. However, the importance of individual agency and the interplay of an individual's resilience and attitude to risk taking cannot be overlooked when examining life and career transitions.[34] Individual agency is based on the interaction of individual and relational needs and an ability to capitalise on opportunities for career mobility, and aligns to views of career development as self-directed and self-expressive rather than self-sacrificing.[35]

Historically, nurses have viewed career development as synonymous with progression through a hierarchy, as the shape of organisational structures has a direct and significant impact on career opportunities. This has placed what we consider to be an unrealistic emphasis on vertical mobility as the measure of professional success. However, the focus on vertical mobility as the criterion for success and the key contributor to employee attachment and satisfaction represents a tradition that can no longer be supported as organisational and career structures in contemporary healthcare become increasingly less hierarchical. This is consistent with trends in other industries and organisations where research has identified that employees are redefining career success as multidimensional, shaped by the individual and linked to broader factors such as happiness and personal values.[36]

Lateral mobility has been noted as an alternative to vertical mobility. In nursing, this is exemplified by the expansion of the roles and functions within the scope of nurses' clinical practice, which has seen a renewed valuing of clinical practice roles as career development opportunities, rather than the longstanding view that management or education roles constitute career progression in nursing. These increased lateral mobility opportunities substitute for reduced opportunities for upward mobility and are a mechanism for career growth and success. While they can provide an antidote to experiencing a career plateau, more importantly they maintain nursing expertise in direct client care roles.

As we see it, those engaging in professional career development make one of three choices at various stages of their career depending upon personal and professional conditions: (1) remain and consolidate in an existing role; (2) realign and commit to a different role; or (3) remove and commence a new role. Irrespective of which of these choices is made, the motivation for the decision and the methods used to acquire professional career development must be authentic.

EXERCISE 20.3

List factors in your personal life that may have an impact on the realisation of your professional aspirations.

Determining Authenticity

The workplace enables professional career development to remain authentic and congruent with client, personal and workplace needs. Experiences within the workplace establish the curriculum of work. In doing so they define the goal-directed activity of nursing which underpins the direction for professional career development. Authentic development opportunities are active, meaningful and constructive both for nurses and for those with whom they work as clients and peers.

It is not enough to take a minimalist approach to do what needs to be done to keep a job. Authenticity is grounded in contemporary practice and based in sound evidence of what the clientele, the organisation and the health service need with respect to optimal outcomes with minimal risk. Hence, seeking or taking any opportunity for career development needs to be authentic on several levels – organisational, process and personal.

Organisational authenticity can be determined through examining the PEST framework (Figure 20.1) and your particular context of practice, including the strategic plan for the area in which you work.

On matters of process, there is a need to relate policy on human resource management to practice. This applies to applications for positions or for promotion within the workforce or workplace. The manner in which a CV is developed and the claims presented need to be valid so that objective referees can attest to their authenticity.

Personal authenticity suggests an open mindset to the development of yourself and others – not a hidden curriculum. Personal authenticity can be determined through exploring your personal commitment and motivation, your willingness to invest in your professional career, and your ability to be realistic about your accomplishments, goals, expectations and intent. Personal authenticity is an inherently ethical endeavour and should assist in being not only non-maleficent, but in enacting beneficence as you develop your career.

EXERCISE 20.4

Think about your career aspirations. Examine what motivates you. Explore how realistic you are about your accomplishments, goals, expectations and intent.

Enacting Beneficence

The intent of beneficence is to achieve 'good'. In terms of professional career development, this means being able to identify one's own and others' strengths, to avail yourself and others of opportunities, and to operate within – and accept – processes.

The ultimate goal of professional career development in nursing is to achieve increased capacity in the profession in order to be able to respond to complexities in client needs and enhance the profession's ability to address these needs. Professional career development activity should contribute to the maintenance of quality and the reforms necessary to optimise healthcare delivery. Nurses are expected to practise in ways that are safe, competent, culturally appropriate and supported by a sound knowledge base, and that enhance the generation and dissemination of new knowledge and learning.

Frequently, position descriptions and interview processes require demonstration of application of knowledge about ethical practice and personal and professional standards. Individuals, employers, supervisors, education bodies and regulatory authorities have a collective responsibility to ensure that the knowledge and skills base from which a nurse operates are not only extensive enough for the roles and functions of a given position, but also up to date, within the law and directed towards client benefit. This provides a series of safeguards, enhances risk management, and contributes to quality improvement through promoting application of the principles of ethics, which include justice and autonomy, doing good and not doing harm.

As fully developed professionals, nurses should demonstrate that they include ethical behaviour as part of their repertoire for practice. Just as it is an expectation that care should be in the patient's or community's best interest, professional career development should also be in the best interests of the patient/community and profession. Those who seek professional career development should ensure that the processes through which they seek and gain development are ethical. Most workplaces have a range of rules, policies and guidelines shaped by various acts and other legislative frameworks that govern procedures for professional career development. The principles of confidentiality, privacy and equity are enshrined in many of these.

Although both the employer and the individual are responsible for ethical behaviour, nurses, as professionals, should operate ethically in all facets of their working lives. In our experience, many nurses are not fully aware of the governance processes surrounding professional career development and seek opportunity or advancement outside the usual parameters of merit, equal opportunity, objective review and competitive appointment. Nurses should be conscious of the potential for there to be a contradiction between their professional commitment to ethical practice in client care and some of the processes through which they seek and provide professional career development and progression.

Professional development experiences underpin a range of functions in the healthcare environment and are critical to enhanced patient care as well as to developing the confidence and competence necessary for a career in nursing. Engaging in lifelong learning is part of the ethical nurse's repertoire, as lifelong learning is oriented to maximising individual potential in order to optimise practice and performance and reduce and avoid risk.

EXERCISE 20.5

Imagine you are involved in a selection process. What criteria would you use to determine the ethical behaviours of others in both clinical practice and their professional lives?

Engaging in Lifelong Learning

The Nursing and Midwifery Board of Australia has identified the need for continuing professional development (CPD) within its standards. In doing so, it has determined the minimum requirements for demonstration of CPD for registration.[32] The Board defines CPD as

> ... the means by which members of the professions maintain, improve and broaden their knowledge, expertise and competence, and develop the personal and professional qualities required throughout their professional lives.[37]

When transitioning from formal, institutionalised education such as that experienced in universities and other training environments, many people fail to transfer the structure previously provided by the curriculum within that educational experience to their personal professional development in the workplace. Moreover, they fail to recognise that experience, when framed appropriately, results in learning, internalisation and professional development.

A plan for lifelong learning is the formalised and systematic procedure that is the outcome of rational and analytical processes within context analysis and the conduct of appraisal. The lifelong learning plan for career progression is an integrated set of decisions focused on moving from the critical thinking and problem solving that underpin effective clinical performance to strategic thinking and problem framing.

Development activities, including formal learning opportunities, membership of professional associations and collegial networks, experience that is deconstructed through reflective practice, and developmental relationships are all required for professional career development. While there are numerous terms for and approaches to developmental relationships, such as *mentoring, coaching, critical companionship* and *clinical supervision*, we concur with the views of Rock and Garavan[38] on the four key elements that dictate the:

> ... conceptual and operational aspects of developmental relationships. These focus on self-insight, self-efficacy and self-determination; learner motivation and capability; social capital theory; and learning and feedback culture.

Irrespective of the term used to describe a developmental relationship, the key outcome of such a relationship is that nurses are, both personally and professionally, constantly transformed and emancipated from their previous ways of thinking and acting.[39–41]

Considerable intellectual, human and financial investment is made in clinical teaching and professional development in nursing. Effective professional career development requires the ability to develop and demonstrate psychomotor skills, clinical reasoning and decision making, along with attitudinal attributes such as accountability, respect for others and professionalism. Nurses, as lifelong learners, require information fluency, mindset and commitment to nursing. They are required to be knowledge-able, rather than simply knowledgeable. That is, they should be procedurally competent, information-fluent personnel who are able to coordinate client throughput and care processes; make meaningful contributions to systems review; manage consumer expectations, competing value systems and tensions in resource allocation; and be active and influential participants in healthcare teams.

In order to achieve this, nurses should be able to articulate and conceptualise the nature of their discipline in order to develop both themselves and the profession. As knowledgeable, lifelong learners, nurses should seek, and provide to others, professional career development opportunities which:

- incorporate learning opportunities that maximise exploration of the elements of evidence-based practice in nursing
- include discipline-specific application of knowledge to practice
- integrate knowledge from other sources to inform the practice of nursing
- have a spiral effect through continual conceptualisation and reconceptualisation of nursing practice in context
- centralise the concept of inquiry into and about practice
- align 'thinking about nursing' with 'knowing how to nurse'
- result in thoughtful, skilled and efficient nursing actions
- promote the notion of 'ongoing inquiry'.

Nurses who have effective careers are able to question and justify their practice, and to perform nursing actions that best manage nursing situations. They have developed thoughtful, highly skilled and efficient actions, can integrate knowledge from other disciplines with nursing-specific knowledge, and continue with lifelong learning as part of their professional career development. In addition, they are proficient at collecting evidence of their professional career development and presenting this for scrutiny and evaluation.

EXERCISE 20.6

List two activities you are engaged in that provide evidence of your commitment to lifelong learning.

Gathering Evidence

The workplace should be seen as a knowledge-building site – a place in which people heighten their awareness, skills and experience in order to gain insight, take action, review and reflect, and demonstrate tangible outcomes.

In order to demonstrate outcomes that support claims of professional career development, evidence must be collected and presented. The evidence must be of sufficient quality and be related to its intended purpose. We recommend that all nurses maintain a portfolio of evidence about their practice and development. This can be used both to guide personal reflection and analysis of professional career development needs, and to present evidence to others at performance review or when applying for a position.

EXERCISE 20.7

Locate a description for a position to which you aspire. Identify two criteria, and collect evidence to support the extent to which you satisfy these.

A portfolio offers a legitimate basis on which to judge personal competence. It can be a powerful reflective mechanism through which to identify additional education or expansion goals while incorporating critical thinking, reflection and theory–practice integration.[42]

The presentation and organisation of a professional portfolio are critical to its impact and utility. A portfolio is more than a collection of statements of attendance at professional development sessions, or a log of activity. It is a well-structured communication of critical reflection on practice and development that requires continuous investment. Effective portfolio development requires that the 'rules of evidence' are met. That is, the evidence within the portfolio must be current, relevant, accurate, objective and of sufficient scope to support meaningful decision making. It should also be well organised and presented professionally.

The way in which a portfolio is structured and presented can reflect a person's thinking (or lack of thinking) about his or her work and career as a nurse. It should demonstrate an ability to analyse and relate to context, appraise personal professional performance, make judicious decisions regarding personal and professional conditions, commit to authenticity and beneficence, and engage in lifelong learning. It is, after all, the evidence of a CAPABLE professional.

EXERCISE 20.8

Examine your professional career aspirations and apply the CAPABLE framework by asking yourself the key questions related to each element of the framework, as presented below.

Aspects for exploration and alignment	Have I ...
Context	fully explored contemporary economic, social and political issues that have an impact on opportunities for optimal role enactment as a nurse?
Appraisal	critically examined my own performance and accepted accountability for my own actions?
Personal and professional conditions	explored the extent to which individual life and work aspirations and priorities align and are sustainable?
Authenticity	represented myself accurately and realistically and behaved in a manner consistent with codes of conduct and within organisational processes?
Beneficence	ensured that my motivations and expectations are ethical and client-focused?
Lifelong learning	actively sought and engaged in career development opportunities?
Evidence	collected sufficient evidence to support claims I make about my current capabilities and career experience?

CONCLUSION

It is acknowledged that there is no single path or simple recipe for professional career development and that the next decade will see the emergence of new career paths and structures for nurses.

Any approach to career development needs to include an overall understanding of the expectations of the future health workforce, and to identify a set of personal and professional principles and goals to be progressed on a consistent basis. The CAPABLE framework provides an integrated approach to minimise dissonance among career aspirations, educational achievement, personal goals and contemporary workplace needs.

RECOMMENDED READING

Conway J, McMillan M. Connecting clinical and theoretical knowledge for practice. In: Daly J, Speedy S, Jackson D, editors. *Contexts of nursing*. 4th ed. Sydney: Churchill Livingstone; 2013. pp 373–92.

Dagget L. Career management and care of the professional self. In: Masters K, editor. *Role development in professional nursing practice*. 3rd ed. Burlington, MA: Jones & Bartlett Publishers; 2014. pp 167–93.

Phillips C, Kenny A, Esterman A, Smith C. A secondary data analysis examining the needs of graduate nurses in their transition to a new role. *Nurse Education in Practice* 2014;**14**(2):106–11.

Pineau Stam LM, Spence Laschinger HK, Regan S, Wong CA. The influence of personal and workplace resources on new graduate nurses' job satisfaction. *Journal of Nursing Management* 2013 (online). doi:10.1111/jonm.12113.

Zerwekh J, Garneau AZ. *Nursing today: transition and trends*. 8th ed. St Louis, MO: Elsevier Health Sciences; 2014.

REFERENCES

1. Tams S, Arthur M. New directions for boundaryless careers: agency and interdependence in a changing world. *Journal of Organizational Behavior* 2010;**31**:629–46.

2. Lent RW, Brown SD. Understanding and facilitating career development in the 21st century. In: Lent RW, Brown SD, editors. *Career development and counseling: putting theory and research to work*. 2nd ed. Hoboken, NJ: John Wiley & Sons; 2013. pp 1–26.

3. Lent RW, Brown SD. Social cognitive model of career self-management: toward a unifying view of adaptive career behavior across the life span. *Journal of Counseling Psychology* 2013;**60**(4):557–68.

4. Somnez B, Yildirim A. What are the career planning and development practices for nurses in hospitals? *Journal of Clinical Nursing* 2009;**18**(24):3461–71.

5. Li ZK, You LM, Lin HS, Chan SWC. The career success scale in nursing: psychometric evidence to support the Chinese version. *Journal of Advanced Nursing* 2014;**70**(5):1194–203.

6. Greenhaus JH, Kossek EE. The contemporary career: a work–home perspective. *Annual Review of Organizational Psychology and Organizational Behavior* 2014;**1**:361–88.

7. Savickas ML. Life design: a paradigm for career intervention in the 21st century. *Journal of Counseling & Development* 2012;**90**:13–19.

8. Amundson NE, Harris-Bowlsbey J, Niles S. *Essential elements of career counseling*. 3rd ed. Upper Saddle River, NJ: Pearson; 2014.

9. Castellano W. *Practices for engaging the 21st century workforce: challenges of talent management in a changing workplace.* Upper Saddle River, NJ: Pearson; 2014.

10. Miskelly P, Duncan L. 'I'm actually being the grown-up now': leadership, maturity and professional identity development. *Journal of Nursing Management* 2014;**22**:38–48.

11. Ahmed SW, Wolf KA. Evolution to revolution: positioning advanced practice to influence contemporary health care arenas. In: Ahmed SW, Andrist L, Davis S, Fuller V, editors. *DNP education, practice, and policy: redesigning advanced practice roles for the 21st century.* New York: Springer Publishing Company; 2013. pp 3–18.

12. Veras M, Pottie K, Deonandan R, Welch V, Ramsay T, Tugwell P. Health professionals in the 21st century: results from an inter professional and multi-institutional global health competencies survey (a pilot study). *British Journal of Medicine & Medical Research* 2014;**4**(10):2002–13.

13. Ten Hoeve Y, Jansen G, Roodbol P. The nursing profession: public image, self-concept and professional identity. A discussion paper. *Journal of Advanced Nursing* 2013;**70**(2):295–309.

14. Lis GA, Hanson P, Burgermeister D, Banfield B. Transforming graduate nursing education in the context of complex adaptive systems: implications for master's and DNP curricula. *Journal of Professional Nursing* 2014;**30**(6):456–62.

15. Yoder-Wise PS. *Leading and managing in nursing.* 5th ed. St Louis, MO: Elsevier Health Sciences; 2014. p xiii.

16. Buchan J, O'May F, Dussault G. Nursing workforce policy and the economic crisis: a global overview. *Journal of Nursing Scholarship* 2013;**45**:298–307.

17. MacWilliams BR, Schmidt B, Bleich MR. Men in nursing. *The American Journal of Nursing* 2013;**113**(1):38–44.

18. Rajacich D, Kane D, Williston C, Cameron S. If they do call you a nurse, it is always a 'male nurse': experiences of men in the nursing profession. *Nursing Forum* 2013;**48**(1):71–80.

19. Pool I, Poell R, ten Cate O. Nurses' and managers' perceptions of continuing professional development for older and younger nurses: a focus group study. *International Journal of Nursing Studies* 2013;**50**(1):34–43.

20. Laschinger HKS, Wong CA, Macdonald-Rencz S, Burkoski V, Cummings G, D'amour D, et al. The influence of personal and situational predictors on nurses' aspirations to management roles: preliminary findings of a national survey of Canadian nurses. *Journal of Nursing Management* 2012;**21**(2):217–30.

21. Chang PL, Chou YC, Cheng FC. Designing career development programs through understanding of nurses' career needs. *Journal of Nurses in Staff Development* 2006;**22**:246–53.

22. Savickas ML. Life design: a paradigm for career intervention in the 21st century. *Journal of Counseling & Development* 2012;**90**(1):13–19.

23. Mintzberg H. *The rise and fall of strategic planning.* New York: The Free Press; 1994.

24. Moore DT. Analyzing the curriculum of experience. In: Moore DT, editor. *Engaged learning in the academy.* New York: Palgrave Macmillan; 2013. [Chapter 3]. Online. Available: <www.palgraveconnect.com/pc/doifinder/10.1057/9781137025197>.

25. Savickas ML. Career construction theory and practice. In: Lent RW, Brown SD, editors. *Career development and counseling: putting theory and research to work.* 2nd ed. Hoboken, NJ: John Wiley & Sons; 2013. pp 147–83.

26. Clarke M. The organizational career: not dead but in need of redefinition. *International Journal of Human Resource Management* 2013;**24**(4):684–703.

27. Kanter E. Careers and the wealth of nations: a macro-perspective on the structure and implications of career forms. In: Arthur M, Hall D, Lawrence B, editors. *Handbook of career theory.* Cambridge, UK: Cambridge University Press; 1989. pp 506–22.

28. Scottish Executive. *Modernising nursing careers: setting the direction.* Edinburgh: Scottish Executive; 2006.

29. Sullivan Havens D, Warshawsky NE, Vasey J. RN work engagement in generational cohorts: the view from rural US hospitals. *Journal of Nursing Management* 2013;**21**(7):927–40.

30. Alsop A. *Continuing professional development in health and social care: strategies for lifelong learning.* 2nd ed. Chichester, UK: John Wiley & Sons; 2013.

31. Sykes H, Temple J. A systematic review to appraise the evidence relating to the impact and effects of formal continuing professional education on professional practice. *Journal of Nursing Education and Practice* 2012;**2**(4):194.

32. Nursing and Midwifery Board of Australia. *Continuing professional development registration standard, 2010.* Online. Available: www.nursingmidwiferyboard.gov.au/Registration-Standards.aspx.

33. Hall D. Careers and socialization. *Journal of Management* 1987;**13**:301–21.

34. Schoon I. *Risk and resilience: adaptations in changing time.* Cambridge, UK: Cambridge University Press; 2006.

35. LaPointe K, Heilmann P. No sacrificing dupes: the construction of meaning and agency in media narratives of career change. *Academy of Management Proceedings* 2013;**1**:12147.

36. Abele-Brehm AE. The influence of career success on subjective well-being. In: Keller AC, Samuel R, Bergman MM, Semmer NK, editors. *Psychological, educational, and sociological perspectives on success and well-being in career development.* Dordrecht: Springer Netherlands; 2014. pp 7–18.

37. Nursing and Midwifery Board of Australia. *Continuing professional development: frequently asked questions, 2014.* Online. Available: www.nursingmidwiferyboard.gov.au/Codes-Guidelines-Statements/FAQ/CPD-FAQ-for-nurses-and-midwives.aspx.

38. Rock A, Garavan T. Reconceptualizing development relationships. *Human Resource Development Review* 2006;**5**:330–54.

39. Freire P. *The pedagogy of oppression.* Harmondsworth, UK: Penguin; 1972.

40. Mezirow J. A critical theory of self directed learning. *New Directions for Continuing Education* 1985;**25**:17–30.

41. Faulk DR, Parker FM, Morris AH. Reforming perspectives: MSN graduates' knowledge, attitudes and awareness of self-transformation. *International Journal of Nursing Education Scholarship* 2010;**7**:Art 24.

42. Green J, Wyllie A, Jackson D. Electronic portfolios in nursing education: a review of the literature. *Nurse Education in Practice* 2014;**14**(1):4–8.

CHAPTER 21

Transition into practice: the regulatory framework for nursing

Amanda Adrian and Mary Chiarella

LEARNING OBJECTIVES

When you have completed this chapter you will be able to:

- ▲ explain the way in which a 'protective regulatory jurisdiction' functions
- ▲ identify how the elements of a regulatory authority's safety and quality framework provide a strong guide for registered nurses in their daily practice
- ▲ discuss the registered nurse's responsibilities in relation to the following:
  - › competence to practise
  - › recency of practice
  - › professional indemnity insurance
  - › criminal record checks
  - › mandatory reporting
- ▲ reflect on the importance of both technical and non-technical skills in relation to patient safety
- ▲ discuss the importance of boundaries for professional practice.

KEYWORDS: protective regulatory jurisdiction, regulatory safety and quality framework, professional conduct and competence, technical and non-technical skills, regulatory oversight

INTRODUCTION

Registration as a registered nurse brings with it considerable professional rights as well as obligations. Graduation from your nursing program is the foundation for your professional practice as a registered nurse. Registration is the formal regulatory recognition that you have successfully demonstrated competence at a sufficient level to commence your professional career as a nurse. It is the fact that you are registered that enables you to call yourself a registered nurse. Only when you are registered are you able to do this, as the title is protected.[1]

The testamur that states you have successfully graduated from a nursing program is only part of the evidence required for registration.

While you have to demonstrate competence to practise at the beginning of your career to become a registered nurse, it is expected that you will continue to grow and develop professionally. To this end, you are expected to exhibit the level of competence appropriate to a registered nurse with the level of skill, knowledge, attitude and experience at the equivalent stage of your professional career.[2]

This chapter focuses on the elements of professional regulation that contribute to the quality and safety of healthcare for the community, and the obligations of and guidance available to registered nurses to develop professionally, practise ethically and be able to demonstrate continuing competence throughout their professional career.

THE CONCEPT OF A PROTECTIVE JURISDICTION

In Australia, New Zealand and many other countries of the world there is an increasingly sophisticated government-supported regulatory system for many different health professionals, not just nurses. In Australia, in 2014, there are 14 categories of health practitioners regulated, as set out on Box 21.1.

The primary purpose of the Australian (and most other) regulatory schemes is to protect the community from people who are not 'suitably trained and qualified to practise in a competent and ethical manner'.[3]

The area of law that governs the regulation of their conduct and practice is known as a 'protective jurisdiction' and is part of the legal system known as 'administrative

---

BOX 21.1 Categories of health practitioners regulated in Australia as at October 2014

1. Nurses and midwives
2. Aboriginal and Torres Strait Islander health practitioners
3. Chinese medicine practitioners
4. Chiropractors
5. Dentists and allied dental personnel
6. Medical practitioners
7. Medical radiation practitioners
8. Occupational therapists
9. Optometrists
10. Osteopaths
11. Pharmacists
12. Physiotherapists
13. Podiatrists
14. Psychologists.

Source: *Australian Health Practitioner Regulation Agency (AHPRA)*, AHPRA and National Boards 2013/2014 Annual Report, *2014. p 1.*

law'. Administrative law is defined as 'the legal principles governing the relationship between the government and the governed'.[4] The legislation – and therefore the agencies, boards and other instruments created by it – all exist to protect the community from the risk of harm. This is sometimes rather a surprise for health professionals, who imagine that their registration is intended to protect the interests of the professions. In some ways, of course, health professionals are protected if they heed the advice and work within the regulatory frameworks, but that is a byproduct of the protective jurisdiction, not its intent. This form of occupational regulation provides:

- a barrier to entry to the professions by untrained persons
- the establishment of codes and standards for professional education, conduct, ethics and practice
- mechanisms for these codes and standards to be enforced
- an avenue for consumers to have complaints against nurses and midwives addressed.[5]

The criteria for which health professions ought to be included in the scheme were determined recently again in Australia in 2008 through the Intergovernmental Agreement for a National Registration and Accreditation Scheme for the Health Professions, where it was agreed that a profession was to be included in the scheme if

1. it was supported by a majority of jurisdictions; and
2. it could be demonstrated that the occupation's practice presents a serious risk to public health and safety which could be minimised by regulation.[6]

Nurses and midwives have been regulated in Australia and New Zealand since the end of the 19th century and early 20th century because it was clearly identified that the intimacy and therapeutic nature of nursing and midwifery practice, if not practised ethically and with the necessary knowledge, skill, care and judgement, could pose a risk to people.[7]

THE DIFFERENCE BETWEEN STUDENT REGISTRATION AND PROFESSIONAL REGISTRATION

When you enrolled in your nursing program of study with the intention of becoming a registered nurse, the university or college you enrolled in had to ensure that the particular education program you were enrolled in was accredited and approved by the National Board for the entire period you were enrolled in the program.

The Nursing and Midwifery Board of Australia (NMBA), the National Board for the professions of nursing and midwifery created under the *Health Practitioner Regulation National Law* ('National Law'), does not accredit these education programs. Instead, the NMBA has delegated this responsibility to the Australian Nursing and Midwifery Accreditation Council (ANMAC), 'an external accreditation entity'[8] independent of the NMBA.

ANMAC has a number of delegated functions under the National Law, including developing accreditation standards for nursing and midwifery education programs leading to registration or endorsement.[9] These accreditation standards must be approved by the NMBA before they can be used to assess and accredit education programs that the education provider can offer as leading to registration or endorsement.[10,11] The accreditation standards that govern the conduct of education programs leading to registration as a registered nurse set out the requirements for universities and colleges covering matters such as:

- the governance of the education program, including what education providers may offer the program and what is the minimum level of qualification that must be achieved for registration as a registered nurse
- the conceptual framework that underpins the program
- the way the program is developed and structured
- the content of the education program
- varied and appropriate approaches of student assessment
- the teachers, facilities, equipment and teaching resources available to students
- the management of workplace experience
- managing risks for the program and students, and quality improvement.[12]

ANMAC is also responsible for accrediting all nursing and midwifery education programs leading to registration or endorsement in Australia using the accreditation standards to assess the programs.[13] Once again, it is the responsibility of the NMBA to approve the programs accredited by ANMAC as qualifications for the purposes of registration or endorsement.[14]

A third delegated function carried out by ANMAC is the monitoring of accredited education programs to ensure the university or college continues to comply with the accreditation standards during the period of accreditation,[15] which is usually 5 years. Universities or colleges risk having conditions placed on their accreditation status, or having accreditation revoked, if they do not continue to meet the approved accreditation standards.

To ensure that these obligations under the National Law can be met between the two independent organisations, a regulatory partnership exists between the NMBA and ANMAC enabling both organisations to carry out their separate regulatory functions. This partnership is based on good communication and understanding of the separation of the powers of each agency while meeting the common objectives of the National Law of protecting the community and ensuring a flexible and sustainable health workforce in Australia.[16]

In Australia the NMBA also requires that nursing students undertaking an accredited and approved university or college program are registered. Registration as a student of nursing is quite different from registration as a qualified nursing health professional. It is not your responsibility to ensure your registration as a student. It is your education provider that has to notify the NMBA of the list of students undertaking the pre-registration program on the day of census for the university. This notification must occur prior to any students undertaking clinical placements or other activities where students may 'have contact with members of the public'[17] and where there is 'potential risk that contact may pose to members of the public'.[18] While the emphasis remains on protection of the community, as it does for the individual professional registration of you as a registered nurse, registration as a student is primarily a notification and risk management strategy for the National Board, the education provider and any clinical services provider where students may be on clinical placement. Most student matters are still managed by the education provider. However, the university or college is required to notify the NMBA of any impairment or criminal matters relating to a student that may pose a risk to the public.

MEETING THE REGISTRATION STANDARDS

When you have successfully completed your education program and wish to apply for registration as a registered nurse, the onus is on you to provide the evidence that, in addition to your academic qualifications, you meet all the relevant practice standards to practise as a new graduate and beginning practitioner. On initial registration, these standards are the English language standard,[19] the professional indemnity insurance standard[20] and the criminal history registration standard.[21]

Renewing your registration each year requires you to attest that you are continuing to practise competently and ethically, and to meet the initial standards for registration. However, in addition you are required to maintain and develop your professional knowledge, skills and expertise by also meeting the recency of practice[22] and continuing professional development standards.[23]

Many regulatory authorities also provide guidance for health professionals to practise safely and ethically and meet the expectations of the community and the professions. This is one of the four functions of a regulatory authority, the others being accreditation of programs, setting standards for practice, and managing complaints or notifications about registered health professionals.[24] This guidance in Australia is set out in a safety and quality framework and includes a number of key documents.

ELEMENTS OF A SAFETY AND QUALITY FRAMEWORK FOR PRACTISING NURSES

Safety and quality frameworks may consist of different documents and descriptions in different countries, but they are generally made up of similar fundamental components. In most, there are strong statements about the standards expected of the nurse or midwife in relation to professional conduct, ethical behaviour, practice standards, decision-making framework and boundaries of professional practice.

Professional Conduct

Professional conduct is the manner in which a person behaves while acting in a professional capacity as a nurse or midwife. It is generally accepted that, when performing their duties and conducting their affairs, professionals will uphold exemplary standards of conduct, commonly taken to mean standards not generally expected of lay people or the 'ordinary person in the street'.[25] The *Code of Professional Conduct for Nurses in Australia*[26] forms one of the key elements of the safety and quality framework for the nursing profession in this country. The purposes of the Code are to:

- outline a set of minimum national standards of conduct members of the nursing profession are expected to uphold
- inform the community of the standards of professional conduct it can expect nurses in Australia to uphold, and
- provide consumer, regulatory, employing and professional bodies with a basis for evaluating the professional conduct of nurses (p 1).[26]

The conduct statements contained in the *Code of Professional Conduct for Nurses in Australia* are set out in Box 21.2.

BOX 21.2 Conduct statements

1. Nurses practise in a safe and competent manner.
2. Nurses practise in accordance with the standards of the profession and broader health system.
3. Nurses practise and conduct themselves in accordance with laws relevant to the profession and practice of nursing.
4. Nurses respect the dignity, culture, ethnicity, values and beliefs of people receiving care and treatment, and of their colleagues.
5. Nurses treat personal information obtained in a professional capacity as private and confidential.
6. Nurses provide impartial, honest and accurate information in relation to nursing care and healthcare products.
7. Nurses support the health, wellbeing and informed decision making of people requiring or receiving care.
8. Nurses promote and preserve the trust and privilege inherent in the relationship between nurses and people receiving care.
9. Nurses maintain and build on the community's trust and confidence in the nursing profession.
10. Nurses practise nursing reflectively and ethically (p 1).[26]

Each of the conduct statements is accompanied by a series of explanations to further clarify its meaning.

Ethical Behaviour

Ethical behaviour is the necessity to 'respect, promote, protect and uphold the fundamental rights of people who are both the recipients and providers of health care'.[27] A *Code of Ethics for Nurses in Australia* forms another of the key elements of the safety and quality framework for nurses in Australia. Like the *Code of Professional Conduct*, the *Code of Ethics* addresses the ethical challenges that confront nurses in their professional and personal lives as a registered nurse. The purposes of the *Code of Ethics for Nurses in Australia* are to:

- identify the fundamental ethical standards and values to which the nursing profession is committed, and that are incorporated in other endorsed professional nursing guidelines and standards of conduct
- provide nurses with a reference point from which to reflect on the conduct of themselves and others
- guide ethical decision making and practice, and
- indicate to the community the human rights standards and ethical values it can expect nurses to uphold (p 1).[27]

The *Code of Ethics for Nurses in Australia* contains a number of value statements, each with explanatory notes. These are set out in Box 21.3.

BOX 21.3 Value statements

1. Nurses value quality nursing care for all people.
2. Nurses value respect and kindness for self and others.
3. Nurses value the diversity of people.
4. Nurses value access to quality nursing and healthcare for all people.
5. Nurses value informed decision making.
6. Nurses value a culture of safety in nursing and healthcare.
7. Nurses value ethical management of information.
8. Nurses value a socially, economically and ecologically sustainable environment promoting health and wellbeing (p 1).[27]

Each of the value statements is accompanied by a series of explanations to further clarify its meaning.

In other countries such as New Zealand and Singapore, the codes for professional conduct and ethics have been combined. Both approaches have strengths and weaknesses, and it is a policy choice for the relevant regulatory authority.

Standards for Practice

Standards for practice are the core competency standards by which performance is assessed to obtain and retain registration as a registered nurse or midwife. They cover the application of knowledge, skill, judgment and care in the practice of nursing or midwifery. In Australia, these standards have traditionally been known as 'national competency standards'. However, as they are being reviewed and updated by the NMBA, they are referred to as 'standards for practice'.[28] The purpose of these standards is to provide an evidence base to describe the core standards for practice for each professional group within nursing and midwifery. The standards are regularly updated and reviewed, and can be used by educators, governments, nursing and midwifery professionals, employers and regulators to prepare and assess the performance of a nursing and/or midwifery professional. It is critical that you examine your own practice against the standards for practice each year when you renew your registration. This reflection can assist you in developing your continuing professional development (CPD) program for the next year.

Decision-making Framework

Nurses, particularly registered nurses, often lead a team of health professionals and other workers. This team may include other registered nurses, enrolled nurses and assistants in nursing, as well as other staff such as porters and care assistants. In addition, nurses work closely with other health professionals such as medical practitioners, physiotherapists, pharmacists and other allied health staff. Work sometimes flows seamlessly between these groups based on issues such as the context of practice and patient needs. However, it is sometimes difficult for nurses to make decisions as to when to make and accept delegations of care, and the purpose of the decision-making framework (DMF) is to provide advice and guidance in relation to making and accepting delegations.

Nonetheless, the DMF makes clear that:

> These template tools establish a framework for decision making that is based in competence. They do not condone or authorise the substitution of less qualified health workers for nurses or midwives when the knowledge and skills of nurses or midwives are needed. No nurse or midwife may be directed, pressured or compelled by an employer, or other person, to engage in any practice that falls short of, or is in breach of, any professional standard, guidelines and/or code of conduct, ethics or practice for their profession.[29]

Boundaries of Professional Practice

Professional boundary violations have been a recurrent source of notifications to regulatory bodies for many health professions in the past;[30] as a result, the combined nursing and midwifery regulatory authorities commissioned research into an advisory document to assist nurses and midwives to make decisions in relation to managing professional boundaries. Two separate sets of advice were developed for nurses and midwives because it was felt that there were different challenges for each profession. The advisory document for nurses makes the point that:

> These guidelines are designed to be read in conjunction with the above codes and provide more detailed guidance and discussion in relation to the sometimes challenging area of managing professional boundaries; that is, identifying and differentiating the boundaries between professional relationships and personal relationships. In doing so, these guidelines aim to protect the community by helping to prevent distress, confusion, harm or abuse of people being cared for by nurses. It is intended this resource will stimulate reflection, stimulate discussion and guide decision making in all aspects of the relationship that is established when care is provided by nurses to people in the course of their professional role in all practice settings.[31]

Application of the Safety and Quality Framework to Clinical Practice

These documents have been developed to assist nurses in their daily practice. They are not prescriptive but principle based, and their intent is to enable nurses to reflect on the complex and sometimes difficult professional and ethical issues they encounter in clinical practice. It is strongly recommended that you familiarise yourself with these documents. Should you ever be called to account for your practice, these are the documents that will inform the standards against which you would be judged.

REGISTERED NURSE RESPONSIBILITIES IN RELATION TO REGULATORY STANDARDS AND MANDATORY NOTIFICATIONS

Each year when nurses come to renew their registration, they complete a statutory declaration (this is usually online for the majority of health professionals in Australia) whereby they confirm that they comply with the continuing professional development standard, the recency of practice (RoP) standard and the criminal history registration standard. They also agree not to practise unless they know they have adequate professional indemnity insurance arrangements.[32] All of these standards can be subject to audit, and indeed the report for the first audit is now available.[33] Although not a requirement on initial registration, on renewal registered nurses are expected to have undertaken 20 hours of CPD every year, relevant to their context of practice,[23] and must have undertaken the full-time equivalent of 3 months' practice within the past 5 years in order to claim they have met the recency of practice requirements.[22]

All registered health professionals in Australia and employers have a legal obligation to make a mandatory notification if they have formed a reasonable belief that a health practitioner has behaved in a way that constitutes notifiable conduct in relation to the practice of their profession.[34] 'Reasonable belief' is a term commonly used in legislation, including in criminal, consumer and administrative law. While it is not defined in the National Law, in general, a reasonable belief is a belief based on reasonable grounds.[35]

Notifiable conduct by registered health practitioners is defined as:

- practising while intoxicated by alcohol or drugs
- sexual misconduct in the practice of the profession
- placing the public at risk of substantial harm because of an impairment (health issue)
- placing the public at risk because of a significant departure from accepted professional standards.[36]

The Australian Health Professional Regulatory Agency (AHPRA) has detailed information about notifiable conduct on its website.[37]

CONCLUSION

During your nursing education program you will study a number of subjects dealing with law and ethics. While emphasis is often placed on the law surrounding matters such as negligence, consent and other legal doctrines and ethical dilemmas, it is important to recognise that the safety and quality framework for clinical practice has comprehensive guidance that will ensure you attain and maintain ongoing competence to practise and will, if adhered to, concomitantly reduce the risk of committing legal and ethical misdemeanours. Obviously you may still be exposed to situations requiring difficult decisions. In addition, you may still witness others making or not making decisions that will challenge you professionally, or which may have legal implications and may raise ethical dilemmas. The protective jurisdiction for the regulation of health professionals is primarily there to protect the community from harm. However, if you can demonstrate that you practise nursing according to the codes, standards and guidelines, you will also generally be protected from any regulatory censure.

CASE STUDY 21.1

RN1 was a registered nurse. She had been registered after successfully graduating from a Bachelor of Nursing course in late 1997.

RN1 had been employed in mental health, surgical and disability services in different health services over the period since registration. She was working on a general medical unit in a regional hospital at the time when the following incidents occurred, which led to a series of incident reports being made by a senior nurse manager (SNM), an enrolled nurse (EN) and RN1's nursing unit manager (NUM). The reports led to complaints being made to the nursing and midwifery regulatory authorities.

The allegations against RN1 were that:

- she had accessed healthcare records for patients for whom she had no role in providing care
- when the NUM was not on the shift, RN1 spent her time on the computer, leaving the EN to manage the patients.

During the course of the investigation and tribunal hearing, the NUM commented favourably on RN1's clinical skills and experience. She also stated that she was aware that RN1 was 'under a lot of stress because [she] came to us with some difficulties from another hospital that were unresolved at the time'.[38]

REFLECTIVE QUESTIONS

1. Using the relevant codes, standards and guidelines that are part of the safety and quality framework for registered nurses in Australia, identify potential breaches of these instruments that may lead to a finding of unsatisfactory professional conduct or professional misconduct being made against RN1.
2. If you were working as a registered nurse and were a witness to RN1's conduct, what would your responsibilities be?
3. What other resources should be available to assist you in situations such as this?

CASE STUDY 21.2

RN2 was a registered nurse who had been registered for several decades. For the past four years, she had been working in a residential aged care facility. Mrs GR and Mrs ST were residents at the facility.

A complaint was made to the nursing and midwifery regulatory authority alleging that:

Incident 1

- RN2 was on duty during day shift when a resident, Mrs GR, experienced shortness of breath and her son requested that she be transferred to the hospital by ambulance.
- There was a delay of a half to three-quarters of an hour before Mrs GR was given oxygen. RN2 had failed to comprehensively assess Mrs GR's medical condition, attend to her health and physical needs in a timely fashion, and comprehensively document her observations and treatment of Mrs GR.
- Mrs GR's family members said that RN2 behaved in a discourteous and insensitive way when dealing with their care concerns, including when talking in their presence to another health professional who supported the calling of an ambulance for Mrs GR. She had said, 'We've spoken about this lady before. She's on her way out.'
- When sending Mrs GR to hospital, RN2 referred to the 'tonne of paperwork' that now had to be done before the ambulance arrived.

Incident 2

- RN2 was on duty during day shift on another day, when she behaved in a discourteous and insensitive manner towards Mrs ST's family members when dealing with their care concerns relating to Mrs ST. When they requested that a commode that was covered in faeces be removed and cleaned, she responded: 'Well, you do what you have to do.'[39]

REFLECTIVE QUESTIONS

1. Using the relevant codes, standards and guidelines that are part of the safety and quality framework for registered nurses in Australia, identify the areas that may give guidance in relation to RN2's professional conduct in these situations.
2. If you were a witness to RN2's conduct when on a clinical placement in a residential aged care facility, what action should you take?
3. Is the outcome likely to differ if there is a one-off complaint or incident, as opposed to a series of incidents and complaints?

CASE STUDY 21.3

RN3 was a registered nurse providing care to Ms AL, a young woman admitted involuntarily to a mental health unit with a history of bipolar disorder, with periods of mania and depression marked by psychotic symptoms. Ms AL's condition was characterised by sexual disinhibition, intrusiveness, and a preoccupation with males and sexual relations. After Ms AL was discharged to a group home, she began ringing RN3 and he went to visit her and, according to Ms AL, had sexual relations with her on at least five occasions. The phone calls became so frequent, RN3 discussed the matter with his nursing unit manager but did not reveal the sexual nature of the relationship.[40]

REFLECTIVE QUESTIONS

1. Using the relevant codes, standards and guidelines that are part of the safety and quality framework for registered nurses in Australia, identify the areas that may give guidance in relation to RN3's professional conduct in this situation.
2. Would the situation be different if Ms AL did not have mental health conditions?
3. What are our professional obligations if we know of a colleague or friend who is a registered nurse having a personal relationship with a person who is/has been in their care?

RECOMMENDED READING

Chiarella M, Staunton P. *Law for nurses and midwives.* 7th ed. Sydney: Harcourt Publishers Group (Australia) Pty Ltd; 2012. [Chapter 8].

Johnstone MJ. *Bioethics: a nursing perspective.* 5th ed. Sydney: Churchill Livingstone; 2008.

Nursing and Midwifery Board of Australia. *Code of ethics for nurses in Australia, 2013.* Online. Available: www.nursingmidwiferyboard.gov.au/Codes-Guidelines-Statements/Codes-Guidelines.aspx#codesofethics.

Nursing and Midwifery Board of Australia. *Code of professional conduct for nurses in Australia, 2013.* Online. Available: www.nursingmidwiferyboard.gov.au/Codes-Guidelines-Statements/Codes-Guidelines.aspx#professionalconduct.

Other nursing standards and guidelines available through the Nursing and Midwifery Board of Australia at: www.nursingmidwiferyboard.gov.au; and the Australian Nursing and Midwifery Accreditation Council at: www.anmac.org.au.

REFERENCES

1. Section 113 of the *Health Practitioner Regulation National Law Act* as in force in each State and Territory in Australia; hereafter referred to as the National Law.
2. Nursing and Midwifery Board of Australia (NMBA). *Framework for assessing national competency standards for registered nurses, enrolled nurses and midwives*, 2013. Online. Available: www.nursingmidwiferyboard.gov.au/Codes-Guidelines-Statements/Codes-Guidelines/Framework-for-assessing-national-competency-standards.aspx [Viewed 12 October 2014].
3. Section 3(2)(a) of the National Law.
4. Butt P, editor. *Butterworths' concise Australian legal dictionary*. 3rd ed. Sydney: LexisNexis Butterworths; 2004.
5. National Nursing & Nursing Education Taskforce. Towards consistent regulation of nursing and midwifery practice in Australia: a select analysis of the legislation and professional regulation of nursing and midwifery in Australia. A report prepared by Amanda Adrian & Associates for the National Nursing and Nursing Education Taskforce; 2006, p 22; citing Department of Human Services Victoria. Regulation of the health professions in Victoria: a discussion paper. Melbourne: 2003. p 17.
6. Council of Australian Governments. *Intergovernmental agreement for a national registration and accreditation scheme for the health professions*, 2008. Online. Available: www.ahpra.gov.au/documents/default.aspx?record=WD10%2F36 [Viewed 12 October 2014].
7. Chiarella M. *The legal and professional status of nursing*. Edinburgh: Elsevier; 2002.
8. Section 43(1)(a) of the National Law.
9. Section 46 of the National Law.
10. Section 47 of the National Law.
11. 'Endorsement of registration' is an additional step to initial registration. For example, a registered nurse may be endorsed as a nurse practitioner if he or she meets the qualification requirements outlined in section 95 of the National Law.
12. Australian Nursing and Midwifery Accreditation Council. *Registered Nurse Accreditation Standards*, 2012. Online. Available: www.anmac.org.au/accreditation-standards [Viewed 15 October 2014].
13. Section 48 of the National Law.
14. Section 49 of the National Law.
15. Section 50 of the National Law.
16. Section 3(2) of the National Law.
17. Section 87(2)(a) of the National Law.
18. Section 87(2)(b) of the National Law.
19. NMBA. *English language skills registration standard*, 2011. Online. Available: www.nursingmidwiferyboard.gov.au/Registration-Standards.aspx [Viewed 12 October 2014].
20. NMBA. *Professional indemnity insurance arrangements standard*, 2011. Online. Available: www.nursingmidwiferyboard.gov.au/Registration-Standards.aspx [Viewed 12 October 2014].
21. NMBA. *Criminal history registration standard*, 2010. Online. Available: www.nursingmidwiferyboard.gov.au/Registration-Standards.aspx [Viewed 12 October 2014].
22. NMBA. *Recency of practice registration standard*, 2010. Online. Available: www.nursingmidwiferyboard.gov.au/Registration-Standards.aspx [Viewed 12 October 2014].
23. NMBA. *Continuing professional development registration standard*, 2010. Online. Available: www.nursingmidwiferyboard.gov.au/Registration-Standards.aspx [Viewed 12 October 2014].

24. Chiarella M, White J. Which tail wags which dog? Exploring the interface between health professional regulation and health professional education. *Nurse Education Today* 2013. Online. Available: www.nurseeducationtoday.com/article/S0260-6917(13)00046-4/fulltext.

25. Johnstone M, Kanitsaki O. *Professional conduct: a report to the Nurses Board of Victoria.* Melbourne: RMIT University; 2001. Quoted in: Australian Nursing and Midwifery Council. *Code of professional conduct for nurses in Australia,* Canberra: 2008. p 1. This document was re-branded in 2013 and issued through the Nursing and Midwifery Board of Australia with copyright held by the NMBA. Online. Available: www.nursingmidwiferyboard.gov.au/ Codes-Guidelines-Statements/Codes-Guidelines.aspx#professionalconduct [Viewed 18 August 2014].

26. NMBA. *Code of professional conduct for nurses in Australia,* 2013. Online. Available: www.nursingmidwiferyboard.gov.au/Codes-Guidelines-Statements/Codes-Guidelines .aspx#professionalconduct [Viewed 12 October 2014].

27. Australian Nursing and Midwifery Council, Royal College of Nursing and the Australian Nursing Federation. *Code of ethics for nurses in Australia.* Canberra: 2008. p 1. This document was re-branded in 2013 and is issued through the Nursing and Midwifery Board of Australia. Online. Available: www.nursingmidwiferyboard.gov.au/Codes-Guidelines-Statements/Codes-Guidelines.aspx#codesofethics [Viewed 18 August 2014].

28. At the time of writing the nurse practitioner and enrolled nurse standards have been rebadged as standards for practice. The registered nurse standards are under development, and the midwife standards review has been postponed until 2015.

29. NMBA. *National framework for the development of decision-making tools for nursing and midwifery practice* – September 2007 – rebranded, 2013. Online. Available: www .nursingmidwiferyboard.gov.au/Codes-Guidelines-Statements/Codes-Guidelines .aspx#professionalconduct [Viewed 12 October 2014].

30. Chiarella M, Adrian A. Boundary violations, gender and the nature of nursing work. *Nursing Ethics* 2013;27 August.

31. NMBA. *Professional boundaries for nurses,* 2010. Online. Available: www. nursingmidwiferyboard.gov.au/Codes-Guidelines-Statements/Codes-Guidelines. aspx#professionalconduct [Viewed 12 October 2014].

32. All these standards are available at www.nursingmidwiferyboard.gov.au/Registration-Standards.aspx.

33. NMBA. *Nursing and midwifery audit report phase 3,* 2014. Online. Available: www.ahpra. gov.au/Registration/Audit.aspx#prac [Viewed 12 October 2014].

34. Section 141 of the National Law.

35. AHPRA. *Mandatory notifications,* 2013. Online. Available: www.ahpra.gov.au/Notifications/ Who-can-make-a-notification/Mandatory-notifications.aspx [Viewed 12 October 2014].

36. Section 140 of the National Law.

37. www.ahpra.gov.au/ [Viewed 12 October 2014].

38. *HCCC v Burggraaff* [2012] NSWNMT 2. Available: www.austlii.edu.au/au/cases/nsw/ NSWNMT/2012/4.html [Viewed 11 December 2014].

39. *Nursing and Midwifery Board of Australia v Hancock* [2011] SAHPT 13 (31 May 2011). Available: www.austlii.edu.au/cgi-bin/sinodisp/au/cases/sa/SAHPT/2011/13.html?stem=0&syn onyms=0&query=Nursing_and_Midwifery_Board_of_Australia [Viewed 11 December 2014].

40. Burke – NT121202RPB. In: Adrian A, Chiarella M, editors. *Professional conduct: a case book of disciplinary decisions relating to professional conduct matters.* 2nd ed. Sydney: Nurses and Midwives Board of New South Wales; 2010. pp 339–40.

INDEX

Page numbers followed by '*f*' indicate figures, '*t*' indicate tables, and '*b*' indicate boxes.